feeding the whole family

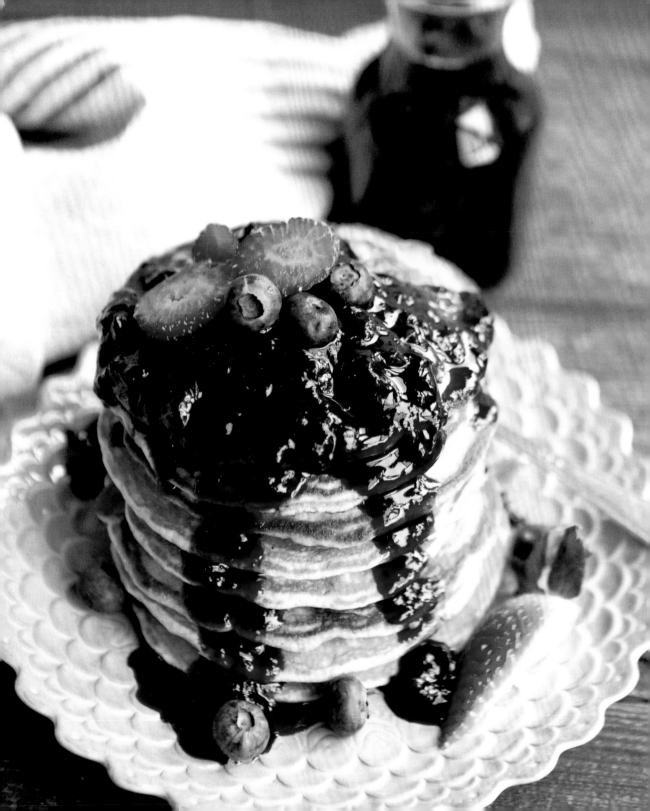

feeding *the* whole family

Cooking with Whole Foods: More than 200 Recipes
for BABIES, YOUNG CHILDREN, and their PARENTS

CYNTHIA LAIR

Foreword by
HILARY MCCLAFFERTY, MD, FAAP

Photography by Michael Kartes

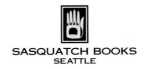

SASQUATCH BOOKS
SEATTLE

To Michael and Grace

First edition: LuraMedia, Inc., 1994
Second edition: Moon Smile Press, 1997
Third edition: Sasquatch Books, 2008

Printed in China

Published by Sasquatch Books

20 19 18 17 16   9 8 7 6 5 4 3 2 1

Editor: Susan Roxborough
Production editor: Emma Reh
Photographs: Michael Kartes
Design and illustrations: Joyce Hwang
Food styling: Danielle Kartes
Copyeditor: Michelle Hope Anderson

Library of Congress Cataloging-in-Publication Data is available.

ISBN: 978-1-63217-059-0

Sasquatch Books
1904 Third Avenue, Suite 710
Seattle, WA 98101
(206) 467-4300
www.sasquatchbooks.com
custserv@sasquatchbooks.com

- - - - - - - - - - - - - - - - - - - -

The information in this book has been prepared thoughtfully and carefully. It is not intended to be diagnostic or prescriptive. Those who read the book are encouraged to use their own good judgment and to consult with their chosen health practitioner when planning their family's diet.

contents

- -

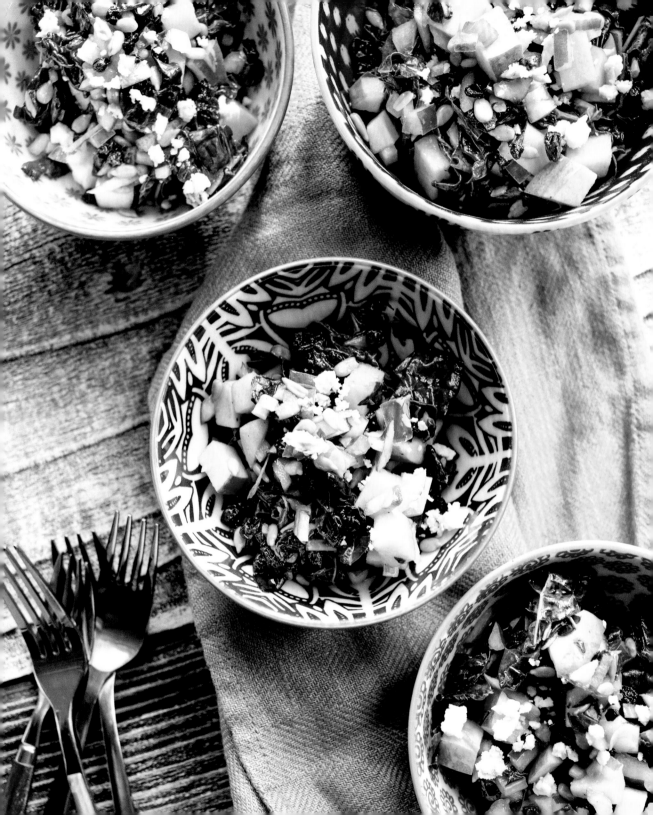

recipe list

bustling breakfasts

fresh-baked breads & muffins

lively lunch boxes

soothing soups

vivacious vegetables

substantial suppers

EGG, FISH, CHICKEN & BEEF DISHES

simple sweet desserts

COOKIES

FRUITS, NUTS & PIES

CAKES & TOPPINGS

daily drinks & brews

refreshing relishes & convenient condiments

kitchen remedies for children

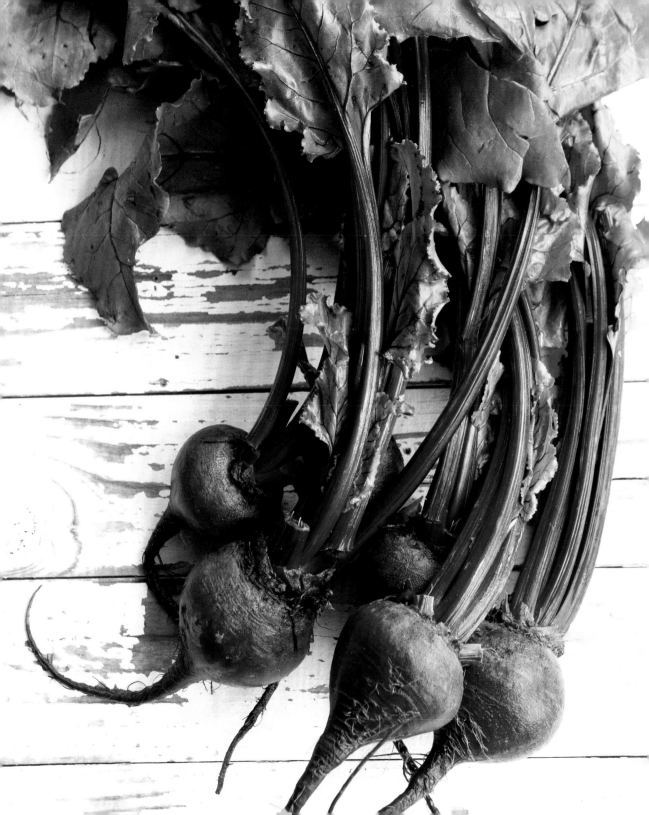

foreword

-- -- -- -- -- -- -- -- -- -- -- -- --

In my role as fellowship director at the University of Arizona Center for Integrative Medicine, I am responsible for teaching physicians, advanced nurse practitioners, and physician assistants about the many topics that encompass integrative medicine. Nutrition is one of the most important topics, not only because of its enormous impact on health, but because, paradoxically, physicians receive almost no education on practical nutrition during medical training. When I had the pleasure of reading Cynthia Lair's material in 2014, I knew that she had an important message to share with our fellows that could help fill this educational gap. In her roles as the founder of Bastyr University's Bachelor of Science in Nutrition and Culinary Arts program and as assistant professor for the School of Nutrition and Exercise Science at Bastyr University, she has perfected her teaching approach to engage the adult learner in both the science and creative pleasure of preparing healthy foods.

As a nutrition scientist, she has had to stay abreast of the rapidly evolving research in nutrition science. During her standing-room-only talk on fermented foods at the University of Arizona Center for Integrative Medicine's 2015 Nutrition and Health Conference, it was apparent that she had tapped into a topic of great interest and relevance to the assembled crowd of health-care professionals. Cynthia's ability to provide up-to-date scientific knowledge while confidently demystifying meal planning and preparation is rare indeed. In this fourth edition of *Feeding the Whole Family*, Cynthia again moves directly to the heart of the matter, thoughtfully combining the most current nutrition science with clear, delicious, and thoughtful practical applications of her craft.

As a pediatrician and a mother, I am especially appreciative of the skill Cynthia brings to the challenges of feeding young children and adolescents whole, healthy foods. Her knowledge of the challenges in pediatric nutrition and her practical advice and innovative approaches to addressing obstacles at every age and stage of development are impressive and sorely needed by parents and by clinicians caring for children. The alarming rise in the prevalence of pediatric obesity alone highlights the critical need for clinicians and parents to work together to blend the science and day-to-day know-how that will help lay a strong foundation for healthy habits. One of the strongest elements of Cynthia's work is her grasp of the importance of the home setting in health. Study after study has shown that the child who eats family meals is at lower risk of obesity, is likely to be better nourished in terms of variety and freshness of foods, and is likely to have stronger social connections. I can think of no worthier work than improving a family's and child's health by teaching parents and clinicians about the magic of great nutrition. We are very fortunate to have Cynthia Lair as our expert guide.

—HILARY MCCLAFFERTY, MD, FAAP
Tucson, Arizona

embracing the gray

- - - - - - - - - - - - - -

A loving gesture of nepotism kicked off the life of this book. My mother-in-law, Lura, owned a small publishing company—their specialty, New Age, feminist, and spiritual books. She had no business taking on a cookbook for new families, and her tiny staff had huge doubts. But Lura was a determined woman, and the first edition of *Feeding the Whole Family* was birthed.

When she sold her business and retired, she granted the rights back to me. After many rejections from publishers, in a naive act of hope, I self-published this book. The learning curve was ridiculous. Rules about the Library of Congress, bar codes, trim size, binding, blue lines, and distribution filled my days, while figuring out an accounting system and a plan to sell the books being printed on borrowed money kept me awake at night. When a semitrailer truck backed into our driveway and unloaded *pallets* with boxes, my mouth went dry, and my face lost color. *Who is going to sell these books*, I thought, *and how?*

My steady husband helped stack the cartons with a confidence that I lacked. I scheduled talks, wrote articles, and learned how to design a website (in those days you had to write in code!). I sold fifty-five thousand copies of the book out of my garage. By 2007, weary of carting my hand truck to the post office, I reached out to Sasquatch Books, who welcomed *Feeding the Whole Family* enthusiastically. Combined, we have sold over eighty thousand copies.

When I wrote the third edition for Sasquatch Books, I was struck by the various "camps" people had parked themselves in with regard to diet. Students in my cooking classes labeled themselves "dairy-free" or "pescatarian"—and defended their regime passionately. Sadly, this trend toward dogmatism around food has become even more pronounced as I update *Feeding the Whole Family* for its fourth edition. Imagine a teaching kitchen where some students are die-hard paleos, others strict vegans, and some can't or won't eat a speck of gluten. What does a cooking teacher teach to this group? Okay, braised greens. But using which fat? Committing to a new diet trend based on nutritional science is risky business, as the science is not only young but rapidly shifting. Wasn't it just a decade or so ago that we were shunning butter?

How we characterize food to our children has an impact. It even sets the stage for how children begin to form their worldview. Though binary thinking—this is good, this is evil—eases anxiety about life's complex issues, it leads to inflexibility. Professor Jim Dawes, who wrote the book *Evil Men*, says, "We must train people to occupy the 'grey space' of uncertainty; to feel the anxiety of not knowing the answer to complex problems and be okay with that." Instead of glorifying kale or demonizing doughnuts, can we talk about the pros and cons? Eat some of both? Stay open to opposing ideas? Model the okay-ness of gray space and ask questions instead of giving pat answers?

I remain committed to honoring any truths behind popular diet trends, while hanging on tight to the tried-and-true foods served at family tables for centuries. "All nations welcome" applies to my classes and this book. Bring me your vegetarian, your gluten-free, your meat craver. There's something here for you. I promise. Let's work together.

Along with nourishing food, serve up tolerance rather than dishing out rights and wrongs. Garnish everything with gratitude. Provide a dining space where children see, hear, and experience the pleasure inherent in sharing good food.

—CYNTHIA LAIR, 2016

Careful the things you say
Children will listen
Careful the things you do
Children will see and learn
Children may not obey, but children will listen
Children will look to you for which way to turn
To learn what to be

—INTO THE WOODS
"*FINALE: CHILDREN WILL LISTEN*"
Lyrics by Stephen Sondheim

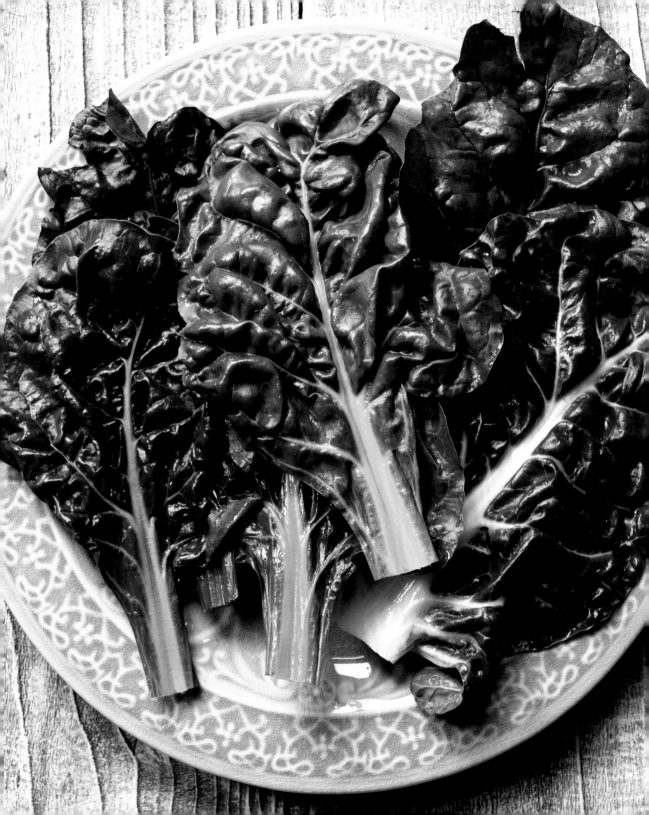

wholesome family eating

- - - - - - - - - - - - - - -

WHEN MY DAUGHTER WAS YOUNG, my husband or I read aloud to her each night. The Little House on the Prairie books, set in this country in the late 1800s, were a favorite. Food on the Ingalls family table was, for the most part, grown, raised, caught, or shot. Corn mush and rabbit stew made a regular appearance. Day after day, Laura and Mary ate corn mush or, if lucky, bread made from wheat flour they ground themselves. My daughter and I felt so relieved when summer came to the prairie and we read about the girls picking fresh blackberries. Only a hundred plus years ago, humans survived on surprisingly limited food choices.

In the summer I sometimes visit my family who live in my hometown, Wichita, Kansas. My sister's house is near a sprawling suburban supermarket where every imaginable kind of food can be purchased. People push giant grocery carts piled high with packages of every color, shape, and size. Besides the vast array of mostly packaged or ready-to-eat foods, there's a post office, a paperback book section, video rentals, a banking facility, dry cleaners, a prescription drug counter, and free colon cancer screening tests— all in the same store! The number of choices and amount of stimuli in the store overwhelms me. The question "What should we eat for dinner?" had thousands of answers. And not many of them involved cooking.

If I don't have my priorities in place, a trip to the grocery store can be like getting lost in the woods. Not only do I function better with a list in hand, but I need clear criteria to decide how to spend hard-earned family dollars.

In this book I have carved out my own interpretation of the more-than-ample information available about nutrition using research and data from today as well as common sense from my grandparents' time. The information isn't meant to be the final word. Start your own journey uniting food and health. Find food that lights up your family's eyes while keeping their bodies in prime condition.

In 1988 Ronald Reagan delivered a farewell speech that included this message: "And let me offer lesson number one about America: All great change in America begins at the dinner table." Though Mr. Reagan referred to talking with children about what it means to be an American, I prefer to nab the quote out of context. Yes, Mr. Reagan, great change certainly does occur at the dinner table. What we choose to eat and how we eat it most definitely transform family lives.

WHAT DO WE MEAN BY WHOLESOME?

The word "wholesome" conjures up happy images. We think of rosy-cheeked children running and playing in the sunshine, or a tidy house with clean cotton sheets on the beds, a simple wood table for meals, and the smell of apple pie in the oven. The word can also suggest something about a person's character, hinting at openness, honesty, and a wealth of common sense. "Wholesome" linked to foods calls up adjectives such as "health-giving," "fresh," and "naturally produced." We might picture a pot of freshly made vegetable soup, a basket of apples, or the local farmers' market with its bounty of colorful produce. Sounds good.

As parents, we want our children to have a wholesome upbringing to establish a steady base from which they can eventually contribute to the world. The primary way to fulfill that intention is by providing nourishing food for our children to eat. Yet much of the information about how to do that is conflicting. We are easily swayed by the latest fad diets or glorified food substance rather than relying on foods that have sustained families for centuries.

Food manufacturers leap on any evidence uncovered in research no matter how small the study or where the study's funding came from. The media machine has us believing we won't survive without some particular nutrient or that a revered food will be the death of us. Fear is set in motion. Money is made, but it's doubtful that anyone's health is preserved.

In our culture we maintain a very mechanistic view of nutrition. We dissect food in an attempt to quantify its contents. Charts are formed to show us how an average carrot contains a certain number of calories, so many milligrams of this, international units of that, and grams of such and such. Then we take an "average" eight-year-old weighing so many pounds and walking this many miles a week and decide how many units of each of these macro- and micronutrients they use up. After the data is gathered, someone attempts to crunch the numbers and make recommendations for how many units of each of the nutrients needs to be poured into the model child to make sure the machine works. That's one way of thinking about it.

It is true that knowing something about the nutrient content of food can be helpful in determining what is wholesome. Be aware, however, that we have identified and named only a tiny percent of all the miraculous nutrients that foods are composed of. In the early nineteenth century, protein, carbohydrates, and fat were named as compounds all foods were made up of. The second wave of discovery about nutrients came when vitamins and minerals were identified. We found that for the macronutrients to metabolize in the body, certain vitamins and minerals had to also be present. More recently, another set of nutrients in food plants were uncovered: polyphenols. There are hundreds of these compounds, and they give plants the things they need to manufacture not just vitamins, minerals, and various antioxidants—but flavor! And now the microbiome has come into play. Feeding our microbiota turns out to be as important to our health as what we feed ourselves.

Consider, too, that feeding a child has to be more than a math quiz. Vitamins and minerals and grams of whatever are good to know about, but we have to take their invisible presence on faith. When you eat kale, your taste buds can't compute how many milligrams of calcium, vitamin A, and vitamin C are present. We need to expand our criteria for how to choose and ingest food, employing not just data and research reported by the media but our senses. Sight, smell, touch, taste, and intuition are equally important.

Study a raspberry. Who could make such a voluptuous, tasty thing? Who designed it to gently pull off the vine when it is ripe to perfection, to have all those succulent rosy-red pockets of juicy flavor? Only sun, water, and fertile soil can make this good fruit. Humans depend on simple whole foods like the raspberry, as well as other plants and the animals that eat the plants, to create the tissue and blood and milk that form our children and our grand-children. Let's begin by defining the concept of a "whole food" as the first step on the path to wholesomeness.

WHY CHOOSE WHOLE FOODS?

Until the last century humans have survived on whole foods found in nature. As industrialization and agribusiness made headway, refined food became not only available but popular. Our attraction to these fractionated foods stems from the desire for convenience rather than true appetite. A whole food harvested in season, with very little transportation time to the market, is at its peak in flavor. The good taste and rich color of a food is an indication that nutrients are present. The fiber that comes as a natural part of whole foods makes us feel fuller and more satisfied with smaller serving sizes, and it feeds the friendly bacteria in our gut! Deep in our cells, we know that whole, fresh, natural foods are the best nourishment for body and soul.

our children deserve the best

One need only look at the health statistics of our children to realize that the way we currently eat isn't working. The sobering 2013–14 Centers for Disease Control and Prevention (CDC) report shows no improvement in obesity rates. Among youths aged two to nineteen, 17.2 percent of children were obese in 2014, compared with 17.1 percent in 2003. An additional 15 percent of all US children are considered overweight. Adult obesity has risen from slightly over 32 percent in 2003–04 to almost 38 percent. With obesity comes a higher prevalence of diabetes, hypertension, and orthopedic complica-tions in our children, not to mention the devastating psychosocial effects.

While we know that poor diet and exercise may not be the only culprits involved in generating these numbers, lifestyle factors definitely contribute.

Over 9 percent of our children (6.8 million) have been diagnosed with asthma. Allergies, particularly food allergies, affect one in every thirteen children (under eighteen years of age) in the United States. That's roughly two in every classroom. Eight percent of our children between three and seventeen have been diagnosed with ADHD, the larger percentage being boys. Overuse of antibiotics, which compromise gut health, and the chemicals and additives in commercially made foods are two suspects. While these maladies cannot be ascribed to diet alone, why not feed our children the best food possible to give them a better chance for a healthy body and mind?

Eating less and moving more has been the conventional advice. A more modern strategy endorses serving our children higher-quality food. Empty calories from highly refined foods like sugar contribute to weight gain and little else. Synthetic sweeteners, such as Splenda—as well as pesticides, hormones, antibiotics, preservatives, dyes, fillers, stabilizers, and other chemical concoctions found in our food—are used to increase profits. Optimistically, they are just foreign substances your body has to eliminate or store. Realistically, they can set the stage for malfunction. Nutrient-rich, fiber-rich whole foods are more nutritious and filling per calorie. Every calorie of a peach or bowl of oatmeal is usable in a positive way. Home cooking represents another less measurable but important form of quality. Make a commitment to the future and teach children to enjoy wholesome food.

the desire for wholeness comes from within

Eating whole foods can help feed our desire for connection. This spiritual benefit is magnified when the entire family shares the same food. Not only are the individuals enriched and nourished but family ties are strengthened. In one of my classes, a student asked if a chicken leg was a whole food. "Don't you have to eat all of the chicken for it to be a whole food?" she asked. I posed the question to my friend and mentor, Annemarie Colbin, who wisely told me that, yes, you would have to eat the whole chicken . . . over time. She reminded me that when tribal people killed a buffalo, the whole buffalo was

WHAT IS A WHOLE FOOD?

To determine whether a food is whole or not, one must be awake when making food choices. Before we put a bite in our mouths, before we heat it up, before we even decide to toss it into our grocery cart, there needs to be a moment, a second, when we consider where the food came from. What was its life like before it came to be on this grocery store shelf? Foods that are in boxes can be pretty mysterious. For simple whole foods, foods that don't require a list of ingredients, imagining their journey from field to store is easier. I have found that the best way to determine whether a food is whole or not is to ask these questions:

1. Can I imagine it growing?
It is easy to picture a wheat field or an apple on a tree but tough to picture a field of marshmallows. I know of no streams where one can scoop up a bucket of diet soda, no trees where one can pick Froot Loops.

2. How many ingredients does it have?
A whole food has only one ingredient—itself. No label of ingredients is necessary on simple foods like apples, salmon, and wild rice.

3. What's been done to the food since it was harvested?
The less, the better. Many foods we eat no longer resemble anything found in nature. Stripped, refined, bleached, injected, hydrogenated, chemically treated, irradiated, and gassed, modern foods have literally had the life taken out of them. Don't check out before you reach the checkout counter. Read the list. If you can't pronounce it or can't imagine it growing, don't drop it into your cart. If it is something that you could not possibly make in your kitchen or grow in a garden, be wary.

4. Have any of the edible parts of the plant been removed?
Is this product "part" of the food or the "whole" entity? Juice is only a part of a fruit. Oil is only part of the olive. Are all of the food's edible parts present? When you eat partial foods, your body in its natural wisdom will crave the parts it didn't get.

5. How long has this food been known to nourish human beings?
Putting something on toast or in tea that the FDA approved last month begs caution. Time and again, the rush to put a new manmade "food-like substances" on market has had questionable long-term effects. Most whole foods have been served at the dinner table for centuries.

Good Answers: *1) Yes 2) One 3) Not much 4) No 5) Since my great-great-grandma's time*

used, much of it as food, the rest for other practical needs. Not only is the ritual of a shared meal important but each member of the tribe had consumed a part of something that had recently been a powerful whole. On some level this unifies the tribe.

The intention of this book is to encourage families to share meals consisting of whole foods. That is why it is recommended that babies and children eat the same foods that their parents are eating. There is ample support in this country for developing individualism. What is sometimes missing, what we often long for, is connectedness. We have an opportunity to help satisfy this yearning every day at the dinner table by choosing whole foods and by sharing those foods as a family.

Once confident in knowing what a whole food is and why whole foods are the wisest choice, we can begin to formulate what a diet consisting mostly of whole foods would look like. The Map for Whole Foods Eating (page 9) represents the proportions of basic whole foods to create a well-balanced diet. Quality is stressed more than quantity. Therefore, calories, grams, serving sizes, and other numbers are not listed.

High-quality foods *are* more expensive, but consider this: at the start of World War I, Americans spent nearly half their paycheck on food purchases; today the figure is 6 percent! Americans spend less of our cash on food than any other country—half as much as households in France. As Michael Pollan, Marion Nestle, and others who study our food system have pointed out, food is cheap in our country because the true costs aren't folded in. We pay for our insistence for cheap food through climbing health-care costs, environmental degradation, lax safety measures, and disgraceful labor practices. And if you count the money taxpayers send to the government for farm subsidies— around $292.5 billion between 1995 and 2012—cheap food might not be such a bargain after all. The United States spent $8,233 on health per person in 2010, the highest in the world. Norway, the Netherlands, and Switzerland are the next highest spenders, at $3,000 less per person. Maybe if we spent more on food, we could lower our health-care costs. Sound like a plan?

WHO'S WHO IN THE MAP?

the sun

The image of the sun reminds us of our dependency on it for our livelihood. Without the energy from the sun, human life could not be sustained. We depend on the sun for our food; we depend on our food for life.

Messages suggesting regular exercise and going outdoors are represented within the image of the sun. Moving improves the body, mind, and mood and helps children work up an appetite. Bones are strengthened by regular walking, running, or other weight-bearing exercise. When children are encouraged to experience the joy of movement through playing outside, walking, and hiking, they not only develop strong bodies, but their imagination is exercised. Spending time outside improves the parent's energy too. Go outside at least fifteen minutes a day unless you are ill; thirty minutes is even better. Throw on a sweater, slicker, snowsuit, or hat and breathe some fresh air. Replace staring at a screen with gazing at a tree or the night sky. Problems that seem big in small rooms diminish outdoors.

fresh, local, organic, seasonal is central

fresh

The chemical composition of food changes radically after harvest simply because it is cut off from its food and water supply, so the least time between harvest and consumption is best. Fresh food, particularly fresh produce, gives us maximum nutrients and flavor.

Frozen food can be good too. Most of the nutrients are retained in foods that are frozen; however, some of the enzymes, color, and flavor will have disappeared. If you're purchasing frozen fruits and vegetables, the texture will have changed. The foods are much less crisp than fresh foods because the cell structure is damaged when the water crystallizes.

Canned foods have the same nutrients as frozen, but the flavor, color, and texture may suffer. One exception is tomatoes, which are picked at maximum ripeness and canned the same day. Often a canned tomato will

MAP FOR WHOLE FOODS EATING

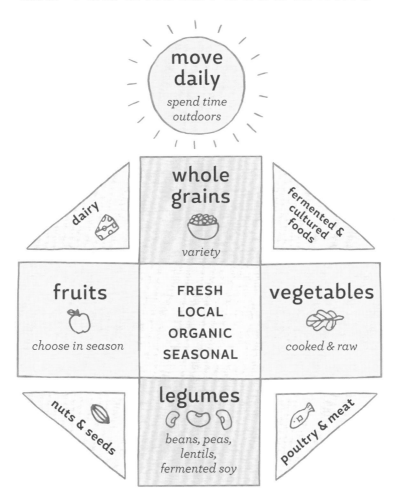

move
daily
*spend time
outdoors*

dairy

whole
grains

variety

fermented &
cultured
foods

fruits

choose in season

FRESH
LOCAL
ORGANIC
SEASONAL

vegetables

cooked & raw

nuts & seeds

legumes

*beans, peas,
lentils,
fermented soy*

poultry & meat

MAIN DISHES (squares): Whole Grains; Vegetables; Legumes; Fruit

SIDE DISHES & TOPPINGS (triangles): Dairy; Cultured and Fermented Foods; Eggs, Fish, Meat, and Poultry; Nuts and Seeds

For most, having side dishes and toppings take a supporting role in the meal is best. However, the proportion of these can be adjusted in the diets of those with elevated needs, such as women who are pregnant or nursing, persons who participate daily in hard physical labor, and children or adults who are regularly involved in aerobic athletic competition.

For those choosing to be vegan, it is important to include nuts and seeds (for fats) and sea vegetables (for minerals).

be superior in flavor to a fresh tomato purchased in February that was transported from thousands of miles away.

local

California produces nearly half of US-grown fruits, nuts, and vegetables. With their current drought fears, we need to diversify where we purchase our produce. Visit your local farmers' market. Make those visits routine. Most farmers who sell their food locally don't artificially treat crops to withstand shipping and extend their shelf life. Have a conversation with some of the nonorganic vendors, and you may find out that some local farmers do not use synthetic fertilizers or pesticides but lack the size or profits to go through the rigorous process to attain organic status. Many ranchers sell their eggs, beef, and pork directly to the consumer on-site or via online stores. The same is true for milk and milk products from healthy cows and goats. Check out EatWild.com and click on your state. Consider subscribing to a CSA (community supported agriculture), where a box of fresh, locally grown produce is delivered or available for pickup every week. As Barbara Kingsolver pointedly reminds us in her essay "Lily's Chickens," "Even if you walk or bike to the store, if you come home with bananas from Ecuador, tomatoes from Holland, cheese from France and artichokes from California, you have guzzled some serious gas. This extravagance that most of us take for granted is a stunning boondoggle: Transporting five calories' worth of strawberry from California to New York costs 435 calories of fossil fuel." Buying locally supports your community, supports your health, and supports the intention of conserving global resources.

organic

Buying organic products is a form of voting. Your organic purchase says that you support the growers and manufacturers who are producing food without the use of the synthetic fertilizers, insecticides, fungicides, herbicides, or pesticides that pollute your body and your world. Buying organic produce, especially locally grown produce, also helps keep you in tune with the seasons. Many believe that organic produce tastes better and contains more nutrients.

We have national standards for labeling food "organic." A label that says "100 Percent Organic" must contain all organic ingredients. If the label simply says "Organic," at least 95 percent of the ingredients are organically produced. When the label reads "Made with Organic Ingredients," at least 70 percent of the ingredients are organic, but the use of the USDA organic seal is prohibited. Organic produce label codes start with the number nine.

Please be aware that before there were national standards set for labeling a food "organic," the term meant that the product had been grown according to strict uniform standards, verified by independent state or private organizations. In constructing national regulations, and now that super chains like Wal-Mart are carrying organic produce, the standards have been watered down some. Large corporations have more lobbying power to get the regulations changed to suit their need for lower prices and bigger profits. This trend may put the small, local farmers out of business, so, whenever possible, buy organic produce at your local farmers' market rather than chain supermarkets.

Make a special effort to use organic products when preparing food for pregnant or nursing moms, infants, and children. Toxins found in the mother's food can cross the placenta to the growing fetus or wind up in breast milk. What may be tolerated by a mature adult may prove harsh to the immature system of a fetus or infant. Regulatory practices used to control pesticides in foods are based on studies of pesticide exposure to the general population, without regard to the special needs of infants. Some of the most pesticide-saturated foods are ones that we routinely give children to snack on, including peanuts, raisins, and potato chips. Nonorganic apples, peaches, strawberries, and celery can contain as many as eighty pesticide residues. Visit the Environmental Working Group's website (ewg.org) to download the latest Dirty Dozen/Clean Fifteen lists. Use your power as a consumer to demand the best for our children, our planet, and the future of both.

seasonal

Choosing food that is in season gives the year rhythm and ritual. It is exciting to wait for local strawberries to appear—which are sweeter and fresher than eating New Zealand berries in January. Anticipation is a wonderful feeling.

I can't wait for corn to be in season locally because it is so sweet it hardly needs to be cooked. By waiting for the local produce to become available, our eating stays in tune with the seasons.

Eating seasonally also puts your body in tune with the climate you are living in. While it may be a cliché to say Californians prefer salads and avocado, there's some sense to it. Avocados and lettuce grow there. Eating raw foods is perfect for living in a sunny, warm climate, whereas Northwesterners need more fat, like salmon, to survive the cold damp of rainy winters. Traveling north of our continent, an even fattier diet is appropriate for surviving the cold. Where do you live? What did the ancestors who inhabited your area grow and eat? Pay attention to your culture as well as your climate when choosing what's best for you to eat.

the squares: main dishes

whole grains

Whole grains and beans are central to the whole foods diet and essential to the vegetarian or vegan diet. Humans have eaten these staple foods for centuries. They represent the beginning of agriculture; planting, tending, and harvesting grains created stability and community. Today, the consumption of grains is an economically viable source of calories. We return to these humble foods at a time when we need a diet rich in nutrients and fiber for better health.

For daily consumption, whole grains are superior to refined grains because the whole product contains protein, fiber, B vitamins, calcium, iron, vitamin E, and *life* (the germ of the grain is the live part). Eating grains in their whole, natural form is satisfying and beneficial. The healthy bacteria in our gut depend on the soluble and insoluble fibers we consume through plants for their livelihood.

As you discover the benefits of whole grains, remember to rotate grains in your diet. When you eat the same grain every day, you are more likely to develop sensitivity to it. If you have brown rice on Monday, try quinoa on Tuesday. Each grain has something unique to offer the body.

Most cereal grains and beans have a phosphorus-containing compound in the outer layers called phytic acid. Phytic acid binds with certain minerals like calcium, iron, and zinc in the intestinal tract, preventing their absorption. A diet based utterly on whole grains and beans and that is also poor in calcium content may cause mineral deficiencies. Most people eat a wide variety of foods, so this is not an issue. Soaking grains and beans activates the seed embryo, which neutralizes much of the phytic acid.

Many natural foods grocery stores offer whole grains, as well as other whole foods, in bulk. Purchasing foods this way is less expensive than buying them in packages and saves waste. There is no difference in the quality. Whole grains can be stored in airtight containers on the shelf. Keep ground grains and flours in the refrigerator or freezer. Their germ has been exposed as a result of grinding, making them more vulnerable. Consider buying some large mason jars for storing grains and beans. You can see what you have and create an interesting display too. If you are keeping grains and beans in glass jars, don't store them in direct sunlight; find a dark, cool place.

legumes

For centuries cultures have combined legumes (beans, peas, lentils, and soy products) with whole grains to create affordable daily fare. Most grains are lacking the amino acid lysine, while most beans lack methionine. Beans have plenty of lysine, grains ample methionine. Together, they are complete. They do not have to be combined at the same meal to get the benefit of complementary amino acids. You carry an amino acid pool of some 80 to 90 grams of complete protein in your body that can be called upon to fill any gaps. Setting aside science, grain and bean combinations provide the basis of many flavorful cuisines around the world.

Beans are rich in protein and complex carbohydrates, high in fiber, low in calories, and contain appreciable amounts of calcium, iron, and other nutrients. The largely indigestible oligosaccharides (carbohydrates that have a handful of simple sugars linked together) found in legumes act as a prebiotic, a food source for the good bacteria in the gut. Beans accept herbs and spices graciously to create hearty, flavorful dishes. Plus, beans are inexpensive and available everywhere—what more could you ask from a food?

Choose from traditional beans such as kidney and pinto or try one of the heritage varieties such as Christmas limas or cranberry beans. Whole dry beans can be purchased in bulk or packaged. Many brands of canned beans are fine, though the flavor and tenderness may be superior if you cook the beans yourself.

SOY FOODS. When the media began reporting scientific research showing health benefits from eating soy products in the 1990s, Americans hopped on the soy wagon. Hence not only the gulping of soy lattes, munching of soy-based candy bars (referred to as "energy bars"), and slicing of tofurkey at Thanksgiving, but the broad acceptance that anything with soy anything in it is good for you. Good news for the soybean farmers who were subsidized $1.5 billion in 2012 by our federal government.

Soybeans have some things to brag about. Farmers like that they are a versatile, inexpensive, and easy-to-grow crop. They are a good non-cholesterol protein source, and a natural source of lecithin, and are concentrated in essential fatty acids, including omega-3.

However, soybeans are also a difficult food for humans to digest. They contain more phytic acid than most grains or beans, which can affect mineral absorption if soy products play too large of a role in the diet. Soybean derivatives such as soy flour, textured soy protein, partially hydrogenated soybean oil, and soy protein isolate certainly raise some concerns. These highly processed soy products, a result of multistage chemical processes, have become a major ingredient in many prepackaged or fast foods. Products made from soy derivatives such as cheese, margarine, burgers, hot dogs, and bacon are a staple in most vegetarian and vegan diets. To me these products do not seem any livelier or healthier than their animal-based counterparts, less so in most cases.

There is a world of difference, both in quality and digestibility, between a dry, soy-based energy bar and handcrafted miso paste teeming with probiotics. The traditional Japanese diet, through centuries of trial and error, found ways to utilize soybeans in a healthful way. Carefully culturing or fermenting the bean, using time as the main ingredient, renders products that not only are easily digestible but also provide beneficial bacteria. Tamari, shoyu, miso, and tempeh add unique flavors and digestibility textures to dishes.

Many Asian societies that traditionally used soy products in their diets also included sea vegetables. If there is any worry about mineral absorption or thyroid deficiencies from eating soy, the plethora of minerals, including iodine, in sea vegetables create balance.

vegetables

Eat both cooked vegetables and raw vegetables every day. Cooking vegetables lessens some of their nutritional value yet makes the food more digestible and the nutrients easier to assimilate. Raw vegetables are rich in nutrients and some enzymes that can't be found in cooked vegetables; however, vegetables such as broccoli and cauliflower are difficult to digest eaten raw. You need both. One way to approach this is to eat mostly cooked vegetables and use raw vegetables as a condiment in the cooler months of the year; reverse this when the weather is warmer.

Eat all colors. Don't form prejudices. Try dark green, light green, white, purple, red, yellow, orange, gold, black, brown; eat vegetables you've never had before. Lean toward nutrient-rich dark-green and orange vegetables, giving them a daily appearance on your plate. However, give peas a chance. Starchy vegetables like fresh corn, peas, and potatoes need not be shunned. They contain many nutrients too. Buy organic and/or locally produced produce whenever possible. Visit the farmers' market.

In a talk given by one of America's renowned food experts, Marion Nestle, she spoke about shopping on the outskirts of the grocery store as a way to choose healthier foods. That's where you will find vegetables and fruit. Use your senses to make your selections: touch avocados; smell melons; look for bright, perky greens. Avoid produce that appears wilted or moldy or where the edges are turning brown.

Store dark leafy greens in open plastic bags in the refrigerator where they will stay moist but still be able to breathe. Keep storage vegetables like onions, garlic, squashes, and potatoes in a cool, dry, dark place—the refrigerator can sometimes be too moist. When in doubt, get clues from where and how the grocery store displays the item.

Not common to most American palates, but worth a taste test, are sea vegetables (a.k.a. seaweed). These jewels from the ocean have a rich and diverse nutritional profile. Ounce for ounce, sea vegetables are higher in minerals than any other class of food because they are grown in seawater where minerals are constantly being renewed. They are a rich source of vitamins A, B, C, and E, as well as calcium and iron. Many trace elements and some key minerals such as zinc and iodine are difficult to obtain in land vegetables today because modern farming methods have depleted our soil. Including sea vegetables in your diet boosts mineral intake.

Sea vegetables are purchased dried in bags in the ethnic or macrobiotic section of natural foods grocery stores. They can be kept indefinitely in a sealed container in a cool, dry, dark place. Most sea vegetables, with the exception of nori, are reconstituted in water prior to using.

fruit

Selecting fruit that is in season helps keep prices low and flavor high. The United States imports fruit from many parts of the world, making it difficult to decipher what's in season. Eating local produce solves the dilemma. Buying produce seasonally reminds us of the rhythm of the passing seasons and keeps us in tune with what's happening outside: strawberries every June, plums in September. Eat seasonal fruit in its whole, fresh state. Include some cooked or dried fruits in your diet, especially in winter.

Drinking juice is not the same as eating a piece of whole fruit. Juice lacks fiber, which aids in slowing the rate of sugar absorption. Plus, juice is not a whole food. Children can get the equivalent of a sugar "high" on straight fruit juice. They may crave juice for quick energy and fill up on it instead of eating more nutritious food. Avoid serving juice with meals, and if it is used as a snack, use it infrequently. Buy organic fruit, especially for babies, children, and pregnant moms.

It's best to store tropical and subtropical fruits, such as pineapple, melon, banana, grapefruit, avocado, and tomato, on the counter at room temperature. These fruits originated in a hot or warm climate and refrigeration can be too cold, causing them to lose flavor. When in doubt, get clues from where and how the grocery store displays the fruit.

the triangles: side dishes & toppings

dairy

The choice to include or exclude dairy products can be confusing, especially when it comes to children. I have been schooled in the ill effects of eating dairy as well as the importance of including this nutrient-rich food. The practice of drinking plain milk, particularly homogenized, pasteurized milk, is fairly recent historically and sometimes causes health problems. For me the evidence seems to validate including small amounts of whole dairy products in the diet. I feel it is important to include dairy in dishes that include nightshades (tomatoes, potatoes, eggplant, and peppers) for balance, as mentioned on page 28. Many who find drinking milk problematic do well eating small amounts of cultured dairy products where the lactose and casein have been transformed, such as yogurt.

Having children drink several glasses of homogenized, pasteurized milk each day is a choice, not a necessity. Children who drink milk with meals may not eat other food, making the variety of nutrients ingested limited. Milk is filling. If you feel it is important to have your child drink cow's milk, do so, but watch for issues that show it is not being digested well, such as frequent runny noses or ear infections. And remember that a glass of milk per day does not make up for an otherwise poor diet.

Because antibiotics, hormones, and pesticides often get stored in the fat of the animal, which is then transferred to the milk, it is wise to purchase organic dairy products. Nonfat or reduced-fat dairy products are no longer whole, natural foods. Their nutritional composition has been altered leaving a disproportionately high water and protein content. Parents should be aware that using low-fat or nonfat milk is inappropriate for children under two years of age. Children need healthy fats in their diet for physical growth and mental development. Many experts agree that consuming a small amount of satisfying full-fat organic dairy rather than large amounts of products with little or no fat may be wiser.

cultured & fermented foods

It is estimated that more than four hundred species of bacteria inhabit our digestive tracts, weighing up to three and a half pounds. These friendly inhabitants regulate our immune system, help keep our intestines clean and free of parasites, and manufacture anti-inflammatory fats, vitamin K, and the B vitamins. Our microbiota can be depleted by taking prescription antibiotics, overusing sanitizers like bleach, and consuming meat or dairy from animals fed antibiotics.

The population of microbiota in our gut affects our health more than we could imagine. Everything from weight issues, immune function, allergies, and mental health seem to be directed by the number, type, and health of the bacteria in our colon. Babies lay the foundation of their microbiome by gathering inhabitants during the journey of vaginal birth and by consuming breast milk as their first food. But keeping the gut population vital needn't and shouldn't stop there!

Is it fermented or cultured? When bacteria and flavor are developed via time (and sometimes salt), we call this fermentation. Sauerkraut, kimchi, unpasteurized pickles, pickled vegetables, miso, red wine, beer, and aged raw-milk cheese fall into this category. When vegetables, such as cabbage or cucumbers, are allowed to undergo this slow aging process, not only are multitudes of friendly bacteria formed but the nutrients in the food become quickly bioavailable. Culturing foods, as implied, involves adding a live culture to a food to promote bacterial growth and flavor change. Examples include tempeh, yogurt, crème fraîche, sour cream, kombucha, and kefir.

Including cultured and fermented foods in the diet has two important benefits: The first is what the bacteria do to the food before it is eaten. Foods that can be difficult for humans to digest, such as milk, soy, and wheat, are transformed through the processes of fermenting and culturing, reducing many of their pesky components. For example, souring milk into yogurt causes lactic acid–producing bacteria to digest and break down both the milk sugar (lactose) and the milk protein (casein), properties thought responsible for digestive problems. Phytic acid, which is present in soybeans and can interfere with absorption of some minerals, is reduced by fermentation.

feeding the whole family

While we might imagine that the bacteria we eat via cultured and fermented food "move in," repopulating the gut, this is not necessarily what they do. Most of the microbiota (bacteria) coming from our food act as transients performing health-giving services as they move through. It is speculated that transient bacteria assist in reinforcing the mucosal layer by nudging intestinal cells to produce certain proteins that act sort of like mortar, reinforcing the lining. The so-called leaky gut comes from the mucosal layer being weak or permeable, and many theorize that this has led to the tremendous increase in allergies and inflammatory diseases. Visiting bacteria also prompt the intestinal cells to release more "defensins," cells that safeguard against invasive bacteria; in other words, they stimulate the immune system to stay effective.

Many whole foods can be cultured or fermented including whole grains, beans, vegetables, dairy, and soy. Some cultures preserve fish and meats by using fermentation (e.g., fish sauce, salami). Including these lively foods as a regular part of the diet acknowledges that the trillions of bacteria living in our gut need support too. Our good health depends on them.

eggs, fish, poultry & meat

Ample protein is needed for growth and repair in the body. Consequently, protein is particularly important for pregnant or nursing mothers, active children, anyone participating in athletics, and persons who do heavy physical labor as part of their employment. Some people can derive all the protein they need from vegetarian sources, while others don't feel right without flesh foods in their diet. For most people, three to four ounces of eggs, fish, poultry, or meat daily is ample, making these foods side dishes rather than the star of the meal. For those with elevated needs, as listed above, more may be needed.

Label reading and questioning your fishmonger or butcher has never been more important. We do not want to support concentrated animal feeding operations (CAFOs) where animals are treated (often inhumanely) as "product." Finding high-quality, respectfully produced meat, poultry, fish, and eggs requires investigation and education. Remember the saying "you are what you eat"? Well, in this case you are what *they* eat. To buy a healthy egg, fish, bird, or animal, find producers who give access to the being's natural diet and who don't employ routine antibiotics or hormones. Visit EatWild.com or CertifiedHumane.com or your local farmers' market to learn more about sustainably raised animal products in your area.

EGGS. The natural diet for a chicken is bugs, worms, and some grains, seeds, and greens. When birds eat this food, they produce incredible eggs. The yolks are golden orange, naturally rich in omega-3 fatty acids, and the whites are viscous, not watery.

Conventional eggs (which have no special labeling) come from factories where two to four pullets as young as nineteen weeks old are put into a wire cage with an area of approximately two feet square. A barn full of these cages is known as a battery of cages. Feeds are allowed to contain antibiotics and are mostly made up of bioengineered corn. Battery cages such as these are banned in some places in Europe.

Though the terms "cage free," "free run," "free roaming," and "free range" sound more appealing, they simply mean that there are no cages in the chicken house and/or that the birds have access to the outside. It doesn't mean they necessarily go outside, nor do the terms tell us anything about the bird's diet. "Omega-3" on the label means the feed given to the birds contains 10 to 20 percent flaxseed, which increases the omega-3 value in the nutrient content of the egg. Organic eggs are pricey, but they guarantee that flocks have *access* to an organic outside area and are fed at least 80 percent organic non-GMO feed. There are no meats or meat by-products, antibiotics, or hormones allowed in the feed, and each bird must have at least two square feet of floor space.

"Pastured" is a new term coined to explain the regimen of keeping birds in an enclosure on wheels, with nests and roosts inside, that is moved once or twice daily to a new piece of grass. The chickens get at least 20 percent of their diet from foraging and eating insects. These are probably the highest-quality eggs you can purchase. You may find pastured eggs at a local farmers' market or by making friends with a neighbor who keeps chickens.

FISH. The highest-quality fish are wild and line caught. This means that the fish lived in its natural habitat, ate its natural diet, and was caught in a sustainable way. The Monterey Bay Aquarium is the watchdog organization in the seafood industry. They do a superb job of letting consumers know with their Seafood Watch guide which fisheries are maintaining our precious oceans and the sea life that live in them.

Fish farming, also known as aquaculture, uses a variety of methods to grow or breed fish or shellfish in marine or fresh water. Fish farms currently provide one-third of all seafood. However, this amount will increase in the future to help meet a growing global demand for seafood that can't be met by wild fisheries alone. Popular seafood such as salmon and shrimp are farm raised in addition to being fished in the wild. Other popular seafood items such as tilapia, catfish, shrimp, and mussels are almost always farm raised.

The upside of farm-raised fish is that more people are eating fish because of its availability and price. The downsides cause concern. Much of our farm-raised fish, particularly "Atlantic" salmon, is genetically modified. Because of the sameness of the fish, disease spreads rapidly and antibiotics must be used. The PCB levels are higher because the fish live in their own waste in an enclosure. Farmed salmon are fed pellets where coloring has been added to obtain the red color in the flesh.

Fish farming can be done responsibly. Trout, for example, are farmed by blocking off a section of river. The water is flowing, allowing natural waste control and providing the trout with more of their natural diet.

Buy fresh or frozen-at-sea (and still frozen) fish caught in a sustainable way using the Seafood Watch guide available at SeafoodWatch.org. When shopping, look for fish that have a shiny semigloss sheen, a fresh smell, and tight flesh. Gaps in the flesh or yellowing are an indication of age. Cook and eat what you have purchased within forty-eight hours if it is not frozen. Store fresh fish in its packaging, resting on a pan of ice, in the refrigerator. Do not attempt to buy fresh fish and freeze it yourself, as the temperature in home freezers does not get low enough and the slow growth of ice crystals will negatively affect the texture.

POULTRY. Many of the terms used on egg cartons are also used for labeling poultry. "Free range" or "free roaming" means that the poultry are free to roam; however, the use of the term "free range," as defined by the USDA, need only mean that the bird has had some access to the outdoors each day. The outdoor area is ideally 50 percent of the size of the barn area, but that is sadly not true in most cases. How much time the bird spends outside depends on the producer and the climate. The USDA allows producers to label meat and poultry products with the claims "no antibiotics administered" or "raised without antibiotics." Claims such as these, or "free range," are defined by the UDSA but are not verified by third-party inspectors.

The term "organic" on poultry lets us know that the birds have been fed organic feed and are antibiotic-free, and no irradiation or genetic modification has taken place. They are raised under conditions that provide for exercise, access to the outdoors, and freedom of movement. Unfortunately, most birds have a very short life and rarely have the time or inclination to hang out in the outdoor area provided. Organic labeling claims are verified by third-party inspectors.

Another option is to research your local community to see if any small farmers are raising poultry to sell. Sometimes purchasing these healthier birds may require a trip to the farm or to a farmers' market.

Remember to always store raw meat or poultry on the bottom shelf of your refrigerator to avoid any cross-contamination that may occur from dripping juices. Wash, rinse, and sanitize the cutting surface and all the utensils (knives, etc.) every time you finish cutting raw meat, fish, and poultry. Household bleach is a good sanitizer. Use a capful (1 teaspoon) for each gallon of *cool* water.

MEAT. The natural diet of cows is grass. Their anatomy and physiology is set up to graze and digest grass. Cows that are allowed to be raised and finished on grass have more omega-3 fatty acids (anti-inflammatory) in their fat. If cattle are fed cornmeal or soy meal in place of grass, they are likely to develop acidosis, requiring antibiotics to cure their ills. The better alternative comes from meat products bearing the label "grass fed."

Cows like to move around as they graze. This is better for the cows and better for the land. Some ranchers offer their cattle hundreds of acres to roam, and it would be quite difficult to maintain that land as "organic"—which is what it would take for their beef to bear the label. So while it is certainly preferable to see the organic label guaranteeing that no hormones or antibiotics were given to the cattle, organic beef is not the only wholesome game in town.

Another good label to shop for is "certified humane raised and handled," which means that cattle have sufficient space and shelter and access to fresh water at all times. They must not be fed hormones or antibiotics and must be treated and handled according to Humane Farm Animal Care (HFAC) standards. Claims are verified by third-party inspectors. See CertifiedHumane .com. Again, checking out ranchers living in your local community may reveal excellent sources.

nuts & seeds

Nuts and seeds are delicious whole foods that contain many beneficial nutrients; for example, almonds are rich in calcium, and pumpkin seeds are high in iron. Nuts and seeds contain high-quality fats. The added calories and healthful fats can be useful for pregnant or nursing moms and active children. Nuts and seeds boast admirable amounts of fiber too (food for your microbiota!). Buy organic nuts whenever possible.

Nuts found in nature are housed in shells—the perfect storage container, protecting the fats from heat, air, and light. Nuts in the shell are not widely available, however. After you purchase raw, shelled nuts or seeds, it is a good idea to mimic nature and keep them in a sealed container in a dark, cold place like the freezer. Be wary of purchasing toasted nuts and seeds unless you are sure of how they were processed: At what temperature? Using what oil?

KITCHEN STAPLES

Whole grains, beans, vegetables, and other starchy whole foods can taste blah on their own. They need salt, fat, herbs, spices, and other natural condiments to bring out their beauty. Sort of like a basic black dress needs the right jewelry or shoes.

salt

"Merlin," the nickname for salt, fits because, when you understand how and when to add it, the results are magical. Salt is essential for bringing bland foods like grains, beans, and starchy vegetables to life. Eggs, fish, poultry, and meat don't taste right without salt. A touch of salt can amplify the sweetness in baked goods. So the question is—what to buy?

A really good sea salt should have no other ingredients on the label than salt—no iodine, anticaking agents, or bleaches. Better to get your iodine from including seafood and sea vegetables in your diet where the iodine is in its natural form. In good sea salts you can usually see tiny flecks of gray or black. These are minerals. Celtic sea salt boasts that 16 percent of the salt is minerals. Another clue is moistness. Solar-evaporated sea salts with minerals still present have a slight moistness.

There are many excellent brands. One resource for salt worth mentioning is Selina Naturally, a purveyor of ingredients of uncommon quality (CelticSalt.com).

fats & oils

For many years Americans were told that hydrogenated fats like margarine were better. Then polyunsaturated vegetable oils were given the big thumbs-up as the answer to high cholesterol. We hear butter is good and then it is bad, but now it's "back." So far no one has bashed olive oil. What is the right fat or oil to cook with?

In the Bastyr Nutrition Kitchen we prefer to cook with traditional fats and oils that have nourished populations for thousands of years. Historically most cultures have cooked with saturated and monounsaturated fats, which are stable and less likely to go rancid. The following are our top picks for use in the whole foods cooking classes at Bastyr and for this book. Whenever possible, organic is preferred.

Butter is stable, has fewer rancidity problems, and maintains its integrity when cooked. Butter contains lauric acid, lecithin, vitamins A and D, and, if the butter comes from cows allowed access to pasture, the possible presence of omega-3 fatty acids increases.

Coconut oil is a saturated fat that is solid at room temperatures lower than 76 degrees F. Its antifungal, antibacterial properties make it the perfect fat for rapidly decomposing foods in the tropics. It is definitely not a local or seasonal food, nor is it a miracle cure-all. Coconut oil has a long shelf life and is a very stable fat. It works nicely in baked goods and holds its integrity during medium-temperature frying.

Cold-pressed extra-virgin olive oil must be mechanically produced with no heat according to standards set by International Olive Oil Council of Madrid. Extra-virgin olive oil comes from the first pressing of the olives and is only 1 percent acid or less. Olive oil contains monounsaturated fats, which are cholesterol-free and help with its stability. The deeper the color, the more intense the flavor will be.

Unrefined sesame oil is a traditional oil from the Asian culture. It is 46 percent monounsaturated and 41 percent polyunsaturated. The poly part is protected from rancidity by sesamol, an antioxidant naturally present in the seed. This oil has a distinct, delicious flavor.

Cold-pressed, unrefined oils are fine for salad dressings and recipes that have low or no heat involved. These oils are fragile, making them unsuitable for baking or high temperatures. They are also usually fairly expensive. Certain food companies produce high-quality unrefined, cold-pressed oils from a variety of food sources; two examples are hazelnut oil and pumpkin seed oil.

Refined vegetable oils are inexpensive because they are sourced from subsidized crops. Most refined vegetable oil manufacturers use chemical solvents to help extract the oil from the seed. The oil is then filtered, refined with alkaline chemicals, steam deodorized at 460 degrees F, and then filtered again. This creates oil that has a long shelf life but few nutrients, no aroma, and very little taste. For occasional high-heat cooking, where the oil is used more as a medium or a lubricant than an ingredient, refined, expeller-pressed grapeseed, safflower, sunflower, or peanut oil work just fine.

sweeteners

The following sweeteners are a little less processed and have a more distinctive flavor, so I prefer them to regular white sugar for baked goods and desserts. Make no mistake, all sweeteners weigh in at around 40 to 50 percent fructose. There's really no such thing as a "healthier" sweetener. Further instructions for how to replace white sugar with these more natural sweeteners are described in Have It Your Way: Flour, Fat, Milk, Sweetener, and Egg Substitutions (page 401). Occasionally a bit of regular white sugar is called for in recipes when the brown color of molasses or maple syrup is undesirable, but the amounts are small.

The generic term *unrefined cane sugar* describes sugar made by simply crushing freshly cut sugarcane, extracting the juice, and heating it in a large vat. Once the juice is reduced to syrup, it is dehydrated and granulated. This product is less refined than white sugar because some of the mineral-rich molasses is present. It resembles brown sugar in appearance and taste, though it is slightly less sweet and often has larger granules.

The procedure to make *barley malt* entails immersing barley in water to encourage the grain to sprout, then drying the barley to halt the progress when the sprouting begins. The water is extracted and then slowly reduced to thick, rich syrup. Barley malt is dark and thick like molasses and has a malt-like taste.

Similar to barley malt, *brown rice syrup* is made from rice that has been soaked, sprouted, and cooked with a cereal enzyme that breaks the starches into maltose. Rice syrup has a light, delicate flavor and looks similar to honey but is less sweet. Both barley malt and brown rice syrup cool to a harder, crispier texture than other sweeteners.

To make *honey*, bees first collect nectar from flowers. The nectar is then pumped out of the body into a hive cell. The cell is sealed and the honey ripens in three weeks. A strong hive will have one queen, a few hundred males, and about twenty thousand female workers. When used to sweeten baked goods and foods, the distinct flavor of the honey shines through. Honey adds a moister quality to baked goods because it loses water to air more slowly than sugar. Do not give babies raw honey.

Forty gallons of sap must be boiled down to obtain one gallon of delicious *maple syrup*. This product is available in grades: A or B. The cooking time and temperature determine the grade. Grade A is lighter and generally used on pancakes and waffles, while grade B has a darker color and flavor, is less expensive, and has a higher mineral content. Grade B is suitable for baking.

herbs & spices

Fresh herbs release their essential oils when they are chopped or rubbed. The tender green plants add not only flavor but some of the nutrients that other green vegetables offer. The woody stemmed herbs, such as rosemary, sage, and thyme, can withstand heat well. More tender leaves, like basil, cilantro, and parsley, need to be added at the end of cooking time or used raw. When fresh herbs are unavailable, substitute 1 teaspoon of dried herbs for each tablespoon of fresh herbs called for in the recipe.

Spices are usually the dried barks, buds, and seeds of plants. Buy them whole and grind them in a small electric coffee grinder before adding to food. The flavor will be about three times as intense as preground spices. Spices respond positively to heat and fat. Toasting or sautéing dry spices helps wake up the flavor, increasing their potency.

If you buy herbs and spices dried or preground be sure to date the package. Throw them out and replace them after 6 to 12 months, as they will lose much of their flavor.

CULINARY MARRIAGES

Three whole foods couples have been paired together in dishes throughout human culinary history. Turns out these duos not only taste good together but balance each other nutritionally. Whenever possible, keep these companions together in the same meal:

whole grains + legumes

Most grains are lacking the amino acid lysine, while most beans lack methionine. Together they provide all nine amino acids.

nightshades + dairy

The nightshade plants (tomato, potato, eggplant, peppers, and tobacco) are high in alkaloids, which according to some may subtly pull calcium from bone. Dairy products have enough calcium to make a baby calf double its bone structure in six months—maybe more calcium than we smaller, slower-growing humans need. Perhaps these two have been kept together in dishes to balance these effects. Who doesn't prefer their potato with a dab of butter or sour cream? Those who eat no dairy products need to be cautious about eating too many nightshade vegetables.

soy foods + sea vegetables

Cultures that include fermented or cultured soy products in their cuisine have also typically included plants from the sea. Soy foods are thought to possibly be demineralizing because of their high phytic acid content, and some claim overuse of soy could possibly lower thyroid function. Sea vegetables are amazingly rich in minerals, including iodine, which stimulates the thyroid. Maybe that's why soy and sea vegetables are usually found together in traditional cuisines.

SETTING THE TABLE, SETTING THE SCENE

In his stellar book *The Omnivore's Dilemma,* Michael Pollan talks about cooking as a way of honoring the things we eat. Conscientiously preparing food is a way of paying respect to the animals and plants that have been sacrificed to serve our needs and of acknowledging the people who have produced the food so that we can enjoy it. Not only can we choose and cook our food thoughtfully, but we can also serve and eat food with care and a spirit of gratefulness.

sit down & breathe

The way in which you eat is equally important as *what* you eat. Marc David has written a comprehensive discussion of this in his book *The Slow Down Diet.* Digestion is remarkably enhanced by sitting down, taking a deep breath, and enjoying each bite. Taking time improves digestion, metabolism, and nutrient uptake. When we wolf down food, in a hurry to get to the next task, the joy of eating disappears. Our bodies aren't relaxed enough to take in the nutrients, and we are left hungry for more, which can lead to overeating. Rule number one for children is to sit down when eating. Even fidgety children can be taught to do this, especially if parents sit down with them.

eating is a visual experience

Eyeing colorful, artfully arranged food nourishes the soul by feeding us beauty. Invite children to express their artistic side with food presentation. Setting the table can be a creative task that very young children are capable of. Let them pick flowers to put in a vase, make placemats out of paper, tie ribbons on napkins, or decide which color of candles would be just right.

Setting a beautiful table need not break the bank. I attended an outdoor wedding where the couple had dyed bedsheets a beautiful lavender tone to fashion matching tablecloths. Mason jars with colored ribbons tied round the top held our beverages, and a potpourri of floral-patterned plates from the thrift shop with a cloth napkin to match completed the look. The food was fabulous, too, but our desire for the food heightened with the images painted via the table settings. Even if the best you can do is order in some Chinese food to go with your leftover brown rice, take the time to set the table. Lay a cheerful tablecloth on the table. Serve the food on colorful plates.

Beauty appears in the way food is arranged on the plate. When you dine out at a fancy restaurant and a plate of food arrives looking like the chef painted the food on the plate, everyone at the table says "Yum!" before they have even tasted it. Arrange food on the plate in a pleasing way. Choose foods that have several colors so that your plate is not all brown or beige. Garnish! Many plain Jane dishes can look like a million dollars with bright-green basil, white sour cream, orange zest, or a sliver of red bell pepper placed just right.

sharing the meal

In a time when families are dealing with two careers, longer working hours, and children with numerous extracurricular activities, the fate of the shared, home-cooked family meal seems in jeopardy. Juggling commitments to make room for shared family meals has rewards. We know that eating meals together increases the enjoyment of the meal, solidifies family bonds, and encourages communication about the day's activities among family members. If we are willing to make the extra effort required to share a common meals, our lives are richer and solidarity is built.

Children love the predictability of events that occur daily and benefit from routines. Family dinner discussion helps expand children's vocabulary skills and increases their success in learning to read. Mealtime is also where children learn many of their social skills, including table manners and the art of conversation.

Much of family history relating to culture and race is passed on to children by parents at the dinner table. Serving traditional meals can illuminate ethnic heritage. These gestures help strengthen the child's identity as a member of a group. Studies show that children who participate in regular family meals have more emotional resilience to help them handle stress and chaos in other areas of life. Marooning babies in high chairs or plopping children in front of the tube to eat robs them of what could be an otherwise enriching experience.

If all that doesn't convince you, consider this: the National Center on Addiction and Substance Abuse at Columbia University released a study showing that teens who regularly dine with their families have a smaller chance of smoking, drinking alcohol, and using drugs; they also earn better grades in school. Set a firm foundation of shared meals when your children are young.

There are also nutritional advantages to eating meals together. Children who dine without parents or siblings eat fewer servings from the necessary food groups. When parents are present, they can observe their child's food intake, ensuring nutritional adequacy. Eating together also gives parents the opportunity to model good eating habits, such as choosing healthy foods, chewing food well, and stopping when full.

family style or plated

When adults plate food at dinnertime, they sometimes overestimate how much small children can eat. In 2011 the Academy of Nutrition and Dietetics advised that child-care providers should serve meals "family style," allowing kids to take what they want from a few dishes served. Research shows that when kids are allowed to serve themselves, they're less likely to overeat. Others claim that family-style eating boosts confidence and independence. More dishes to wash and children repeatedly forgoing certain foods are possible downsides.

Try both styles and see what works best for your family. If you're plating meals, be sure to keep child portions small. Much better to have a child politely request more than to have arguments spark over food left on the plate, right?

table talk

Keep conversation pleasant at mealtime. Encourage each person at the table to "check in." Steer the conversation toward the positive by asking questions such as, "What went well today?" "Did something happen that surprised you?" If you have touchy subjects to bring up with your spouse or children, don't do it while dining. Unpleasant news tightens the stomach, halts digestion, and takes the mind off the enjoyment of eating.

Do not talk about nutrients at the table, particularly with children under five. Most nutrition language is esoteric; there's no way to picture "protein" or "vitamin A" in your mind, because these microscopic structures are invisible to the human eye. Stressing the importance of nutrients can be confusing, even worrisome, for children. Particularly if the concept that the child "won't get enough" to thrive is stressed. Instead, talk about food. Talk about where it comes from, the colors, the history, how it's grown, and how delicious it tastes.

make changes slowly

Step one is to become conscious of what you're putting in your family's mouths. Consider what you are buying at the store. Ask yourself: Does this product deserve my hard-earned money? What's in it? Am I buying it out of habit or because the label looks attractive? Think about your food as you prepare it, as you eat it, and ask: Where did this food originate? Will it add to my vitality? For a while observe what you eat without changing anything.

Take baby steps. Pick one thing to change, such as switching from white bread to whole grain bread or learning to eat the fast-cooking grain quinoa. Make small changes over weeks and months, and create the time and space needed to transition your family to better nourishment one food at a time.

In order to modify old habits, you must feel an intrinsic desire to change. Many people change their diets for health reasons, often the result of a live-or-die situation. But there are reasons to make changes before a crisis occurs. In cooking classes I have heard stories of children who are influencing their parents to eat better. In one class for a local grocery co-op, I had three pairs of mothers and daughters, and all three daughters had instigated the attendance. It is inspiring to see the family align with each other about food and health.

Sometimes people tell me they can't change their family's food habits because one family member simply won't have it. If you're in this situation, talk to the person who objects. Let them know that your motivation comes from love. Perhaps the reluctant family member will agree to one small change—for instance, having a fresh green salad every evening or maybe brown rice instead of white rice once in a while. Go slowly—very slowly. Make changing what and how you eat a gentle, healing process. There is no rush. Lasting changes require intention and patience.

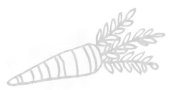

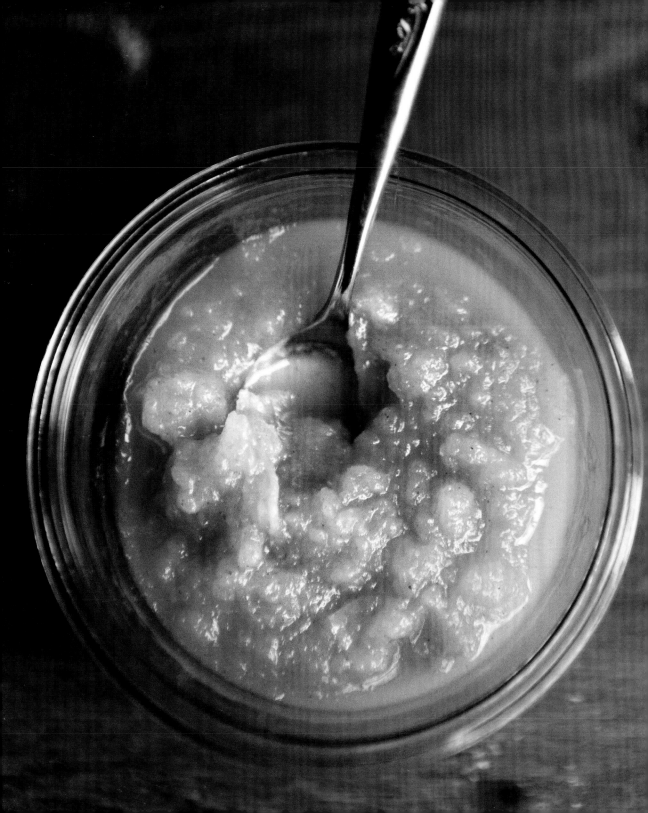

CHAPTER 2

including baby

- - - - - - - - - - - -

WHEN I WAS A BRAND-NEW MOTHER, my two-week-old infant curled her fists up in tight balls and screamed for several hours straight every evening. Her condition was delegated to a catchall term for howling babies: "colic." I worried about my breast milk being okay. I worried about her tiny digestive system. I was exhausted. I felt lost.

I chose to stay right with Grace during her long tirades. I paced holding her, bounced her on a big exercise ball, and just plain hung in there with her. When I could get past my own frustration, I would think about how difficult her transition must have been, from spirit to water baby in my womb to infant out in the world. I would consider how foreign it must be to suddenly find yourself in a helpless, tiny body, a body that requires ingesting food and eliminating waste, wearing clothes, seeing lights, and hearing noise. My heart would go out to this tiny child who seemed to be furious about making this transition. Tears would slide down my cheeks with regularity.

Humans spend their whole lives searching for a sense of belonging and being loved. Giving food is a primal means of expressing love. There is nothing that can duplicate the reassurance that is conveyed when a baby's food is accompanied by the face, hands, voice, breast, or chest of a loving parent.

DOING THE MONTH: POSTPARTUM CARE

The United States, Lesotho, Swaziland, and Papua New Guinea are the only countries that do not mandate paid maternity leave, according to *The Arkansas Journal of Social Change and Public Service*. Most countries offer three months of paid leave for new mothers and many offer benefits for fathers as well. Fingers crossed this changes soon. In the meantime even though pregnancy is considered a distinct condition filled with medical visits, advice, and caution postdelivery, American women are expected to pull on their prepregnancy jeans and have a jog within days of giving birth.

Giving birth demands huge physical exertion. Most women lose nearly 10 percent of their body's blood supply. Experiencing extreme exhaustion postbirth is natural and expected. Most cultures of the world recognize this and make sure the postpartum woman receives ample support and rest. In Chinese culture the thirty days of restful confinement is called "doing the month." During this time moms consume special soups and tonics. Some larger Asian cities have luxury postpartum centers where women of means spend their month of recovery. The *cuarentena* (which translates as "forty") practiced in Mexico prescribes a forty-day resting period for new moms. The Korean postpartum custom *Samchilil* prescribes twenty-one days of rest following birth. Even in the early twentieth century in the United States, it was not uncommon for women to spend a week in the hospital followed by two weeks in bed at home after giving birth. These rituals acknowledge that it takes weeks, sometimes months, to heal from childbirth. This rebuilding time is especially crucial if the mother will be returning to a job and expects to be effective.

Recognize that a woman who has just given birth should be considered a recuperating person. Best advice: Allow others to take care of you. Ask for help. Rest as often and as much as you can. Focus on sleeping and eating and getting acquainted with your new soul mate, defined as "a person with whom you have an immediate connection the moment you meet."

BREASTFEEDING BONUSES

"Affordable Health Care Begins with Breastfeeding." This slogan, promoted by many breastfeeding coalitions throughout the country, rings true. Every year, new studies appear with news that there is a nutrient or immunological factor found in breast milk that cannot be duplicated in the laboratory. Breast milk has been engineered to provide the child with the best chance of survival. We have only begun to discover the myriad ways in which breast milk nourishes and protects both mother and child.

Despite the American Academy of Pediatrics recommendation of six months of exclusive breastfeeding followed by another six months of breastfeeding plus solids, and the World Health Organization's advice of two full years of breastfeeding, less than 25 percent of US moms breastfeed for twelve months. Advocacy is still needed.

The first liquid from the mother's breast after birth is a thick fluid called colostrum, which helps the baby pass meconium, a substance in the baby's bowels that needs to be expelled before ordinary digestion can begin. Colostrum contains much of the immunological properties the newborn needs, ensuring immediate protection. Colostrum also decreases the absorption of bilirubin, reducing the chance of jaundice. The amount of colostrum decreases as mother's milk matures in the ten to fourteen days following birth.

Breast milk is the only food your baby will need for six months. No extra water, juice, tea, or anything else is necessary. Giving a baby a bottle of anything during the first few weeks of breastfeeding may cause nipple confusion. The breast and bottle require different sucking styles. Going from one to the other can result in frustration for mother and baby. In our society, where the need for variety verges on obsessive, it is hard to believe that babies can thrive on the simplicity of breast milk alone. When well-meaning relatives and friends encourage you to feed the baby something else, thank them for their advice. They may be unaware of the bonuses Mother Nature included in breast milk. (See A List of Breastfeeding Pluses, page 40.)

The intricate biological communication established between mother and baby during nursing inspires awe. The milk responds to the needs of the baby. Formula is static, but breast milk is a living, constantly changing food. For example, the milk produced for a premature baby differs from the milk that comes in for a full-term infant. Breast milk even changes within a single feeding. The milk that comes out of the breast at the beginning of the feeding is more watery and satisfies thirst quickly. Toward the end of the feeding, the milk (called the hind milk) becomes richer in fat. Both are vital for baby. Milk composition also varies with infant gender! More nutrition-rich milk is produced for female children when times are hard and for sons when there are fewer struggles. Daughters are a better bet when income level and safety concerns are heightened, as they can perpetuate the family line.

The interaction between the baby's mouth and the mother's nipple signals the mother's body to increase certain nutrients in the milk if needed or restrict substances that appear dangerous. Even the flavor of a woman's breast milk changes in response to what mom has eaten, while formula remains the same. My good friend Susan, a postpartum doula, wonders if the breastfed baby may respond to and accept new foods more readily, as they have already been receiving a variety of tastes. No human-made substance can duplicate the responsiveness of human breast milk.

The "living" part of breast milk also refers to its inherent friendly bacteria or probiotics. The colonization of baby's gut flora, which dictates the efficacy of the immune system as well as a myriad of other vital systems in the body, happens during the first three years of life. The journey through the vagina provides baby with vital bacteria, but the next exposure that helps establish a healthy gut population comes via nursing. Not only does breast milk provide living bacteria for baby's gut, it provides food for the bacteria! Human milk oligosaccharides (HMOs) are complex carbohydrates found only in breast milk. For years, scientists wondered why they were there since humans do not have the capacity to digest them. The special purpose of the HMOs in breast milk is to nourish the 100 trillion bacterial inhabitants in baby's gut. HMOs also seed bacteroides, other important beneficial bacteria. Though formula companies continue to try to mimic breast milk by adding probiotics or galacto-oligosaccharides intended to emulate HMOs, there is little data showing that these additives approximate breast milk in its ability to establish a healthy gut.

Cultural influences have led women to believe breastfeeding is a hardship. Even when women choose to nurse, their husbands, relatives, and friends may pressure them into early weaning because they are socially uncomfortable seeing the child and the mother's breast together. Social conditioning from advertisements by formula manufacturers or guidance from health-care practitioners unfamiliar with the advantages of breastfeeding may perpetuate this message. To raise children strengthened by breastfeeding requires the courage to ignore social stigmas that go against nature.

If you are pregnant, contact your local La Leche League before the birth for additional support. This amazing international organization has a network of regular meetings, counselors, and literature that promote and support breastfeeding. The Childbirth Education Association (CEA) provides breastfeeding classes and early mothering support classes. Breastfeeding is not simply a matter of doing what you've seen many women in your family do before. We are isolated, no longer privy to the shared wisdom of the greater family. Natural ways often need to be explained and justified. Nevertheless, the resources for innate wisdom remain within our reach and within us, but remember that breastfeeding is a learned skill that often requires guidance and practice.

In instances where breastfeeding may not be possible, such as adoption, formula is the preferred second choice. Formula makers continue to simulate nature by adding long-chain fatty acids (for the development of brain and nerves), probiotics (for healthy gut flora), and beta-carotene (the precursor for vitamin A)—components naturally present in breast milk. However, most commercial formulas contain sugar, salt, and cheap fats such as refined oils. Read the ingredient list on the formula packaging carefully and make the most informed choice possible. Organic formula is a step in the right direction. Do not give baby soy or other alternative milk beverages as a replacement for breast milk or formula.

Creative nutritionists, naturopaths, or other health-care practitioners have attempted to invent more lively homemade formulas that usually combine some form of milk with high-quality vitamin and mineral supplements.

Explore your community and see if there is a reasonable alternative that you and your health-care practitioner can agree upon.

Parents have an instinctual need to nourish their children; the premise of this book is based on that drive. Make whatever changes needed, in your lifestyle or thinking, in order to experience the power of breastfeeding. It is a primal aspect of womanhood we need to reclaim and pass on to the next generation.

a list of breastfeeding pluses
for baby

- Colostrum, the first substance from the mother's breast, helps baby pass meconium, reduces the chance of jaundice, and supplies baby with immunological properties.

- Breast milk contains antibodies to illnesses the mother has had, protecting baby against some infections and reducing the risk of allergies.

- Baby can easily absorb the iron in breast milk thanks to the presence of specialized proteins and vitamin C.

- Sucking at the breast enhances good hand-eye coordination and promotes proper jaw and teeth alignment.

- Breast milk naturally contains the long-chain fatty acids necessary for the development of brain and nerves and beta-carotene, which is considered an important vitamin for the healthy growth of cells.

- Probiotics are naturally present in breast milk, and they help babies develop healthy gut flora, bolstering the developing immune system and reducing the risk of autoimmune diseases and obesity.

- HMOs provide nourishment for friendly bacteria in the gut, helping them thrive.

- Breastfeeding provides a "flavor bridge," so that when the flavors present in breast milk from the maternal diet are introduced as solid food, they will be more welcome.

- Covering baby with kisses has a positive effect! Any pathogens on the baby's skin make their way through mom's lymphatic system where antibodies to fight those pathogens are made. Baby then receives the antibodies through mom's milk. Amazing!

for mother

- After birth, immediate breastfeeding helps contract the uterus and reduce the risk of hemorrhaging.
- The hormone oxytocin, stimulated to release via baby's sucking, acts to return the uterus to its regular size more quickly and can reduce postpartum bleeding. This magic hormone also lowers heart rate and blood pressure and stimulates the production of endorphins (which trigger positive feelings). And as if that weren't enough, women with high levels of oxytocin tolerate mundane, repetitive tasks better (like changing diapers!).
- Breastfeeding aids in steady, slow weight loss by using up approximately an extra five hundred calories a day.
- Night feedings are made easier by not having to warm up a bottle.
- Studies show that every year of breastfeeding reduces the risk of breast cancer by 4.3 percent (which now strikes one out of eight women in this country).
- Recent studies also show reduced risk of developing diabetes or becoming obese in mothers who breastfeed.

for everyone

- Breastfeeding gives mother and child a deep sense of security and love, and it encourages physical closeness.
- Breastfeeding saves time and money. Formula feeding can cost as much as $1,500 a year.
- Outings with baby are easier using naturally hygienic breast milk: no bottles, no sterilizing, no heating things up, no formula, and no fuss.

- The community at large benefits from coming into contact with women nourishing their child naturally rather than relying on commercial technology.

FOODS FOR BREASTFEEDING MOMS

Sometimes women who have been very careful about their eating habits during pregnancy may forget, during nursing, that their bodies are still the source of nutrition for their child. The intake of nutrient-rich foods remains important, though it is sometimes harder to remember with a wee one in tow. The substances taken in by the nursing mother have a potent effect on the milk she produces, both positive and not so positive.

Be aware that the alcohol from a single drink consumed by a nursing mother appears in the breast milk in the same concentration as the mother's blood within 30 minutes. Nicotine ingested by a nursing mother who smokes cigarettes passes into the breast milk as well. Foods eaten by mom can sometimes disagree with the breastfed child, especially high-dosage vitamins, supplements high in iron, artificial sweeteners, caffeine, heavily spiced foods, and occasionally milk. Colicky or fussy babies may improve if the nursing mother's diet is changed. Consult with your health practitioner or lactation counselor. Overindulging in caffeine found in coffee, soft drinks (diet or regular), or over-the-counter drugs can result in an overstimulated baby. Many women feel rushed to get rid of weight gained during pregnancy. The nursing period is not an appropriate time to diet, as reducing calories or restricting nutrient groups can compromise the mother's stamina and her milk supply. Breastfeeding, regular nutritious meals, and long walks are the most important factors in finding the way back to your non-pregnant weight.

The postnatal diet of tribal women throughout the world reveals a consistency of custom. Tribal diets focus on grain-vegetable soups, soft-cooked grains and vegetables, greens, and fish soups. Women drink large quantities of warm water and tea to encourage the flow of milk. At one time African women used a grain called *linga-linga* when nursing. The same grain used in Peru was called "quinoa." This grain has an especially high mineral content.

Quinoa has been rediscovered and is now grown and sold in this country. Another grain purported to aid in producing a good milk supply is sweet brown rice, a cousin of brown rice that has a higher fat content. This grain is often eaten in the form of mochi or amazake.

Departing from cultural wisdom and returning to nutritional math, we see that the Recommended Dietary Allowances (RDA) from the National Academy of Sciences proposes that lactating women need an extra seventy to eighty grams of carbohydrates, twenty to twenty-five grams of protein, and three to four grams of fiber, as well as additional vitamins A, C, and E, folate, and vitamin B_{12}. Consuming foods that contain only empty calories, such as soft drinks, candy, pastries, and salty snack foods, are a waste of calories! Keep these foods to a minimum. By eating ample amounts of nutrient-rich whole foods, including those listed on the following page and used in the recipes in this book, meeting the additional requirements of nursing a child can be simple and satisfying.

To get beneficial long-chain fatty acids into mother's milk, it is wise for mom to consume fish, eggs, poultry, and meat from healthfully raised animals, fermented full-fat dairy products, and nuts and seeds. Breast milk rich in beta-carotene, as well as other vitamins and minerals, requires mom to stock up on lots of dark-green and orange vegetables and fruits. All signals point toward whole foods prepared in simple satisfying ways. High-quality breast milk doesn't require you to eat perfectly balanced, home-cooked meals each and every day. Nature provides plenty of leeway. Do your best to eat well and sensibly throughout the day, drink plenty of liquids, sleep when possible, and practice compassionate thinking. Your milk will be blessed food.

better food, better milk

When a woman is pregnant, she requires up to three hundred additional calories during her third trimester, and a whopping five hundred extra calories per day are needed to nurse an infant! Following is a list of foods that have above-average levels of one or more of the following nutrients: protein, calcium, iron, folic acid, vitamin A, and vitamin C. Including cultured or fermented foods such as yogurt or miso helps keep mom's beneficial bacteria primed.

The two most abundant components of breast milk are fat and lactose. Making sure to consume ample fat, as well as carbohydrates and protein, is essential. Meeting these needs tends to be fairly simple for the omnivore. Vegetarian moms including eggs, dairy, and nuts can usually meet these needs. Vegans need to be vigilant and perhaps consider fatty acid supplements.

- Whole grains: quinoa, millet, sweet brown rice
- Legumes: chickpeas, pinto and navy beans, lentils, split peas, fermented soy foods
- Vegetables: anything dark green or orange
- Fruits: oranges, lemons, berries, grapes, grapefruit, apricots, peaches, melon
- Nuts and seeds: almonds, flaxseeds, pine nuts, sesame and pumpkin seeds, walnuts, coconut and coconut milk
- Sea vegetables: dulse, hiziki, arame
- Dairy: organic butter, yogurt, kefir, cultured sour cream and aged cheeses (from grass-fed cows if possible), fresh goat milks and cheeses
- Fish: wild line-caught fish (especially salmon and halibut), cod liver oil or omega-3 supplement
- Poultry: pastured poultry (both the eggs and the flesh)
- Meat: beef, lamb, and pork (from humanely raised animals)

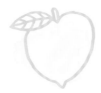

STARTING SOLIDS

Parenthood begins with extreme closeness, the baby living inside the mother. Even if the child is adopted, infants are held against the chest of mom or dad more hours of the day than they are not. We let go of our children slowly, giving them nourishment in many forms to help them literally get on their feet. We want to provide the best food possible for our children so that they can grow healthy bodies capable of fulfilling their wildest dreams.

When we give little ones bland "baby food" prepared by commercial food producers, we rob them of certain opportunities. This trains the child to expect separate meals (special foods) and prefer bland empty calories. Do your child a favor and introduce food with flavor. Feed them versions of the foods you love to eat. Make what you eat good enough to feed your baby.

when

There is no hurry. Look at your baby, not the calendar. Your baby will let you know when it's time to start by giving visible signs of readiness for solid foods. When baby reaches six to seven months of age, here's what to watch for:

- Can baby sit up unattended? Sitting upright is necessary for swallowing thicker substances.

- Is baby able to pick up small objects? This indicates that baby could put a small bit of food in their mouth.

- Does baby show interest in what you're eating? Mimicking your chewing, watching food go in your mouth, or even grabbing for your food are all signs of interest. Baby is ready for solids when they try to intercept the food between your plate and your mouth!

- If you offer baby a little taste of food, are they able to swallow it, or is it pushed back out with the tongue? There is some practice involved here, but the tongue-thrusting reflex is a physiological protection device that begins to diminish around six months of age. Note that some babies may gag or choke easily when first learning to eat. This is not abnormal. If this happens, try diluting the food so that it is more like thick milk or thin cereal.

- Has your baby begun teething? Some cultures regard the appearance of teeth as a sign of readiness for solid food.

Baby's delicate digestive system can become unbalanced by introducing food too soon. Starting solids too early has no benefits unless there are clinical signs that early feeding is critical. Don't be fooled into thinking your baby will sleep through the night by starting solid foods early. Trust your observations. Wait until your child is physically prepared for solids before introducing them.

how

The introduction of solids is formative in how children establish their relationship with food. Make it a joyful occasion, not one approached with fear or trepidation. Again, there is no hurry; the initial step is to introduce new tastes and textures. Your baby is still getting all the nutrition needed from breast milk or formula. The transition to solid food as the primary source of nutrition should be slow.

Once you feel baby may be ready to experiment with solids, here's how to start:

- Invest in a blender and keep it in an easy-to-reach place. Usually, babies ready to begin eating solids have no teeth. Once upon a time mom prechewed food before giving it to baby. Blenders can prechew for us.

- Use one simple whole food. A soft fruit or a cooked sweet vegetable is a good choice.

- Puree the food in a blender or processor, or mash it with a fork. Start with a consistency that is similar to thick milk or thin cereal. Mix the food with a little breast milk or formula. This adds a familiar taste.

- Choose a quiet time of the day that isn't a regular nursing or bottle time. Begin with only a teaspoon of food.

- Talk to your baby about the food and the eating procedure. Later they will be able to respond to cues such as "Open your mouth!" or "Bananas,

Henry?" Don't coax baby into eating something that you wouldn't dream of eating. Tell the truth. Approach the task as a fun experiment.

- Taste a little of the food yourself to model the deliciousness of the food. Offer the food from your finger or from a spoon, or allow baby to grab (messier for you, fascinating for baby).

- Stay with one feeding a day of one simple food. Wait about three to four days before introducing another new food.

- With each new food tried, be aware of allergic reactions such as rashes around the mouth or anus, diarrhea, skin reactions, lethargy, or unusual fussiness. Eliminate, for the time being, any food that causes a reaction and try it again when baby is several months older. For a list of common allergens and other potentially disruptive foods that should be avoided, see Food Intolerances or Sensitivities (page 54).

- After several weeks of one small meal a day, you can increase to two small meals a day. If your baby doesn't seem to enjoy eating solid foods, stop the feedings for a few weeks.

what

Around the globe babies start solids on a variety of foods. In Oceania little ones begin with prechewed fish, grubs, and liver. The Polynesians prefer to start with a pudding-like mixture of breadfruit and coconut cream. Inuit babies are started on seaweed and seal blubber, while Japanese health-care providers recommend a thin rice porridge, eventually made thicker and topped with dried fish, tuna, tofu, and mashed pumpkin.

In American culture whether your baby's first solid food should be a cereal, a fruit, or a vegetable is debatable. If your child is labeled underweight, a health-care practitioner or a relative may encourage you to start with cereals. Others recommend starting baby on fruits and vegetables because these foods digest more easily and quickly than grains. There is some thought that grains are too complex and introducing cereals too early can give babies digestive trouble or lead to allergies. The culprit is likely the overuse of highly refined, flaked baby cereals and the grain fillers (such as modified cornstarch and flour) added to jarred food. Adverse reactions are less likely if freshly made grains are served. It is reasonable to suggest that we may be exacerbating the infant's sensitivity to foods in this culture by early use of antibiotics, disinterest in breastfeeding, and other lifestyle choices. (See Food Intolerances or Sensitivities, page 54.)

Other cultures include fats and proteins as part of baby's beginner foods, whereas American practitioners tend to guide parents toward carbohydrates as starter foods. There are exceptions to every hard-and-fast rule about which foods to introduce when. Starting solids must take into account the food heritage of the parents as well as the health of the infant. Collect information from various sources and choose what makes sense. Parents who serve beginner foods that stay within the realm of simple, whole, fresh foods, and avoid foods on the list of "Not-So-Good" Food for Infants (page 51), will encounter minimal dangers. What matters most is that baby's first eating experience is an enjoyable occasion.

1. START WITH PUREED FRUITS AND VEGETABLES. A safe plan is to serve simple fruits and vegetables for the first few weeks of starting solids. Nice beginning fruits and vegetables include applesauce, avocado, bananas, carrots, sweet potato, peas, and winter squash. Begin with a mashed fruit or vegetable that is the consistency of thick milk or thin soup. Babies will let you know what their favorite foods are. My daughter hated tried-and-true mashed banana but adored sweet potatoes and applesauce.

2. BEGIN TO ADD NONALLERGENIC CEREAL GRAINS. After several weeks of serving pureed fruits and vegetables, you might try cereal. The least allergenic grains, the ones recommended in this book, include brown rice, sweet brown rice, quinoa, and millet. See instructions on how to make Cream of Millet Weaning Cereal (page 77), Toasted Whole Grain Baby Cereal (page 78), or Soaked Whole Grain Baby Porridge (page 80). Begin with cereal that is the consistency of thick milk or thin soup.

Researchers have noted that the introduction of cereals into the infant's diet sharply accelerates the bacterial growth in the gut. One of the great benefits of starting baby on whole grain cereals is the fiber available to feed those burgeoning microbiota.

3. INCLUDE BEGINNER FATS AND PROTEINS. After several weeks of successful eating, you might begin adding a teaspoon or two of organic plain whole-milk yogurt or soft-cooked egg yolks. These offer easily digested high-quality proteins and fats. Start cultured and fermented foods early. Yogurts should list only organic whole milk and a variety of live cultures on the ingredient list—no sweeteners or dried milk solids. Putting a little organic butter on cooked vegetables or soups that you serve to baby is another way to begin adding brain-building fats. Another way to add healthful fat and protein to baby's diet is to puree vegetables and grains with homemade soup stock (see Simple Chicken Stock, page 165).

homemade vs. commercial

Be aware that many commercial baby food manufacturers replace real food with thickening agents (like flour or starches) in their products. This helps their profit margin but does little to nourish your baby. Commercial baby foods are high priced compared to similar regular foods, especially foods such as juices, yogurts, and applesauce. Baby food manufacturers encourage a mystique about their products, making parents believe that commercial baby food has special properties that can't be duplicated in their kitchen. This is clearly untrue. Why pay high prices for nutritionally inferior food for your baby?

Parents can easily prepare safe, nutritious, and economical foods for their infants at home.

Certainly occasional organic jarred food can be used for baby as a convenience, but it definitely lacks freshness and flavor. Instead of training baby to eat bland premade food, help him develop a repertoire of the flavors and textures the rest of the family regularly enjoys. This makes the transition to eating family meals more seamless. Adaptations for how to take part of the food that the rest of the family is eating and prepare some for baby are given at the end of most recipes in this book. Any time you see "FOR BABIES 6 MONTHS & OLDER" at the bottom of a recipe, an idea follows for taking part of the dish and making food for a baby just starting solids.

iron fortification?

How could we have survived as a species so long if babies can't thrive without artificial supplements? Many parents are encouraged to give their baby iron supplements or iron-fortified cereals starting at around six months. Ferrous sulfate, the most common iron supplement, is poorly absorbed and can cause indigestion and constipation. The type of iron used in commercial baby cereal, one of the least absorbable, is used because it sticks to the flakes and won't discolor the cereal.

Your baby was born with a good store of iron, which came from the mother during pregnancy. This is one reason why hematocrit levels are monitored in pregnant women and why women are encouraged to increase their iron intake during pregnancy. During the past century it became common practice to clamp the cord about ten seconds after the baby's shoulders are delivered. However, there has been little scientific research to justify such rapid clamping. Just a two-minute delay in clamping a baby's umbilical cord can boost the child's iron reserves and prevent anemia for months. This was reported by nutritionists at the University of California, Davis, from a 2005 study done in Mexico City, though it has been common knowledge among savvy midwives for many years.

Breast milk contains a small amount of highly absorbable iron to meet baby's needs. Babies can absorb up to 50 percent of the iron in breast milk but only 4 percent of the iron in fortified formula. The vitamin C present in breast milk increases the absorption of the iron. Lactoferrin and transferrin, two specialized proteins in mother's milk, regulate the iron supply to baby. As long as the mother was not anemic during pregnancy, and the umbilical cord was not cut too soon, the breastfed baby should have adequate iron for the first year of life.

Around six months, when solid foods are introduced, baby begins to get iron from sources other than breast milk, formula, or stores accumulated in utero. With the transition to a whole foods diet, most babies need no supplements. If skeptical, you can give your child a baby multivitamin, which may be benign. For extra iron, add sea vegetables (dulse is best) to baby's diet or use cast-iron cookware to prepare baby's food.

safety tips for homemade baby food

- Before using any equipment to prepare baby food, wash it with hot water and soap. Rinse well and dry.

- Never serve baby hot food. Room temperature or slightly warm is fine. Hungry baby, but cereal's too hot? Stir it with an ice cube for quick cooling.

- Microwaving sometimes heats food unevenly. This can create "hot spots" in baby's food or bottle that can burn baby's mouth. Use caution if microwaving or avoid it.

- If you've made a large batch of food, remove a small portion to a separate dish to serve your baby.

- Discard leftover food that has had spoon-to-mouth contact.

- Store leftovers that have not had spoon-to-mouth contact in the refrigerator and use within two or three days.

- Freeze extra pureed food in ice cube trays. Frozen cubes can then be stored in the freezer in plastic bags. For a quick meal, place a cube or two of frozen food in a small dish and heat in a covered pan of boiling water. Use frozen baby food within four weeks.

- Store ground grains for cereals in sterile jars in the refrigerator or freezer.

- Label all stored food.

"not-so-good" food for infants

CAFFEINE. Caffeine is a stimulant, not a food, and can be found in soft drinks and cocoa. Caffeine can cause elevated blood sugar and stimulate the heart and lungs. This kind of stimulation can be jolting to a baby's sensitive system.

CHEMICAL ADDITIVES. Avoid aspartame, saccharin, Splenda (sucralose), all other artificial sweeteners, BHT, artificial flavors and colors, MSG, nitrates, and other additives. The effect of chemical additives on adults is not entirely known. There certainly can be no benefit to introducing substances to your baby's immature system. Read labels.

CITRUS FOODS. The acids in oranges, lemons, and limes as well as strawberries and tomatoes can sometimes cause diaper rash or other signs of intolerance in babies under one year old. These are important Vitamin C foods that can be introduced when baby is more mature. The tiny seeds in strawberries can sometimes irritate an immature digestive tract. Wait on these.

COMMON ALLERGENS. A true food allergy is a reaction by the immune system to a specific protein. Peanuts, cow's milk, and egg whites are the most common, but fish, shellfish, soy, and wheat are also problematic for a few people. If you have a family history of food allergies, it would seem prudent to forgo giving your baby the foods listed above. However, recent studies involving peanut allergies conclude that introducing peanut-containing foods into the diets of babies—including those prone to allergies—is a safe practice and drastically reduces their risk of developing peanut allergies later on. Recommendations on early introduction of other allergens are pending. See Food Allergies and Intolerances (page 53) for more information.

COW'S MILK. Cow's milk is not appropriate for babies under one year old. It can cause bleeding in the intestines that is difficult to detect, resulting in iron-deficiency anemia.

RAW HONEY. Uncooked honey and corn syrup sometimes contains botulism toxins in amounts that are dangerous for infants under one year of age. Barley malt or brown rice syrup can be substituted.

SALT. Seasoning home-cooked foods with sea salt that will later be served to baby is fine. This is a very negligible amount and much different than giving baby processed packaged foods. Avoid giving baby salty snack foods such as pretzels, Goldfish crackers, or potato chips. These heavily salted foods, designed to make you want more, can stress baby's immature kidneys.

SUGAR. A prime source of empty calories, sugar has almost no nutritive value. Eating large amounts of sugary foods can displace more nutritional foods, resulting in vitamin and mineral deficiencies. Refined sugar consumption, including corn syrup, fructose, agave, high fructose corn syrup, and cane sugar, has been linked with tooth decay, heart disease, atherosclerosis, diabetes, obesity, learning difficulties, and behavior problems. Why let your baby develop an early craving for it? For more on sugar, see Sweet Tooth (page 67).

foods babies often choke on

To prevent accidents avoid giving the following foods to babies under one year old. When you're trying any new snack, be sure that your baby is within eyesight and earshot so that you can be quick to help if a problem develops. Have little ones sit down when eating, as choking most often occurs when children are walking or running. A good rule of thumb is to make sure that any food bite larger than marble size can mash quickly and easily with the soft pad of your finger (like baby's gums). The following list includes foods that could be problematic for small mouths and throats.

- Apple chunks or slices
- Grapes
- Hard candy
- Hard cookies
- Hot dogs
- Meat chunks
- Nut butter sandwiches
- Olives
- Popcorn
- Potato chips
- Raw carrot sticks or slices
- Rice cakes
- Whole nuts and seeds
- Whole or unseeded berries

FOOD ALLERGIES & INTOLERANCES

food allergies

A food allergy is a reaction by the immune system to a specific protein in food. The diagnosis can be confirmed by a skin or blood test. The allergy can be expressed in a variety of ways, everything from rashes, vomiting, or wheezing to (in rare cases) anaphylactic shock. A true food allergy is actually quite rare (affecting 2 percent of the population), although nearly 20 percent claim they have a food allergy. When children are suspected of having a food allergy, usually a parent or family member suffers from the same problem. If you discover your child has a food allergy, through testing with a health-care practitioner, the food needs to be avoided. Except in severe cases, the child may outgrow the allergy and the food can be tried again with a health-care practitioner's supervision.

If members of your family have food allergies and you feel your baby may be at risk for developing them, there are preventative tactics. Aim for exclusive breastfeeding for six months and continued breastfeeding for the first year. The probiotics in breast milk and in early food such as plain yogurt help establish a healthy biome in the gut, which is advantageous in preventing allergies. Special baby formulas exist that may be useful in alleviating allergies as well; check with your health-care practitioner.

When you introduce solid foods at six months old, start with low-allergy foods such as rice, millet, squash, sweet potato, and pear as a cautionary measure. For families that suspect food allergies, waiting to introduce cow's milk, eggs, soy, fish, and wheat until the child reaches age three has been the recommended protocol by the American Academy of Pediatrics for nearly fifteen years. But the pediatrician group withdrew those recommendations in 2008 after the number of kids with peanut allergies continued to rise and after several studies began hinting at benefits to introducing allergenic foods during infancy. To date only early introduction of peanuts have been studied. Do not avoid potential allergenic foods unless you have been advised by your health-care practitioner to do so.

food intolerances or sensitivities

A food intolerance or sensitivity is not a true food allergy. This diagnosis is common, yet it is not well understood why the intolerances occur. The skin and blood tests that can be used to determine an allergy to a food protein cannot reveal the more subtle "intolerance" to a food. Symptoms of food intolerance are quite varied. They include skin reactions such as eczema, breathing problems such as runny or stuffed nose, and, for some, headaches, muscle pain, and chronic irritability. The most common prescribed way of determining food sensitivity is to go on a diet that avoids all of the likely foods and then gradually add back the foods one by one to determine which ones are causing the symptoms.

If you find that your child has a food intolerance or sensitivity, by noticing that symptoms improve when certain foods are avoided, here are a few things to consider. Babies are born with a fairly primitive immune system. How the immune system develops and reacts to new foods is influenced by the microbiota in the gut. A few things that destroy the friendly bacteria in our gut include antibiotics (taken directly or from our food supply), chlorinated water, and stress. In our ultraclean society, we sometimes don't develop enough friendly bacteria in our gut to support the immune system, making us more hypersensitive to foods.

Breastfed babies have the benefit of receiving the friendly bacteria present in mother's milk as well as the HMOs that nourish the bacteria. Improving gut flora by including small amounts of yogurt or kefir containing live cultures with baby's food (just a ½ teaspoon will do) can be beneficial. Allowing baby to interact with dirt, plants, other children, and tame animals exposes them to a variety of bacteria, strengthening their immune system.

Antibiotics kill good guys along with the bad guys. Overuse of these seeming wonder drugs has left its mark, contributing to the rise of what Dr. Martin Blaser (author of *Missing Microbes*) calls our modern plagues: obesity, asthma, allergies, diabetes, and certain forms of cancer. Blaser's studies suggest antibiotic use during early childhood poses the greatest risk to long-term health. Surprisingly, most American children have received seventeen courses before the age of twenty! Be cautious about jumping to give your baby antibiotics, especially if the illness is not serious—such as a head cold. If your child has recently taken a round of antibiotics, it might be prudent to follow that with a round of probiotics to help reestablish their intestinal flora. Check with your health-care provider to find the right probiotic supplement to administer.

Some food sensitivities may simply be a symptom of poor digestion. Improve your child's ability to digest their food by making sure that they eat at regular times and sit calmly while they eat, chewing well. Include some cultured or fermented foods in their diet, such as high-quality yogurt, miso soup, or pickles to give the friendly bacteria in their digestive system a boost. Remember that microbiota need food too! Include nuts, seeds, whole grains, and beans in daily meals.

Food sensitivities may also be reflective of overdoing certain foods. Because of the overproduction of soy, corn, and wheat crops in our country, food producers have found ways to stretch their profits by adding cheap oils, sweeteners, starches, and fillers made from highly refined versions of these foods. As a result they are in virtually every processed food product that we purchase. This certainly can lead to consuming the same food, in un-whole, un-fresh forms, over and over and over. Read labels, eat a variety of grains and legumes, and avoid refined forms of soy, corn, and wheat.

Cow's milk is a common food sensitivity for young children. Most often the symptoms are skin or sinus related. Avoiding pasteurized, homogenized cow's milk and focusing on fermented and cultured dairy products may be one solution. These products have some of the more problematic proteins and sugars broken down by friendly bacteria, making the food easier to tolerate. Be wary of replacing everything that comes from a cow (milk, cheese) with products that come from soy foods (see page 14).

Celiac disease represents a much more serious problem. This is a genetic disorder where symptoms include frequent diarrhea and weight loss. Those affected suffer damage to the villi in the intestines when they eat grains that contain gluten, wheat, barley, and rye. Gluten-free flour formulas for baking can be found. (See Have It Your Way: Flour, Fat, Milk, Sweetener, and Egg Substitutions, page 401.) Gluten sensitivity is not the same as celiac disease and is more often self-diagnosed. If you suspect gluten sensitivity, because of a wide array of seemingly unrelated symptoms, begin by eliminating white flour products from the diet. Most commercial breads and crackers contain additives that may bring on symptoms. Recent surveys show that the 36 percent of people choosing gluten-free products are doing so because they believe the products are "healthier" or for "no reason." Many so-called experts blame the grain when in truth the problems more likely come from compromised gut health.

Take time to contemplate how your child is doing on an emotional level. Food intolerances are more common in children who are under stress, either emotionally, physically, or both. Once their life becomes more balanced, the sensitivity may go away.

Food sensitivities are a snapshot representing a period of time, not a life sentence. Some children simply outgrow food intolerances as their bodies get larger and more mature.

Here's good news—this book provides many recipes that are friendly toward families with food allergies or sensitivities! Besides using a wide variety of grains, legumes, and nuts, there are simple instructions for how to make substitutions. (See Have It Your Way: Flour, Fat, Milk, Sweetener, and Egg Substitutions, page 401.)

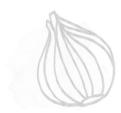

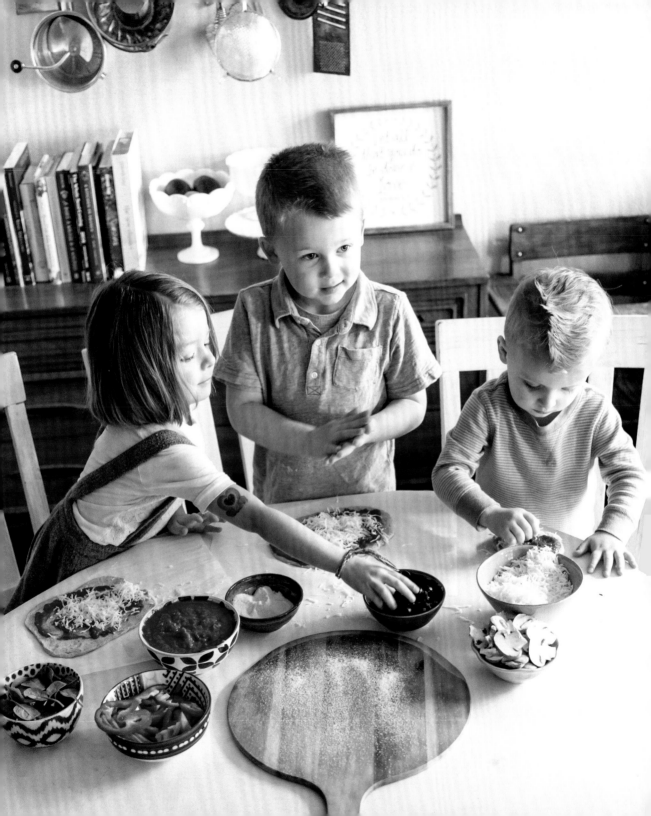

CHAPTER 3

raising healthy eaters

- - - - - - - - - - - - - -

WHEN I PICKED MY DAUGHTER up from kindergarten, she usually wanted to stay and play until all the other children were gone, so I often observed the action. There was a mischievous elflike boy named Jonathan in her class. He would run and hide when the teachers wanted him to come in. He would dart outside without putting his shoes on. Once, he sat down in the mud, delighting in testing boundaries. I formed opinions about him. I thought of him as a "handful." One time I thought that they probably needed an extra teacher just for Jonathan.

I was invited to school to make lunch with the children one Friday and brought pinto beans, tortillas, brown rice, avocados, salsa, cheese, and lettuce to make a burrito lunch line. The kitchen was near the classroom and the children were welcome to help. Some would stop by and assist for ten or fifteen minutes and then drift on to play.

One child stayed right by my side all morning—Jonathan. He mashed beans, peeled avocados, and squeezed limes. He listened and followed instructions and was not only helpful but gleeful about making guacamole. I was humbled. This little elf reminded me about "respect," a word that means "to look again."

Children are remarkably malleable. As soon as we label them, thinking that we can predict their behavior in some way, they surprise us by doing the opposite. Children invite us to experience the world with fresh eyes. They remind us that we do not know what will happen next. Don't presume that Fred will never eat lima beans or that Judy will always want her apple peeled. Stay open to the little bits of magic lurking in every corner.

Maybe you'll discover an elf in your kitchen.

PARENTS AS ROLE MODELS

Parents powerfully shape their child's early experiences with food and eating. The tiniest baby notices every move you make, every forkful that goes into your mouth. Young children are ready to learn about foods of their parents eat; their ability to learn to accept a wide range of foods is remarkable. Parents select the foods of the family diet, serve as models, and impose the feeding practices that develop the child's eating patterns.

A well-intentioned parent may spoon carefully prepared homemade purees into baby while dining on fast-food takeout. What message does this convey? As soon as the child can walk and grab, baby wants what mommy and daddy eat. The primary job of parents is to set a good example. Adherence to the parent's eating habits will wax and wane through various stages of the child's life. Most kids go through rebellious stages (ages three and fifteen come to mind) where rejecting whatever parents do is the course of the day, but the underlying patterns they were shown about food remain. Here are four suggestions to help you become models of healthful eating habits for your children.

1. BECOME AWARE OF HOW YOU FEEL ABOUT FOOD. What are some of your favorite foods? What kind of feelings would surface if you could never have them again? What are some foods you hate? Do you know why you hate them? Many hated foods have their roots in childhood. How closely have you modeled your parent's eating habits? Are vegetables something you're supposed to eat or do you really like them? Is sugar something you deserve if you've been good, had a bad day, or finished your plate?

These unspoken beliefs and preferences transmit loud and clear to children. Changing feelings about certain foods may not come easy, but awareness of those feelings can. Take stock. Figure out which food habits have become unconscious. Make decisions about whether passing them on would be harmful or beneficial.

2. MAKE CONSCIENTIOUS CHOICES ABOUT WHAT FOOD YOU BUY AND HOW YOU SERVE IT. Parents control the supply line. Stock your cupboards with food you feel good about serving. Many child-rearing books encourage parents to set gentle but firm boundaries with children to help them feel safe and protected. This concept applies to eating as well. Be sure to set boundaries that you can follow too. It's not fair to have a strict no-sugar policy while you sneak adults-only ice cream. Boundaries for feeding children that instill positive eating habits with minimum stress are outlined in Guides for Successful Mealtime (page 62). Include pleasurable rituals as part of boundary setting. Maybe Sunday night is "pizza night," where each family member creates their own pizza (see Veggie Lovers' Pizza Party, page 261).

3. MAKE EVERY DAY FOOD APPRECIATION DAY. As soon as your child can talk, you can begin to communicate information about food. Notice the word "food" is used, not "nutrition"! Refrain from nagging them about how they need to eat specific micronutrients, like "You have to drink your milk or you won't get enough calcium!" Studies show the inverse of what you want is more likely to happen—children disliking or avoiding these foods. You can offer simple, brief reasons why you don't want them to eat certain food, such as "This soda has stuff in it that your body can't use; let's buy something else to drink." Or you help children notice how they feel when have skipped meals or eaten too much. More often, talk to them about mouthwatering Poached Pears (page 311) or yummy Split Pea Soup with Fresh Peas and Potatoes (page 176).

Take your children shopping with you. As children reach grade school age, present them with a challenge, such as finding the loaf of bread with the fewest ingredients. Encourage your children to help you cook by slowing down and allowing for the longer preparation time necessary to include a willing participant. Check Involving Your Children in the Kitchen (page 68) for oodles of ideas.

4. LET GO. Learning to bend rules and being flexible are perhaps the most important lessons of parenting. Relaxing around birthday parties and other social gatherings where less-than-optimal foods are offered is easier if what's served at home is nutritionally sound. A woman in one of my classes proudly announced that she baked no-sugar, whole wheat birthday cakes for her child to take to parties instead of allowing the child to share the cake being served. Yikes! Rules that cause a child to feel uncomfortable in social situations are unnecessary and much unhealthier than sugary cake. Research shows that giving children restrictive demands or fear-filled messages such as "No cookies until you eat that broccoli" or "If you don't eat protein, you won't grow" backfire. This type of communication may very well cause children to reject the foods you want them to eat. Overcontrolling certain foods may make them become irresistible, taking on more power than warranted.

Children have a lot to teach us. Have you ever had the experience of offering food to your child all day, having the offer repeatedly refused, then realizing later that they were coming down with a cold? The child's intuition not to eat at that time was right on the nose. My child used to regularly come home from a birthday party and ask to eat nori strips. How did she know that one of the consequences of too much sugar is that it creates a mineral debt in the body and that seaweed contains more minerals than any other food? Many children intuitively request what their bodies need.

GUIDES FOR SUCCESSFUL MEALTIME

We keep infants very close to our bodies. With each year, we give them a little more space to roam and a few more choices to make, even as we continue to provide limits. This slow release also applies to food. An infant feels secure with just breast or bottle. Preschoolers may be able to clearly tell you if they would prefer an apple or a bowl of oatmeal. A ten-year-old can help plan the dinner menu. The goal is to help your child develop a self-regulating intake of wholesome food. Pressuring children doesn't work. Think through these seven guides.

1. PROVIDE EXCELLENT CHOICES. Stock your cupboards and your refrigerator with fresh, healthful, whole food products. When you feel good about all the food in your cupboards, battles are reduced or eliminated. You can't expect to keep junk foods in the house and not be badgered for a taste, especially if your child sees you eating those items. Keep good foods ready and available. Have prepared fruits and vegetables placed at your child's eye level in the refrigerator; more will be eaten. Buy less of foods that you want to limit and store them in harder-to-reach cupboards.

You are the food authority in your home, not your child. A four-year-old cannot plan a balanced meal or decide which kind of peanut butter to buy. Too many choices overwhelm a young child, and yet they strive for independence. Use Ellyn Satter's Division of Responsibility in Feeding (EllynSatterInstitute.org): parents decide what to serve and when and where to serve it, and children decide what and how much to eat from what is served.

2. HONOR RITUAL. How often families eat together and who is present during family meals matters as much as what food is served. Commit to sharing at least one common meal with your whole family each day or several times a week. The family meal is not only a time for nourishment but an opportunity for children to experience social education. Put all electronic devices away. Turn off the television. Emphasize rituals: lighting candles, saying a verse, setting the table with care, serving food a certain way. Consider keeping a regular time for the evening meal. For some pretty convincing reasons on why sharing meals benefits children, check out Sharing the Meal (page 30).

3. WHAT'S SERVED IS SERVED. Do not make the mistake of preparing a separate meal for your child. Serve each person at the table a portion of each dish prepared. If a child refuses to eat one of the foods, you can encourage them to sample one or two bites, but a stronger message is to let them see you enjoy eating the food. Don't oversell with words. Just eat. Another idea is to ask, "What would make this food yummier?" You might get a stubborn "Nothing," but you could receive some helpful information about serving size, appearance, or toppings!

Try serving meals family style rather than plated. This allows children the opportunity to select what and how much they want to eat of the choices provided. Children who refuse to eat anything on the plate should be asked to excuse themselves and told that no other food will be served until break-fast or whatever seems reasonable considering your child's age. If they come whining for food later, consider offering the leftover dinner. One way to avoid the "untouched meal" syndrome is to make sure that each meal has a sure winner: a simple side dish you know your child will like (see Include a Winner at Every Meal, below).

Incorporate a "no-critics-at-the-table" rule. Teach your children that it is inappropriate to shout out harsh or cruel reviews such as, "I hate every-thing!" or "This looks awful!" Remind such reviewers that their words are unkind and ask them to excuse themselves from the dinner table. Suggest more courteous ways for expressing dislike of a food. Let them know they will be welcome at dinner the next night, where they can practice being more considerate. Big tip: children who help prepare the food for a meal are less critical at the dinner table.

4. INCLUDE A WINNER AT EVERY MEAL. Children usually like simple food and will sometimes refuse foods that have multiple ingredients. Honor this by regularly offering carrot sticks, apple slices, baked sweet potato, or unadorned brown rice. Sometimes it takes an elaborate salad with an excit-ing dressing to please an adult, whereas a five-year-old may be happy with undressed, sliced cucumbers. When planning meals, include something sim-ple that you're certain your child will like, even if it's just a side dish of sliced bread or applesauce.

5. DON'T BRIBE, REWARD, OR PUNISH WITH FOOD. Offering or withholding sweets or any other "forbidden" food in exchange for good behavior is a bad idea. This sets up hard-to-reverse psychological attachments to food. Food is something you eat in order to get energy to play and to grow. Eating is a primal need, a joyful daily ritual. Find an arena besides the dinner table to work out power struggles with children.

Avoid tension and save money by not serving desserts every day. Reserve home-baked goodies for occasional snacks or special occasions and avoid constant negotiation about sweets. Let's say doughnuts are the favorite food and you, the parent, feel it is not in the child's best interest to serve them every day. Instead of banishing doughnuts or using them as a trade for fin-ishing math homework (bad idea), set a schedule about how often doughnuts are eaten and stick to it; maybe they become the Saturday breakfast treat. When battles or negotiations arise, you can simply restate the rule.

6. LIMIT (BUT INCLUDE) SPECIAL TREATS AND FAVORITE "LESS-NUTRITIOUS" FOODS. Let's say you've got a child that loves hot dogs. We don't want to shame this nutritionally questionable preference. On the other hand, we don't want to cave and serve them every day, right? What about a monthly hot dog night? Buy the best dogs available and serve them with plenty of other good foods. The same can go for trips to favorite fast-food joints.

Unfortunately, most American celebrations seem to revolve around sugar, particularly sweets aimed at children. Provide some reasonable limits to curb the heavy intake of sugary foods at these times. For example, when given a bag of candy as a "favor" at a birthday party, let the child choose one piece a day to eat. This may work, as sometimes interest wanes after a few days. If your child is over age eight, let them help design the rules.

When your child is ill or has an infection, this is the good time to go ahead and restrict stressful foods. Forgo candy, soda, and salty and fried foods. Bodies recover from illnesses much quicker when they are given nourishing foods that are easy to digest, such as soups and broths. Congee for Recovery on (page 395) fits the bill. Teach your child how to recover from illness.

7. TRUST YOUR CHILD'S PREFERENCES (MOST OF THE TIME). Children have good instincts. If they are being offered a variety of wholesome foods, they will eat what their body needs. Balance is achieved over several days rather than within one twenty-four-hour period. Watch. Often they will hit all the food groups during the week. To eliminate worry about sufficient nutrients, offer a variety of whole foods steadily and consistently.

A child's wonderful intuition can go awry. Refined sugar, foods with chemical additives, and highly salted foods can trigger miscues. Excessive amounts of these substances can mar your child's natural good judgment. Food manufacturers count on this and design food for its "cravability." When heavy doses of unnatural foods have been consumed and children begin expressing cravings for more, parents need to intervene and restore balance.

Remember to respect your child's individuality. For example, children who behave negatively after eating too much sugar may benefit from firmer boundaries. Other children may show so little interest in food that you may not want to set many limits. Some children are natural vegetarians, while others may want or need animal protein. Listen to your child's requests and guide them toward the healthier, whole foods way of fulfilling them.

for parents of picky eaters

Recent studies reveal some interesting information about children who express a narrow idea of what they want to eat. Twenty percent of all children aged two to six are moderate to severe picky eaters. Their heightened sensitivity to certain foods is real. Bitter tastes (like broccoli) can be particularly repellent, a natural biological response.

Picky eaters first judge a food by how it looks! The second level of criteria is texture, and lastly, the flavor. This progression can prove important, as the first two sensory cues are fairly easy to change. The social setting in which the meal is served also has an effect, meaning: don't make the dinner table the family battleground.

More ideas:

- Have your child help plan, shop for, and prepare meals. See Involving Your Children in the Kitchen (page 68).

- Change the look of the food. Examples can be found in Appealing Food Presentation (page 70), "My Child Won't Eat Vegetables" (page 72), and at the bottom of some of the recipes in the recipe section.

- Alter the texture. Cooked, sliced beets may get a thumbs-down but Rosemary Red Soup (page 175) might warrant tasting.

- Don't be tempted to make separate meals for your picky eater. This habit gets old fast and can generate worry or resentment in the family cook. Follow the What's Served Is Served guide (page 63).

- Consider serving meals family style.

- Include one dish at each meal that you know your child will enjoy. Something as simple as carrot sticks or banana slices is fine.

- Stop all snacking two hours before mealtime. That's right. No juice or milk either. Power down any and all screens and encourage physical play. Hungry children are less picky.

- Introduce new foods at snack time, where the atmosphere may be more casual. Characterize trying the new food as an adventure.

- Invite one of your child's friends, a teacher, or coach over for dinner. If your child sees someone they like eat a food they typically shun, they might reconsider!

sweet tooth

Babies and children have an innate preference for sweet foods. We evolved to prefer the sweet taste as a protective functions as it signals energy-rich, safe foods, whereas the bitter or sour taste could indicate the food is toxic. But too much sugar, for children or adults, can be harmful too. Or if that sounds too dramatic, let's put it this way—too much sugar in the diet encourages weight gain and tooth decay, and (for some) triggers cravings.

So how much is too much for children? The American Heart Association suggests that men limit sugar intake to 150 calories a day (9 teaspoons), women to 100 calories (6 to 7 teaspoons), and children should keep it to 62 calories = 16 grams = 4 teaspoons. That's not much room to splurge! Here are a few suggestions to help curb the sugar enthusiasm of the child (or parent) with a persistent sweet tooth.

- Schedule a whole fruit snack break at the time when the sugar cravings usually occur. Coupled with some protein (e.g., apple with cheese, banana with peanut butter) is even better.

- Set some rules about how often a sweet treat is served. Let the child help with the wording of the rule.

- Limit desserts to homemade ones. (This one kicks me out of the sugar den, as I rarely, maybe once a month, have time to make desserts.) When you do make a batch of cookies, plan to share some with the neighbors.

- Be sure the basics are covered: enough sleep, plenty of water, and regular meals. Stress really turns on the sugar crazies.

INVOLVING YOUR CHILDREN IN THE KITCHEN

Children need to feel a sense of belonging. In the days of farms and big families, children were a natural part of doing the chores to get food on the table. Today, children often lose the opportunity to be needed and to contribute to the daily work routine of house and family. In American culture meals are something prepared for children, not by children.

Even children who have just begun to walk can help out in the kitchen. They can learn all sorts of things about food, cooking, nutrition, math, science, and recycling by helping prepare food. Kitchen participation helps teach self-reliance and gives the sense of contributing.

helping your helper

· Use simple, short sentences to describe how the work is to be done while slowly demonstrating the task. Be clear and patient.

· Clear out a low cupboard for your child. Keep pots and pans there so your toddler can play near you, copying you.

· For the preschooler use the space to store unbreakable dishes that they can serve with or use for imaginary house play. Older children may enjoy having their own kitchen tools or ingredients to make simple snacks on a reachable shelf.

· Get a sturdy stool or small chair that your child can move in order to reach the counter and sink.

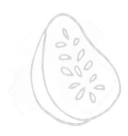

YOUR CHILD'S CONTRIBUTION TO FAMILY MEALS

	FOOD SHOPPING	PREPARATION	SERVING	CLEAN UP
AGES 2-3	Pick herbs or fruit from the garden.	Turn processors on and off. Put muffin cups in muffin tins. Mash bananas or cooked potatoes. Spin the salad spinner. Let you know when the timer goes off. Taste test.*	Set the table. Pick flowers and put them in a vase. Roll napkins into napkin rings. Call the family to dinner.	Take small trash items to the trash can.
AGES 4-5	Help plan lunch box chart (see page 139).	Retrieve items from the refrigerator. Wash fruits and vegetables. Oil pans and baking sheets. Tear lettuce or greens into small pieces. Toss a salad. Measure and pour dry ingredients. Put spread on breads or crackers. Sift flour. Form cookies with hands or cookie cutters. Taste test.* Garnish food.	Create place cards.	Wipe up spills. Clear the kitchen table. Dry and put dishes away. Sort clean silverware into compartments. Sweep the floor with dustpan and brush.
AGES 6-7	Carry groceries into the house.	Grate carrots and cheese Grind grains or nuts in grinder or processor (not removing). Knead dough. Roll out dough with a rolling pin. Taste test.*	Help pack lunch box. Make placemats with paper and markers/crayons. Put candles on the table and light them (with adult help).	Wipe table or placemats. Load dishes in the dishwasher. Take trash and recycling to outside bins.
AGES 8 & UP	Help with menu planning. Unload grocery bags and put things away.	Make snacks. Peel carrots, cucumbers, and potatoes. Stir cooking food. Taste test.* Make salad and/or salad dressing. Scramble eggs. Flip pancakes. Use electric mixer.	Table, platter, and plate food presentation. Serve and refill water.	Put away leftovers. Unload dishes from the dishwasher. Clean countertops. Dust and/or mop the floor.

*   Taste test: I wrote the first version of Feeding the Whole Family when my daughter was three. As a somewhat insecure chef, I constantly offered her a spoonful of creations to test. "Does it need salt?" "Would more lemon juice help?" "Do you like it?" Unbeknownst to me, I was creating an eager diner and a talented cook. I highly recommend employing children to taste test; the benefits are far-reaching.

raising healthy eaters

APPEALING FOOD PRESENTATION

When the eyes behold colorful, artistic, or tantalizing food, the mouth begins secreting enzymes to digest the food, and the lips curve into a smile. Food presentation can be important for young children. Your child may refuse a sandwich unless it's cut in a certain shape or has the crusts removed. You may be able to delight a child into eating something new by putting a face on it or cutting it into a heart shape. Dust off your imagination and expand on the following food presentation ideas for young ones. I once cut a sheet of nori into paper dolls for my three year old. Decorating food can bring humor and light to your and your child's day.

decorate food

• Stock a variety of cookie cutters and use them to cut sandwiches and pancakes. Find cutters in the shapes of your child's favorite animals. International markets sometimes have small, strong cutters for making vegetables into beautiful shapes. These can be fun for turning zucchini or carrot slices into flowers.

• Serve brown rice, potatoes, or other foods with a large ice cream scoop or packed into a ramekin, then inverted. Use different heights to draw interest.

• Make food friendlier by putting a face on it. Use raisins, small pieces of vegetables, small crackers, or whatever you can dream up to fashion eyeballs, noses, and mouths. Bowls of soup, mashed potatoes, or plates of rice suddenly become funny personalities for your child to devour. Apple slices make sweeping smiles; olives make 3-D eyeballs.

use delightful dinnerware
& playful packaging

- You might try buying a special plate, cup, or even silverware for your child. This can be as extravagant as a complete Winnie-the-Pooh set or simply "Jack's yellow plate." Having personal dinnerware can enhance your child's enjoyment of meals. Children also derive security from being able to count on the same bowl or spoon every day. Serving red zinger tea in a special cup or plopping a crazy straw into a smoothie can make all the difference.

- Lunch box packaging can have charm too. Your child may love having lunch packed in a recyclable paper bag with a silly face drawn on the outside. Another child may prefer a basket with a lid and ribbons tied on the handle. Asian markets sell interesting merchandise designed for packing food to go. Sometimes you can find beautiful bento-box style travelers that have colorful little compartments inside.

- Fun surprises hidden inside a lunch box need not be sweets. How about a marble, a seashell, an envelope with a note or stickers inside, a little pad of paper, or a tiny pencil? There are many ways to convey a loving message.

tell a story

Can you turn a plate of spaghetti into a pail of hay for a pretend lamb in your kitchen? Maybe a bowl of yellow split pea soup can be a bowl of melted gold for your pirate? Pretend play is very important to the young, and people of all ages love a good story. Why not use it to everyone's advantage? Make up a wild tale about what magic kingdom the beans came from or how the carrot just barely escaped Mr. Rabbit. This will make the food impossible not to devour (or at least taste).

"MY CHILD WON'T EAT VEGETABLES"

In almost every class that I have taught for parents, someone raises their hand to say, "My husband/daughter/son hates vegetables. What should I do?" This is a common worry, especially now that MyPlate (ChooseMyPlate.gov), the current nutrition guide published by the US Department of Agriculture, suggests that half of our plates be dedicated to fruits and vegetables.

· First, check out your own thoughts about vegetable eating. Make sure that you love them, like them, or at least appreciate them before asking your children to eat more of them. What you are thinking transfers to your child, even if it's unspoken.

· Next, help your child create a relationship with vegetables. One excellent way to improve your child's interest in vegetables is to let them help you plant and harvest a small vegetable garden. If you don't have space for a garden, go visit one. Let them see, touch, and even smell vegetables being grown.

· Bring your child with you to the grocery store and let them pick out fruits and vegetables that look good to them.

· Invite your child to help you prepare vegetables. Look at One-Trick Vegetables (page 191) to find tasty vegetable dishes your child can help make. Let your child make beautiful arrangements on the plate using the bright colors of the vegetables.

With children who eat their fair share of whole grains, fruits, and beans, relax some; these foods contain a wide variety of vitamins and minerals present in vegetables. Remember that children naturally gravitate toward the sweet taste. Roasting carrots or braising brussels sprouts in apple juice sweetens them. Make sure ample whole fruit is available each day. Remembering that beauty is in the eye of the beholder, here are some ways to prepare and serve vegetables that may appeal to your child.

JUICES: Students who take my classes report great success in getting children to drink various vegetable juices. Carrot juice is a favorite, especially mixed with a little apple juice. But remember, juice is not a whole food; the fiber is gone and the sugars become highly concentrated. Dilute vegetable and fruit juices; one half juice, one half water.

SMOOTHIES: Carrots, kale, spinach, and all sorts of vegetable goodness can be tossed into a blender with some yogurt, milk, or banana to create a drinkable meal. Check out the Peachy Green Smoothie (page 90).

DIPPERS: You can use raw vegetables as dippers for your child's favorite dip. Bean dips, guacamole, and tofu dips can be scooped up on a carrot stick, celery stick, or slice of zucchini. To make vegetables easier to chew and digest, as well as enhance their flavor, blanch them (see Blanched Broccoli, page 191).

SOUPS: Children who refuse a serving of vegetables will often eat the same vegetable in a soup. If vegetables in their whole form are a turnoff, puree the soup (see Rosemary Red Soup, page 175, or Golden Mushroom–Basil Cashew Cream Soup, page 177).

MUFFINS: You can add vegetables to muffins and other baked goods (as in Sweet Potato Corn Muffins on page 115). Zucchini, corn, squash, carrots, and sweet potatoes taste great in a muffin mix.

SANDWICH SPREADS: When pureeing beans or tofu or avocado into a tasty sandwich spread, add in some fresh vegetables. Parsley, cilantro, fresh basil, red bell pepper, or green onions work well to enhance flavor and nutritive value. Add corn, grated zucchini, or chopped green bell peppers to burritos, tacos, or wraps.

SINGLE-INGREDIENT SALADS: Sometimes it's just the sight of combined ingredients that turn kids off to salads. Experiment by offering a single raw vegetable or raw vegetables in separate piles, not mixed together. Try different shapes and sizes. Grated beets or radishes, finely sliced cabbage, zucchini, summer squash, or daikon (white radish) or matchstick carrots or cucumbers can be fun to pick up with small fingers.

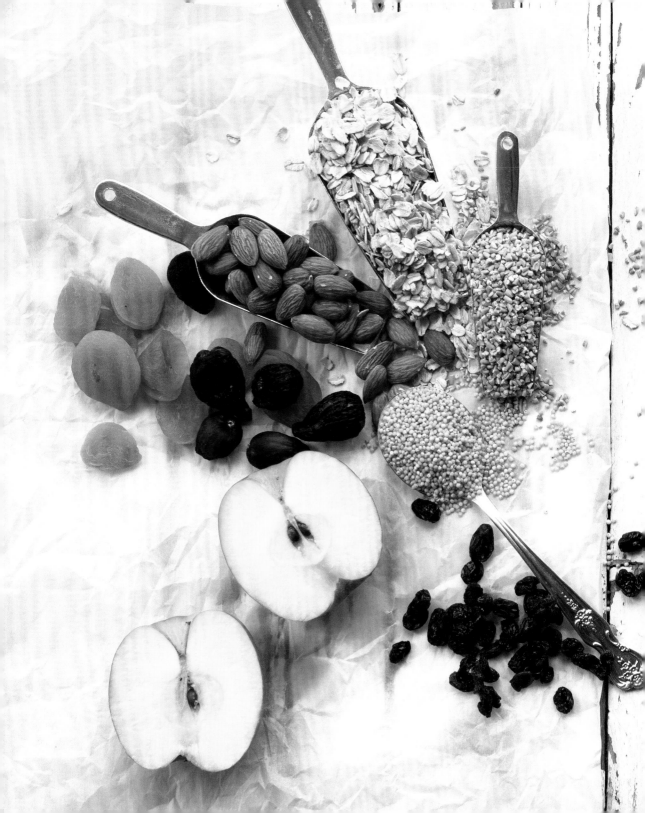

CHAPTER 4

- - - - - - -

bustling breakfasts

L ike some wives on the TV show *Mad Men*, my mom seemed to subsist on coffee and cigarettes. I can't remember her eating breakfast, just sitting with legs crossed sipping coffee and smoking. Maybe that's why as a child I was a disinterested breakfast eater. Instead of coffee, my cup was filled with astronaut-endorsed Tang. Most mornings, I was nagged politely to "just eat a few bites" of Cheerios swimming in milk or buttered cinnamon toast. As the time to walk to school grew closer, my mother would sigh as she looked at the barely touched food and say, "You better get going."

I had the same apathy about lunch and dinner, depending on what was served. Partly I was holding out for candy to appease my relentless sugar cravings. Mostly I was fortifying my image as the pickiest of all picky eaters. Once I was labeled as such, I felt I had to play the role. Color me stubborn.

Imagine my surprise when my own child dove into breakfast each morning with gusto. Maybe it was because my husband and I were enjoying breakfast? Or that I had never thought, let alone spoke, of her as being "picky"? Who knows.

The real takeaway here is hope. Though I was a sick-too-often, gangly child who wouldn't eat, I survived to become a healthy adult. And I grew up to be a cooking teacher and a cookbook author—imagine that! By the time I was approaching high school, my appetite kicked in, my need to be the pickiest eater turned off, and I tried all kinds of once-shunned foods.

If your child has no passion for breakfast, keep the faith. Do your best to resist rolling your eyes or using the "P" word. Pull a stool to the stove where you and your child can gaze at a twirling egg as it poaches. Have your child find the peach with the rosiest blush at the store. You never know who or what might flip the breakfast switch on.

cream *of* millet weaning cereal

Even if baby's first foods are fruits and vegetables, at some point you will want to introduce complex carbohydrates for more calories. A thin home-made cereal, made from a benign grain like millet, is perfect. To aid the digestion of the grain, soaking is essential. This tricks the grain into thinking it is being called upon to sprout, which releases enzymes. Grinding the grain and adding a dot of digestive herbs further enhance its digestibility.

1 In the bowl of a blender, put 1 cup of the water, the millet, 1 tablespoon of the breast milk, and the fennel seeds. Cover and let it sit overnight in the refrigerator. The good bacteria in the milk, along with the soaking time, help begin initial breakdown and digestion of the grain.

2 In the morning, turn the blender on high to completely pulverize the grain in the liquid. In a small saucepan over medium heat, add the millet mixture, the remaining 1 cup water, and the salt and bring it to an active simmer. Reduce the heat to low immediately, stir well with a whisk, and cover. Let the cereal cook for about 10 minutes, stirring often, until the mixture thickens.

3 Let it cool until just warm. Prepare a small bowl with a few tablespoons of cereal and the remaining 1 tablespoon breast milk stirred in (for the familiar taste). Put the remaining cereal in a separate bowl for the caregiver and dress with fresh fruit, yogurt, or maple syrup.

4 Enjoy warm morning cereal together.

PREPARATION TIME:

8 to 10 hours (for soaking);
15 minutes (for cooking)

MAKES 2 CUPS

2 cups water, divided

½ cup millet

2 tablespoons breast milk or formula with probiotics, divided

3 whole fennel or cumin seeds

⅛ teaspoon sea salt

Fresh fruit, yogurt, or maple syrup (optional)

bustling breakfasts

toasted whole grain baby cereal

Making your own baby cereal is nutritious, economical, and quite delicious. The grains listed below were chosen because they are the least allergenic and the easiest to digest. The grain is also toasted for better digestibility and flavor. For babies just starting solids, the cereal should be the consistency of soup. Make the consistency thicker as baby gets older. I hesitate to call this "baby cereal" because this cereal is for everyone!

PREPARATION TIME:

8 to 15 minutes (for toasting); 5 to 12 minutes (for cooking)

MAKES 1 CUP DRY CEREAL MIX OR 4 ADULT-SIZE SERVINGS

Choose one:

1 cup short-grain brown rice
1 cup millet
1 cup quinoa
1 cup sweet brown rice

Sea salt

1 In a fine mesh strainer, put the grain, then rinse and drain.

2 To toast the grain in the oven, preheat the oven to 350 degrees F. Spread the grain on dry baking sheet and toast in the oven until it gives off a nutty aroma, 12 to 15 minutes.

3 Alternatively, you can toast the grain on the stovetop: in a large skillet over medium heat, put the grains and toast, stirring constantly, until the grains are dry and give off nutty aroma, 5 to 8 minutes.

4 Let the grains cool and store them in a labeled, sealed container. You can toast a big batch of several different grains at one time and store them in separate jars. This will keep baby and family stocked with ready-to-make cereal for many moons.

5 For maximum nutrition, in a small electric grinder or blender, grind the amount of grain that you'll be using into a powder just prior to cooking.

6 For a baby-size portion of cereal, in a small pot over medium heat, mix together 2 to 3 tablespoons of the ground grain, ½ to ¾ cup of water, and a pinch of salt and bring it to a boil. Reduce the heat to low and simmer, covered, stirring frequently, until a porridge-like consistency is achieved, about 5 minutes.

7 For four adult-size portions of cereal, in a small pot over medium heat, mix together 1 cup of the ground grain, 3 to 4 cups of water, and ½ teaspoon salt and bring it to a boil. Reduce the heat to low and simmer, covered, stirring frequently, until a porridge-like consistency is achieved, 10 to 12 minutes.

A NOTE ON COMMERCIAL BREAKFAST CEREALS

Quite a variety of organic, whole grain, fruit-sweetened cereals are available in grocery stores everywhere. Many resemble the familiar sugary, refined cereals of the 1950s. The promises on the packaging (added protein!) can't cover up the fact that these foods are akin to sweetened kibble.

What may have once been a whole grain is now dried, baked, flaked, and dried again. Products like these are pretty lifeless, and without the added sugar they would have very little flavor. If you choose to use them, always add something fresh and lively to the meal—like whole fruit or toasted nuts.

Dependency on boxed cereals for breakfast always begs the question of which milk to use.

soaked whole grain baby porridge

Soaking opens up tough grains and saves cooking time. As your child gets older, you can use a higher ratio of yogurt to water. Be sure to buy high-quality yogurt with active cultures and forgo brands that add nonfat milk solids to thicken the product. Add fresh fruit and toasted nuts to porridge for older children and parents.

PREPARATION TIME:

8 to 12 hours (for soaking);
15 minutes (for cooking)

MAKES 2 ADULT-SIZE SERVINGS OR 6 TO 8 BABY-SIZE SERVINGS

½ cup millet or short-grain brown rice

½ to 2 teaspoons plain whole milk yogurt

1 cup water

Pinch of sea salt

1 Put the millet in a blender. In a small bowl, dilute the yogurt in the water. (Use ½ teaspoon of yogurt for babies 6 to 10 months; for older babies you can use a bit more.) Cover the millet with the yogurt water and let it sit in the refrigerator for 8 to 12 hours or overnight.

2 In the morning, in the blender, puree the millet and liquid until smooth. Add more water if necessary to get a porridge-like consistency.

3 In a 1-quart pan over high heat, put the millet mixture and the salt and bring it to a boil. Reduce the heat to low, cover, and simmer until slightly thickened, about 5 minutes.

ancient grain raisin cereal

These grains meld to make a creamy cereal with an earthy flavor. Amaranth, which was grown by the Aztecs, has an impressive nutritional profile, high in protein and calcium. The grain's appearance resembles tiny yellow, brown, and black seeds and has a flavor similar to unsweetened graham crackers. Serve with maple syrup, yogurt, or nuts on top.

1 In a fine mesh strainer, put the barley, millet, oats, and sesame seeds; rinse and drain. In a large bowl, combine the grain mixture, polenta, and amaranth.

2 To toast in the oven, preheat the oven to 350 degrees F. Spread grain mixture on a dry baking sheet and toast until it gives off a nutty aroma, 12 to 15 minutes. Alternatively, you can toast the grain on the stovetop: in a large skillet over medium heat, place the grain mixture, stirring constantly, until it gives off nutty aroma, 5 to 8 minutes. Let the grain mixture cool. Store the cereal mixture in a sealed container, where it will keep for 1 to 2 months.

3 To make the cereal, in a small electric grinder or blender, grind the cereal mixture. In a small pan over medium-high heat, combine the ground cereal, water, raisins, salt, and butter, stirring constantly as you bring to boil. Reduce the heat to low, cover, and simmer, stirring frequently, until a porridge-like consistency is achieved, 10 to 15 minutes.

PREPARATION TIME:

15 to 20 minutes (for toasting); 15 minutes (for cooking)

MAKES 5½ CUPS DRY CEREAL MIX OR 27 SERVINGS

1 cup hulled barley

1 cup millet

1 cup whole oats

½ cup sesame seeds

1 cup polenta

1 cup amaranth

3 cups water

⅓ cup raisins

½ teaspoon sea salt

1 tablespoon unsalted butter

FOR BABIES 6 MONTHS & OLDER: Toast 1 cup of millet separately and use the toasted millet to make Toasted Whole Grain Baby Cereal (page 78).

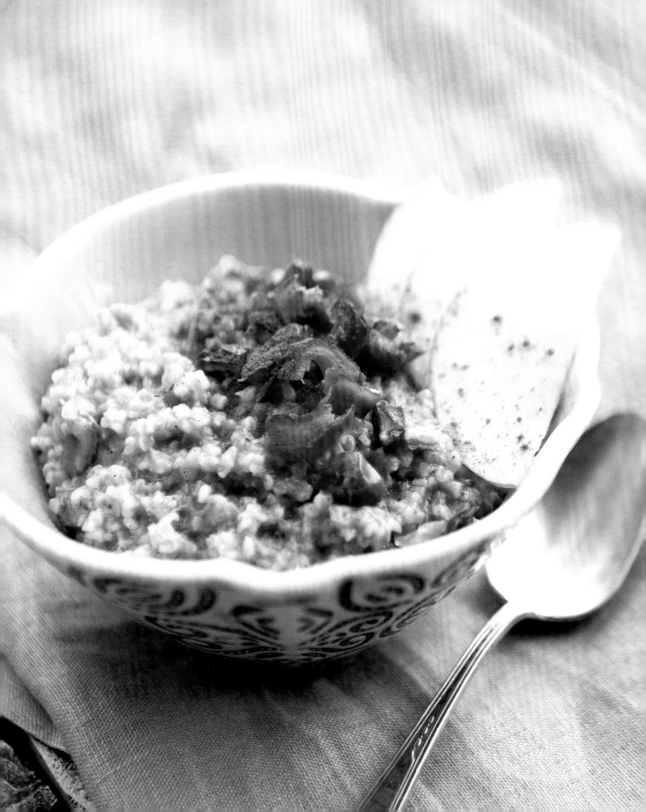

steel-cut oats *with* dates & cinnamon

Steel-cut oats, sometimes called Irish oatmeal, have a heartier flavor and a chewier texture than rolled oats. Serve this oat cereal with sliced apples and Tamari-Roasted Cashews (page 373).

1 In a 2-quart pan over high heat, put all of the ingredients. Stir briefly and bring it to a boil. Reduce the heat to low, cover, and simmer until all the water is absorbed, 20 to 25 minutes. Alternatively, soak the oats in a 2-quart pan with the water for 8 to 12 hours or overnight. In the morning, add the dates, butter, cinnamon, and salt, bring to boil, reduce the heat to low, and simmer, stirring constantly, for 5 minutes.

FOR BABIES 10 MONTHS & OLDER: Puree the cooked cereal briefly before serving.

PREPARATION TIME:

25 minutes

MAKES 4 TO 6 SERVINGS

3 cups water

1 cup steel-cut oats

4 pitted dates, cut into small pieces

1 tablespoon unsalted butter

½ teaspoon ground cinnamon

½ teaspoon sea salt

old-fashioned oatmeal

Whole oat groats that have been heated until soft and pressed flat are called rolled oats. Old-fashioned oats (as opposed to "quick-cooking" oats) are less processed and have more flavor.

PREPARATION TIME:

25 minutes

MAKES 2½ TO 3 CUPS

3 cups water

1 cup rolled oats

½ teaspoon sea salt

1 In a 2-quart pan over medium-high heat, add the water, oats, and salt. Bring the pan to a boil, reduce the heat to low, cover, and simmer until all the water is absorbed, 20 to 25 minutes. Stir and serve immediately.

FOR BABIES 6 MONTHS & OLDER: Creamy oatmeal made from rolled oats is a fine food for weaning infants. To make sure the porridge is thin, run some of it through the blender before giving it to baby.

sunny coconut millet
with peaches

One summer day for breakfast we added ripe peaches to millet, and the combination became a favorite. As the season of fresh fruit unfolds, shift to apricots, pears, or plums.

1 In a fine mesh strainer, put the millet, rinse, and drain. In a 2-quart saucepan over high heat, combine the millet, peaches, water, milk, butter, salt, and nutmeg and bring it to a boil. Reduce the heat to low, cover, and simmer until all water is absorbed, 20 to 25 minutes.

FOR BABIES 10 MONTHS & OLDER: Remove some cooked millet, puree, and serve.

PREPARATION TIME:

30 minutes

MAKES 4 SERVINGS

¾ cup millet

1 peach (or other seasonal fruit), sliced

1 cup water

1 cup whole milk (or milk alternative)

1 teaspoon unsalted butter

½ teaspoon sea salt

¼ teaspoon ground nutmeg

orange hazelnut muesli

Muesli, prepared the night before, proves handy for camping trips and hurried breakfasts. Soaking and not cooking the rolled oats gives them a chewier texture.

PREPARATION TIME:

5 minutes; 6 to 8 hours (for soaking)

MAKES 4 SERVINGS

2 cups rolled oats or rolled barley (or a mixture)

⅓ cup hazelnuts, chopped

⅓ cup raisins

½ teaspoon ground cinnamon

½ teaspoon sea salt

2 cups boiling water

1 teaspoon orange zest

½ cup freshly squeezed orange juice (from 2 oranges)

Sliced pears or apples, for topping (optional)

Plain or vanilla yogurt, for topping (optional)

1 In a large bowl, place the oats, hazelnuts, raisins, cinnamon, and salt. Pour the boiling water over the mixture and stir. Add the zest and juice to oat mixture and stir again. Cover the bowl with a plate or cloth and allow the moisture to soften the oats for 6 to 8 hours or overnight. It will be ready when you wake up! To serve, in a bowl, place your desired amount of muesli and top with the pears and yogurt.

FOR BABIES 6 MONTHS & OLDER: Top the muesli with fresh fruit. Steam some apple or pear slices until soft. Puree and serve.

maple butter nut granola

We can't live without a jar of this at the ready. Sure, it makes a delightful breakfast, but this crunchy mix often poses as a snack, even a dessert, in our house.

1 Preheat the oven to 325 degrees F.

2 In a 9-by-13-inch baking dish, combine the oats, seeds, almonds, cinnamon, cardamom, and salt and mix well.

3 In small pan over low heat, melt the butter, then add the maple syrup and nut butter and stir or whisk to blend. Remove the pan from the heat and stir in the extracts.

4 Slowly pour the wet ingredients over oat mixture, using a spatula to fold and evenly coat the oat mixture.

5 Spread the mixture into a baking dish (with a lip) or a shallow roasting pan and bake until the granola is dry and golden, about 45 minutes, turning the granola every 15 or 20 minutes so that it toasts evenly. Turn the oven off and leave the pan in the oven as it cools. This will add crispness to the cereal.

6 Store the finished granola in an airtight jar where it will keep for 2 weeks.

FOR BABIES 10 MONTHS & OLDER: Use some of the rolled oats to make your baby a bowl of warm oatmeal (see recipe on page 84).

PREPARATION TIME:

70 minutes

MAKES 8 CUPS

3½ cups rolled oats

¾ cup sunflower seeds

½ cup pumpkin seeds

¾ cup almonds, coarsely chopped

½ teaspoon ground cinnamon

½ teaspoon ground cardamom

½ teaspoon sea salt

½ cup (1 stick) unsalted butter, melted

½ cup maple syrup

1 tablespoon nut butter

1 teaspoon vanilla extract

¼ teaspoon almond extract

potato pancakes (latkes)

Jeff Basom was the chef for Bastyr University's renowned cafeteria for over a decade. I wouldn't know half of what I know about whole foods cooking, including this yummy method of pancaking potatoes, had it not been for Jeff's tutelage. Serve with Homemade Applesauce (page 376) and cultured sour cream.

PREPARATION TIME:

1 hour

MAKES 12 LATKES

3 medium baking potatoes, halved lengthwise

2 teaspoons sea salt, divided

3 tablespoons unsalted butter

1 medium onion, cut into ¼-inch dice

¼ cup unbleached flour

½ teaspoon freshly ground black pepper

2 large eggs

1 tablespoon high-heat vegetable oil, such as safflower or peanut, for frying

1 Bring an 8-quart pot filled with water to boil over high heat. Add the potatoes and 1 teaspoon of the salt to the boiling water and boil until they are nearly done—when pierced with a fork, the center will still feel slightly undercooked—6 to 8 minutes.

2 Cool the potatoes until you can easily handle them. Peel, then grate on the largest holes of a box grater. You should have 4 to 5 cups of grated potato. Put them in a large bowl and set aside.

3 In a large skillet over medium heat, add the butter then onions and sauté until the onions turn golden, about 6 to 8 minutes. Reduce the heat to low and slowly stir in the flour.

4 Add the onion-flour mixture to the grated potatoes. Mix in the remaining 1 teaspoon salt a little at a time to taste. Add the pepper. In a small bowl, whisk the eggs. Fold the eggs into the potato mixture until even. With your hands, form the mixture into twelve 3- to 4-inch patties.

5 In a large skillet over medium to high heat, heat the oil. Fry the patties on both sides, until a deep golden-brown crust forms, 2 to 3 minutes on each side. (Do not crowd the pan; you may need to cook the latkes in batches.)

FOR BABIES 6 MONTHS & OLDER: These latkes are delightful served with Homemade Applesauce (page 376), which can be served to baby.

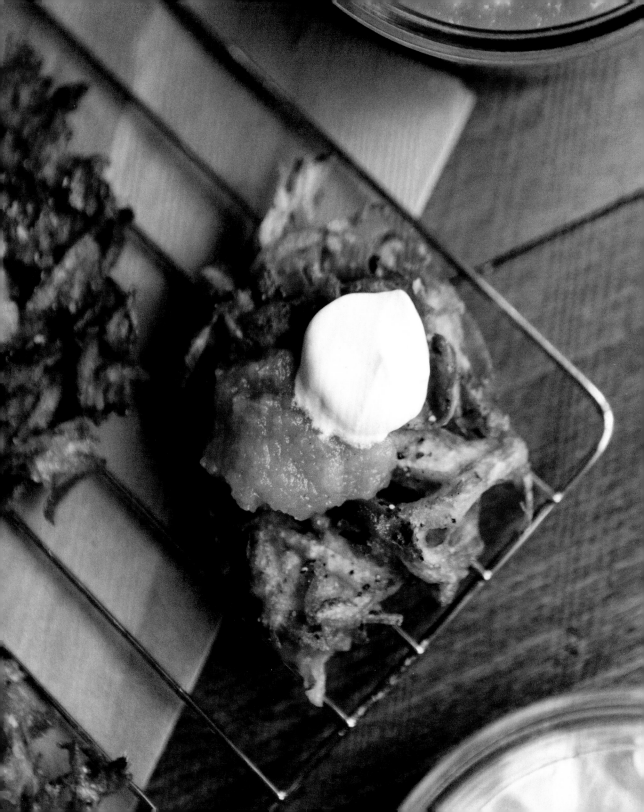

peachy green smoothie

Peaches are ripe in late summer, which is the appropriate time to forgo a warm breakfast and dive into something cooling!

PREPARATION TIME:

5 to 7 minutes

MAKES 3 CUPS

2 medium to large peaches, sliced (about 1 cup)

1 medium banana

2 cups loosely packed baby spinach leaves

½ cup whole milk Greek vanilla yogurt

2 whole pitted dates

1 cup (12 to 14) ice cubes

¼ to ½ cup water

1 In a blender, place the peaches, banana, spinach, yogurt, dates, ice, and ¼ cup of the water and blend on high speed. Check for desired consistency. Add more water if you prefer it a little thinner.

FOR BABIES 6 MONTHS & OLDER: What could be nicer than some ripe peach given a ride in the blender?

strawberry jam &
almond butter–filled mochi

Mochi is made from sweet brown rice that has been cooked, pounded into a paste, and then compressed into dense bars. When broken into squares and baked, it puffs up like a cream puff and gets gooey inside. Mochi comes plain or in several flavors; cinnamon-raisin mochi is the breakfast favorite at our home. Children love this warm chewy breakfast treat.

1 Preheat the oven to 400 degrees F.

2 Put the mochi on a lightly buttered baking sheet and bake until the mochi puffs up, 10 to 12 minutes.

3 Remove the baking sheet from oven and let the mochi cool for a few minutes. Make a slice on one side of each mochi square and slip 1 teaspoon each of jam and almond butter inside each square. Serve immediately.

FOR BABIES 6 MONTHS & OLDER: Mochi is a little too sticky and chewy for a mouth with few teeth. Make some baby cereal out of sweet brown rice (see Toasted Whole Grain Baby Cereal, page 78) so you can both benefit from this unique type of rice.

PREPARATION TIME:

15 minutes

MAKES 6 SERVINGS

1 (12-ounce) block mochi, cut into 2-inch squares

6 teaspoons Old-Fashioned Strawberry-Honey Jam (page 380)

6 teaspoons almond butter

sprouted essene bread
& butter *with* nectarines

The Essenes were a sect of monks from early Biblical times who prepared sweet, moist, flourless bread by slow-baking sprouted wheat. Some who struggle with wheat flour products find the sprouted version A-OK. Look for Essene bread or sprouted bread in the refrigerated or frozen food section at your natural foods store.

PREPARATION TIME:

12 to 15 minutes

MAKES 4 SERVINGS

4 one-inch slices Essene bread

2 teaspoons salted butter

4 nectarines, sliced

1 Preheat the oven to 300 degrees F.

2 Put the bread slices on a dry baking sheet and warm them in the oven for 5 to 10 minutes. (Alternatively, if your toaster has wide slots, you can use it to warm the bread.)

3 Butter the warm bread and serve with the nectarines.

FOR BABIES 6 MONTHS & OLDER: Puree the nectarine slices with a little water and serve.

feeding the whole family

pantry pancake mix

Using this nice variety of whole grains creates hearty hot cakes or waffles. If you need to make your pancakes gluten-free, substitute the barley and whole wheat flour with one of the gluten-free flour mixes on page 402.

1 In a large bowl, stir together all the ingredients. Store the mix in an airtight container in the refrigerator, where it will last for 2 to 3 months.

PREPARATION TIME:

10 minutes

MAKES 6 CUPS

2 cups barley or Kamut flour

2 cups whole wheat pastry flour

1 cup buckwheat flour

1 cup cornmeal

3 tablespoons baking powder

1 teaspoon ground cinnamon

½ teaspoon sea salt

bustling breakfasts

buttermilk banana pancakes

Buttermilk, a cultured dairy product, adds a rich, slightly sour flavor to baked goods. For a dairy-free version, substitute soy, rice, or nut milk with one tablespoon lemon juice added to it. One-half cup water stirred into one-half cup yogurt also works as a buttermilk substitute. These pancakes get silly-good with Strawberry-Blueberry Sauce for Pancakes and Waffles (page 374).

PREPARATION TIME:

25 to 30 minutes

MAKES 10 PANCAKES

1 egg

1½ cups Pantry Pancake Mix (page 93)

1 cup buttermilk

½ cup water

High-heat vegetable oil, such as safflower or peanut, for the griddle

1 medium ripe banana, thinly sliced

1 Separate the egg; put the egg white in one bowl and the yolk in another. Whip the egg white until stiff peaks form. Set aside.

2 In the second bowl, combine the egg yolk, pancake mix, buttermilk, and water. Using a whisk or electric mixer, mix thoroughly. Add the whipped egg white to the batter and gently fold it in.

3 Heat a griddle to medium high and coat the surface with small amount of the oil. Pour ¼ cup of the batter onto the griddle to form each 5-inch pancake. Lay the banana slices on the top surface of each sizzling pancake. Cook for about 1 minute. When tiny bubbles form and the edges of the pancakes firm up, flip them with a spatula and cook the other side for 1 more minute. The pancake should be freckled brown. Repeat with the remaining batter.

4 Keep the cooked pancakes in a warm oven until ready to serve.

FOR BABIES 6 MONTHS & OLDER: Reserve some ripe banana. Mash and serve.

VARIATION FOR CHILDREN: Put the batter in a squeeze bottle and squeeze the batter onto the griddle in shapes such as letters, numbers, or animals.

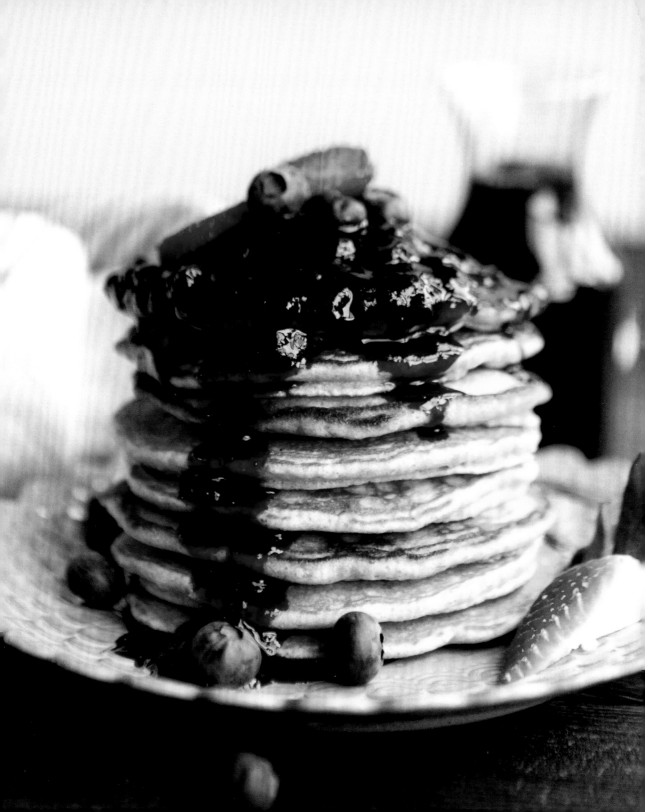

ben's friday morning pancakes

This unique pancake has no flour or wheat but uses highly digestible soaked whole grains. A former student, Ronit Gourarie, adapted this recipe and routinely served these beauties to her son, Ben, every Friday. Homemade Applesauce (page 376) or Strawberry-Blueberry Sauce for Pancakes and Waffles (page 374) on top add color and natural fruit sweetness.

PREPARATION TIME:

6 to 8 hours (for soaking); 15 minutes (for cooking)

MAKES 6 TO 8 PANCAKES

¾ cup water

⅔ cup steel-cut oats

½ cup whole milk plain yogurt

⅓ cup unroasted buckwheat groats

1 egg

2 tablespoons unrefined cane sugar

1 teaspoon baking powder

½ teaspoon freshly grated or ground nutmeg

¼ teaspoon sea salt

High-heat vegetable oil, such as safflower or peanut, for the griddle

1 In the bowl of a blender, combine the water, oats, yogurt, and buckwheat groats. Cover and let soak overnight for 6 to 8 hours.

2 Add the egg, sugar, baking powder, nutmeg, and salt to the soaked grains and blend on high until smooth.

3 Preheat a griddle or frying pan and lubricate with oil. Pour about ¼ cup batter per pancake onto griddle to form each pancake. Cook for 2 minutes. When tiny bubbles form and the edges of the pancakes firm up, flip them with a spatula and cook the other side for about 2 more minutes. Repeat until all the batter has been used.

4 Keep the cooked pancakes warm in the oven until ready to serve.

FOR BABIES 6 MONTHS & OLDER: Try a few teaspoons of plain whole milk yogurt stirred into pureed fruit.

FOR BABIES 10 MONTHS & OLDER: Cut the pancakes into small pieces and serve.

scrambled tofu & pepper breakfast burrito

Any vegetables can be substituted for the green and red bell peppers; however, this combination has colorful eye appeal.

1 Preheat the oven to 250 degrees F.

2 Put the tortillas in a covered baking dish or wrap in aluminum foil and place in oven to warm.

3 In a 10-inch skillet over medium heat, heat the oil. Add the cumin, coriander, turmeric, and cayenne and stir briefly. Add the onion and garlic and sauté until the onion has begun to soften, about 5 to 7 minutes. Add the peppers and salt and sauté until the peppers wilt. Stir in the tofu, then fold in the cilantro.

4 Place about ⅓ cup of the tofu mixture in a line down the middle of each warm tortilla. Bring the bottom of the tortilla up over the tofu mix, pull it in tight, and then roll it up. Repeat with the remaining five tortillas.

5 Serve the burritos warm with salsa on the side.

FOR BABIES 10 MONTHS & OLDER: Reserve some of the crumbled tofu, heat briefly in a lightly oiled skillet, and serve.

PREPARATION TIME:

15 to 20 minutes

MAKES 6 SERVINGS

6 whole grain tortillas

1 tablespoon extra-virgin olive oil

½ teaspoon ground cumin

½ teaspoon ground coriander

½ teaspoon ground turmeric

⅛ teaspoon cayenne

½ medium onion, finely chopped

2 cloves garlic, minced

¼ red bell pepper, chopped to a small dice

¼ green bell pepper, chopped to a small dice

1 teaspoon sea salt

1 pound firm tofu, crumbled

¼ cup chopped fresh cilantro

Salsa, for serving

swirling poached eggs

Invite children to hop on a stool and watch the egg transform as it swirls in the water. Young ones two to four years old can grab the spoons and help make the vortex. Serve the poached eggs on top of Butter-Braised Kale (page 198); Peasant Kasha, Potatoes, and Mushrooms (my favorite, page 274); soft polenta; or toast.

PREPARATION TIME:

10 minutes

MAKES 2 SERVINGS

2 eggs, divided

¼ teaspoon rice or apple cider vinegar

¼ teaspoon sea salt

1 Break one egg into a small bowl.

2 Fill a 2-quart pan with water to twice the depth of an egg and bring the heat to medium. The water needs to be almost but not quite simmering; it should look like carbonated water with tiny bubbles forming but not breaking the surface. Add the vinegar and salt to the water.

3 Reduce the heat to low. Swirl the water along the edge of the pan with a wooden spoon, creating a vortex in the center of the water. Drop the egg into the well formed in the middle. The swirling water will collect the egg.

4 Turn the heat off or reduce it to very low and let the egg stand 3 (for a fairly liquid yolk) or 4 (for a more syrupy texture) minutes. Remove the egg with a slotted spoon.

5 Repeat with the remaining egg.

FOR BABIES 6 MONTHS & OLDER: A teaspoon of soft-cooked egg yolk provides an excellent source of high-quality fat.

green eggs, no ham

Use eggs from happy hens that have been allowed to dine on bugs and worms (pastured eggs). This natural diet increases the yolk's anti-inflammatory omega-3 fat content. Green eggs can be spooned into a corn tortilla with salsa to make a breakfast taco.

1 In a 10-inch skillet over medium heat, put the chard and move it around the pan until the leaves have wilted. You don't need to add water to the pan, as the water clinging to the leaves should provide enough moisture. Remove the leaves, drain, and chop into bite-size pieces. Set aside. Wipe the skillet clean.

2 In a medium bowl, whisk together the eggs and milk. Add the salt and pepper. Reheat the skillet over medium heat. Add the butter; when it sizzles but doesn't brown, add the eggs. Using a heatproof rubber scraper, gently stir the eggs as they cook, lifting the curds from the bottom of the pan and folding. When the eggs are nearly cooked, sprinkle in the chard and cheese and fold them evenly into the cooking eggs.

3 Remove the eggs from the pan when they appear light and fluffy but still shiny and slightly wet. Serve immediately.

FOR BABIES 6 MONTHS & OLDER: Remember that egg whites are inappropriate for infants under 1 year of age. Some of the soft-cooked Swiss chard, cut into tiny bits, works for baby.

PREPARATION TIME:

10 minutes

MAKES 2 TO 3 SERVINGS

2 to 3 large Swiss chard leaves, de-stemmed and torn into large pieces

4 eggs

2 tablespoons milk or water

½ teaspoon sea salt

Freshly ground black pepper

1 tablespoon unsalted butter

¼ cup grated Parmesan cheese (optional)

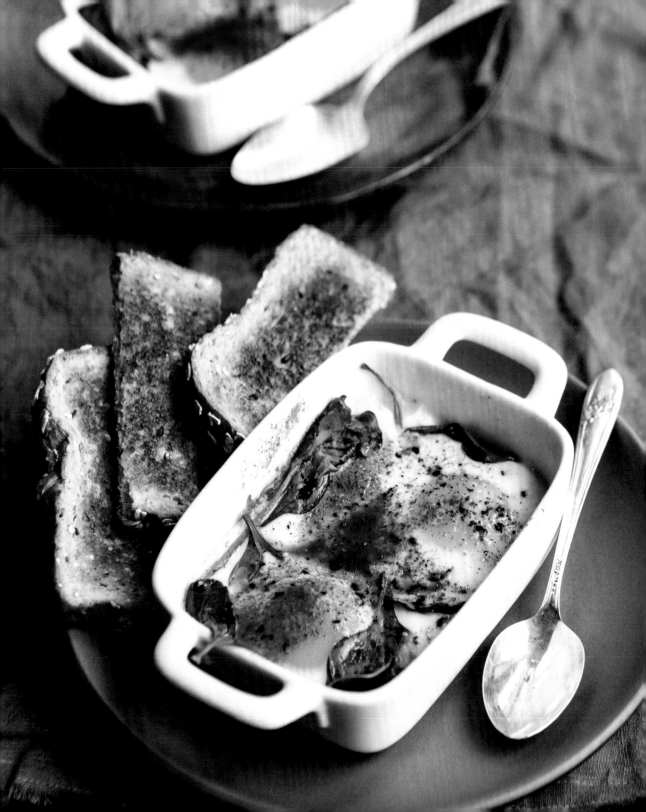

baked eggs *with* spinach & paprika

Greens and eggs make a symbiotic couple. In this recipe the sought-after nutri-
ents in the greens are enhanced by the fat from the butter and egg yolk. Baking
eggs takes about eighteen minutes—the right amount of time to take a quick
shower and get dressed! Serve the eggs with toast, brown rice, or kasha (see
Whole Grains from Scratch, page 242, for whole grain cooking instructions).

1 Preheat the oven to 350 degrees F.

2 Coat the bottom and sides of four 4-inch ramekins
with the butter. Lay a few spinach leaves in the bottom
of each ramekin, tearing larger ones into small pieces.
Crack an egg into each ramekin and season with salt,
pepper, and a dusting of paprika.

3 Put the ramekins in an 8-by-8-inch baking dish and
fill the dish with a ½-inch layer of hot water. Put the dish
in the oven and bake the eggs until the whites become
opaque, about 18 minutes.

4 Remove the baking dish from the oven and serve the
eggs immediately.

FOR BABIES 6 MONTHS & OLDER: A teaspoon of
soft-cooked egg yolk along with a tidbit of spinach is
just lovely.

PREPARATION TIME:

25 minutes

MAKES 4 SERVINGS

1 teaspoon unsalted butter

12 to 15 baby spinach leaves
(about 1 cup loose)

4 eggs

Sea salt and freshly ground
black pepper

Sprinkle of ground paprika

bustling breakfasts

huevos rancheros

Choose peppers wisely. Serranos are superhot, jalapeños can be pretty hot, and habaneros are quite mild. Using the product "fire-roasted chopped tomatoes with green chilies" proves handy, as some or all of the chili peppers can be omitted.

PREPARATION TIME:

30 minutes

MAKES 4 SERVINGS

1 tablespoon extra-virgin olive oil

½ medium onion, chopped

3 cloves garlic, minced

2 habanero chili peppers, diced

1 jalapeño or serrano chili pepper, diced

1 (16-ounce) can chopped tomatoes

½ teaspoon sea salt

½ teaspoon chili powder

1 tablespoon unsalted butter

4 corn tortillas

4 eggs

Jack cheese, grated, for serving

Cultured sour cream, for serving

Ripe avocado, for serving

Cooked black beans (see page 244 for cooking instructions), for serving

1 In a large skillet over medium heat, heat the oil. Then add the onion and give it time to soften and caramelize, 7 to 10 minutes. Next add the garlic, chilies, tomatoes, salt, and chili powder. Bring the sauce to a simmer over medium heat, reduce the heat to low, cover, and cook for about 10 minutes, or until ingredients no longer appear raw.

2 In a second 10-inch skillet or griddle, melt ½ tablespoon of the butter. Add two tortillas and warm them for about 30 seconds on each side. Repeat with the remaining butter and tortillas. Set aside, covered, in a warm place.

3 Crack an egg into a small bowl. Make four wells in the simmering sauce and gently pour the egg into one of the wells. Repeat this with the remaining three eggs. When all four eggs are nestled in the sauce, cover the skillet and allow the eggs to poach in the salsa sauce for 4 minutes, or until the whites are opaque.

4 Place each tortilla on a plate with an egg and sauce on top. Serve with the cheese and sour cream on top of the egg and the avocado and beans on the side.

FOR BABIES 6 MONTHS & OLDER: Some mashed avocado provides healthful fats and vitamins in a delicious, digestible form.

tempeh, avocado &
lettuce breakfast sandwich

Tempeh is made by adding a culture to cooked soybeans. The cultures activate growth, turning the beans into a solid cake that can be cut and sliced. This high-protein food can be baked, boiled, fried, or steamed.

1 In a small bowl, mix together the oregano, thyme, and basil and set aside. In a 10-inch skillet over medium-high heat, add 1 to 2 tablespoons of the oil and then half of the tempeh strips. Let the oil get hot but not smoking. Fry the tempeh until browned, about 30 seconds on each side. The oil should be hot enough that the surface of the tempeh browns quickly. Sprinkle half of the herbs over the tempeh as it fries. Remove the tempeh to a paper towel. Repeat the process with the remaining 1 to 2 tablespoons oil, tempeh, and herbs. Sprinkle the fried tempeh with the tamari.

2 While the tempeh is frying, spread four slices of the bread with mayonnaise and avocado slices. Place the lettuce leaves on the remaining four slices of bread. Top the avocado with the fried tempeh slices and put the sandwiches together.

FOR BABIES 6 MONTHS & OLDER: Avocado! Mash and serve.

PREPARATION TIME:

7 to 10 minutes

MAKES 4 SERVINGS

½ teaspoon dried oregano

½ teaspoon dried thyme

½ teaspoon dried basil

2 to 4 tablespoons unrefined coconut oil or Homemade Ghee (page 383)

1 (8-ounce) package tempeh, cut into ¼-inch strips

1 tablespoon tamari (soy sauce)

8 slices whole grain bread, toasted and buttered

1 tablespoon mayonnaise

1 ripe avocado, sliced

4 leaves romaine or butter lettuce

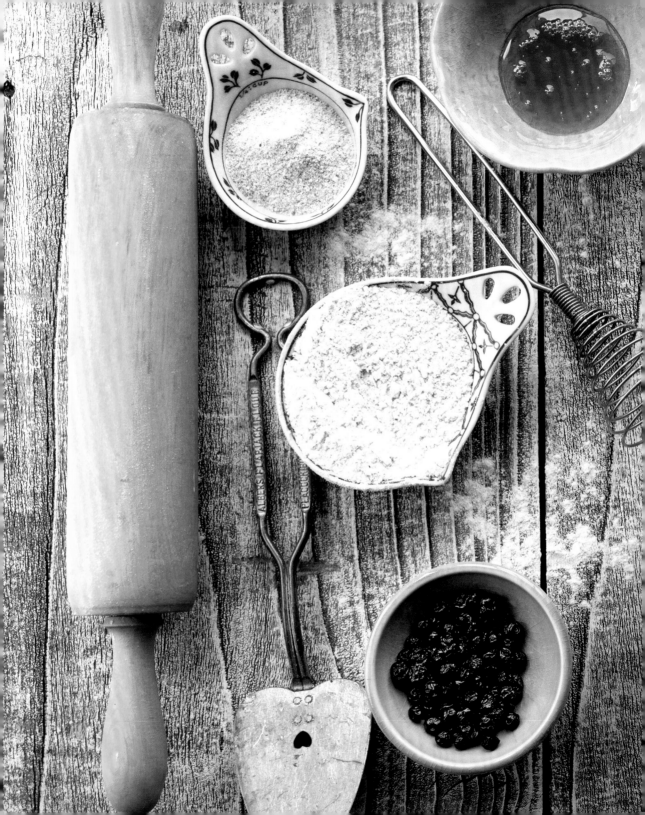

- - - - - - - - - -

CHAPTER 5

fresh-baked breads & muffins

My aunt Phyllis grew up as a Mennonite, a Christian religious sect that began in German- and Dutch-speaking countries in Europe. They were also known as the "Anabaptists" because of their defining rejection of infant baptism, believing that church membership and baptism should only happen when individuals are old enough to willingly and publicly acknowledge belief in Jesus and his teachings. Their ideas went against the ruling Roman Catholic views.

Because of their beliefs, many Mennonites were forced to flee Europe. Some immigrants settled in colonial America and came to be known as the Pennsylvania Dutch. A new wave of immigrants arrived in the late 1800s and settled in the Midwest to tame the plains and become farmers. The Mennonites held a firm belief in the separation of church and state and were known for their opposition of slavery.

When Phyllis was a girl, her family lived on a farm in Kansas. She once told me that her grandfather and father were quite proud to bring hard red winter wheat (the perfect type for baking bread) to Kansas. Naturally, their family meals always included freshly baked bread.

Bread is one of the oldest known prepared foods. Evidence of bread making has been found among thirty-thousand-year-old relics in Europe where starch residue on rocks used for pounding grass kernels into flour was revealed. Religious ceremonies throughout the world use bread as a sacred symbol of the gifts received from our bountiful earth.

Yet this revered staple food has fallen into ill repute in recent years. The consumption of gluten-containing grains, like wheat, is being blamed for a wide range of ills, from headaches and bloating to bad moods. How can this food, "the staff of life" for thousands of years, have suddenly become so tainted? Is it the way bread is being made? Are they using a different type of wheat than the one Phyllis's grandfather brought to Kansas? Botanists say no. Is it the pesticides used on the crops? The additives used in commercially made bread? Maybe the phenomenon has something to do with gut health and not the wheat. There is no conclusive explanation.

Certainly if your body feels better without gluten, respect the evidence, but don't throw the book at homemade bread without good reason.

———

"[Bread making is] one of those almost hypnotic businesses, like a dance from some ancient ceremony. It leaves you filled with one of the world's sweetest smells . . . there is no chiropractic treatment, no Yoga exercise, no hour of meditation in a music-throbbing chapel that will leave you emptier of bad thoughts than this homely ceremony of making bread."

—M. F. K. FISHER and JOAN REARDON,
The Art of Eating: 50th Anniversary Edition

whole grain honey oat sandwich bread

Baking fresh bread is the perfect rainy-day activity for a parent or caretaker and small children. Each step takes only ten to fifteen minutes of attention with ample space for other play between steps. This edible creation cultivates patience and a sense of accomplishment.

PREPARATION TIME:

10- to 15-minute increments over 6 hours; 45 to 55 minutes (for baking)

MAKES 1 LOAF

1 teaspoon active dry yeast

1¼ cups warm water, divided

1 pound (about 3 cups) whole wheat flour

1¼ teaspoons sea salt

½ cup cooked oatmeal

1 tablespoon honey

1 tablespoon extra-virgin olive oil

For the glaze:

½ teaspoon extra-virgin olive oil

½ teaspoon water

½ teaspoon honey

1 In a small bowl, add the yeast and ¼ cup of the warm water to awaken it. This typically takes 5 to 10 minutes. Make sure the yeast is active and bubbly before proceeding. In a large bowl, place the flour and salt and stir.

2 In a blender or food processor, put the oatmeal, honey, oil, and the remaining 1 cup warm water and blend. Pour the oatmeal mixture into a separate large bowl. Stir in the yeast and water and 1 cup of the flour mixture. Stir well and let the mixture rest for 10 to 15 minutes until you see the mixture begin to bubble (it's alive!). Begin adding the remaining flour, stirring until it becomes too difficult, and then begin kneading, first in the bowl and then transfer the dough to a floured surface.

3 Knead the dough—fold, push, turn, and repeat—until it begins to feel smooth and springy, 10 to 15 minutes. Test the dough; if you pull on an edge, it should stretch and not easily break.

4 Clean and lightly oil the bowl and put the kneaded dough ball in it. Cover the bowl with plastic wrap, a damp towel, or a plate and leave it for 3 to 4 hours in a warm place to rise (70 to 72 degrees F is perfect).

5 After a few hours, the dough should have doubled in size. Remove it from the bowl to a floured surface and deflate the dough by pressing it flat. Form it into a ball again, return it to the bowl, cover, and let it rise again for 1½ to 2 hours.

6 Lightly oil a loaf pan with high-heat oil. Set aside.

7 To deflate the dough and shape it into a loaf, press all of the air out of the dough, patting and pushing it gently with the palms of both hands, creating a square shape. Fold the flattened dough into a triangle and press it down again. Fold two corners into the center and press it down again. Fold the top point into the body of the dough and press it down again. Pick up the dough with both hands and begin rolling it into itself. This stretches the outside of the dough and creates a tight roll with no air pockets. Seal the seam by flattening it with the heel of your hand. The dough should now be in a loaf shape. Place the dough in the prepared loaf pan seam side down.

8 To make the glaze, in a small bowl, mix together the oil, water, and honey, then brush it onto the top of the dough. Cover the loaf pan with a loose plastic bag and let the dough rise for an additional 30 minutes.

9 Test the bread for readiness. If you press the dough and it has a little spring but doesn't pop back immediately, it's ready to bake.

10 Preheat the oven to 400 degrees F.

11 Lower the temperature to 350 degrees F once the loaf is in the oven. Bake the loaf until the internal temperature of the loaf, using an instant-read thermometer, is 190 degrees F, 45 to 55 minutes.

12 Let the bread cool at least 30 minutes before slicing.

FOR BABIES 6 MONTHS & OLDER: The leftover oatmeal used to start this bread (hopefully) started out as food for baby!

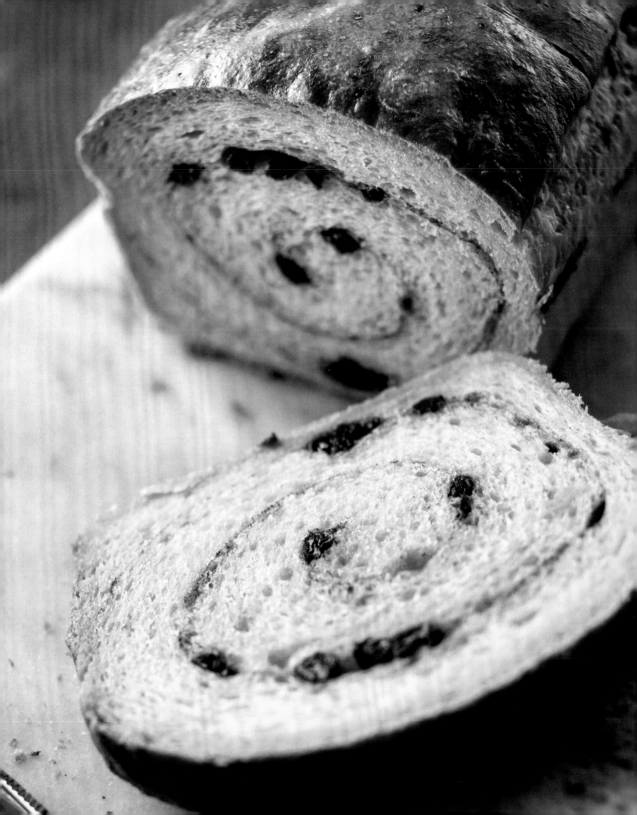

raisin–sweet potato breakfast bread

When this bread is sliced, the insides show off a pretty swirl of raisins and spices. And yes—whole white wheat flour comes complete with bran, germ, and endosperm. It's made from a type of whole grain wheat that doesn't have the genes that give its bran color. Whole wheat bread flour, made from traditional hard red wheat, can be easily substituted.

1 In a small bowl, add the yeast and ¼ cup of the warm water to awaken it. This typically takes 5 to 10 minutes. Make sure the yeast is active and bubbly before proceeding. In a large bowl, stir together the flour and salt.

2 In a blender or food processor, put the sweet potato, 1 tablespoon of the honey, the oil, 1 teaspoon of the sugar, and the remaining 1 cup warm water and blend. Pour the mixture into a separate large bowl. Stir in the yeast and water and 1 cup of the flour mixture. Stir well and let the mixture rest for 10 to 15 minutes until you see the mixture begin to bubble (it's alive!). Begin adding the remaining flour, stirring until it becomes too difficult, and then begin kneading, first in the bowl and then transfer it to a floured surface.

3 Knead the dough—fold, push, turn, and repeat—until it begins to feel smooth and springy, 10 to 15 minutes. Test the dough; if you pull on an edge, it should stretch and not easily break.

4 Clean and lightly oil the bowl and then put the kneaded dough ball in it. Cover the bowl with plastic wrap, a damp towel, or a plate and leave it for 3 to 4 hours in a warm place to rise (70 to 72 degrees F is perfect).

5 After a few hours, the dough should have doubled in size. Remove it from the bowl to a floured surface and

PREPARATION TIME:

10- to 15-minute increments over 6 hours; 45 to 55 minutes (for baking)

MAKES 1 LOAF

1 teaspoon active dry yeast

1¼ cups warm water, divided

1 pound whole white wheat flour (about 3 cups)

1¼ teaspoons sea salt

½ cup peeled baked sweet potato

1 tablespoon plus ½ teaspoons honey, divided

1 tablespoon extra-virgin olive oil

1 tablespoon unrefined cane sugar or brown sugar, divided

High-heat vegetable oil, such as safflower or peanut, for oiling the pan

1 large egg, beaten, divided

¾ cup raisins

1 teaspoon ground cinnamon

½ teaspoon ground allspice

fresh-baked bread & muffins

continued

deflate the dough by pressing it flat. Form it into a ball again, return it to the bowl, cover, and let it rise again for 1½ to 2 hours.

6 Lightly oil a loaf pan with a touch of vegetable oil. Set aside.

7 To deflate the dough and shape it into a loaf, press all of the air out of the dough by pushing or lightly rolling the dough to create a rectangle about 6 inches wide and 20 inches long. Spread half of the beaten egg on the full surface of the dough. Sprinkle the dough with the raisins, cinnamon, allspice, and the remaining 2 teaspoons sugar. Lightly press the raisins into the dough. Starting at the end nearest you, roll up the dough like a rug. Pinch the sides and the long seam to seal. Place the dough in the prepared loaf pan seam side down.

8 In a small bowl, mix the remaining egg and the remaining ½ teaspoon honey together, then brush it onto the top of the loaf. Cover the loaf pan with a loose plastic bag and let the dough rise for an additional 30 minutes.

9 Preheat the oven to 400 degrees F.

10 Test the bread for readiness. If you press the dough and it has a little spring but doesn't pop back immediately, it's ready to bake.

11 Lower the temperature to 350 degrees F once the loaf is in the oven. Bake until the internal temperature of the loaf, using an instant-read thermometer, is 190 degrees F, 45 to 55 minutes.

12 Let the bread cool for at least 30 minutes before slicing.

FOR BABIES 6 MONTHS & OLDER: The leftover sweet potato used to start this bread probably came from a whole baked sweet potato. The other half was, is, or will be food for baby.

lemon-cranberry scones

There's nothing like warm, freshly made scones for breakfast. The buttermilk can be replaced with one-half cup whole milk with one-quarter cup plain yogurt whisked in. If dairy is an issue, replace buttermilk with coconut milk.

1 Preheat the oven to 350 degrees F and lightly oil or line with parchment paper a baking sheet.

2 In a large bowl or food processor, mix together the flour, sugar, baking powder, baking soda, and salt. If the sugar seems coarse, grind it in a coffee mill or blender before proceeding. Cut in the butter with a fork or add it in bits while pulsing the food processor until the mixture is crumbly or pebbly. Transfer the flour mixture to a large bowl if a food processor was used.

3 Add the cranberries and zest and stir to combine. Pour in the buttermilk and extract and stir until the mixture holds together. Then gather the dough onto a floured surface and knead it a few times. Pat the dough out into an 8-inch circle and cut it into eight wedges. Place the wedges on the prepared baking sheet and bake for 25 minutes. Cool the scones on a rack.

FOR BABIES 10 MONTHS & OLDER: Soak 2 teaspoons of dried cranberries in boiling water for 5 to 10 minutes to soften them. Add a few cranberries to baby's cereal while cooking or as you run the cereal through the blender.

PREPARATION TIME:

45 minutes

MAKES 8 SCONES

2 cups whole wheat pastry flour

¼ cup unrefined cane sugar or brown sugar

2 teaspoons nonaluminum baking powder

½ teaspoon baking soda

½ teaspoon sea salt

6 tablespoons chilled unsalted butter

¾ cup dried cranberries

1 tablespoon lemon zest (from 1 medium lemon)

¾ cup buttermilk

½ teaspoon lemon extract

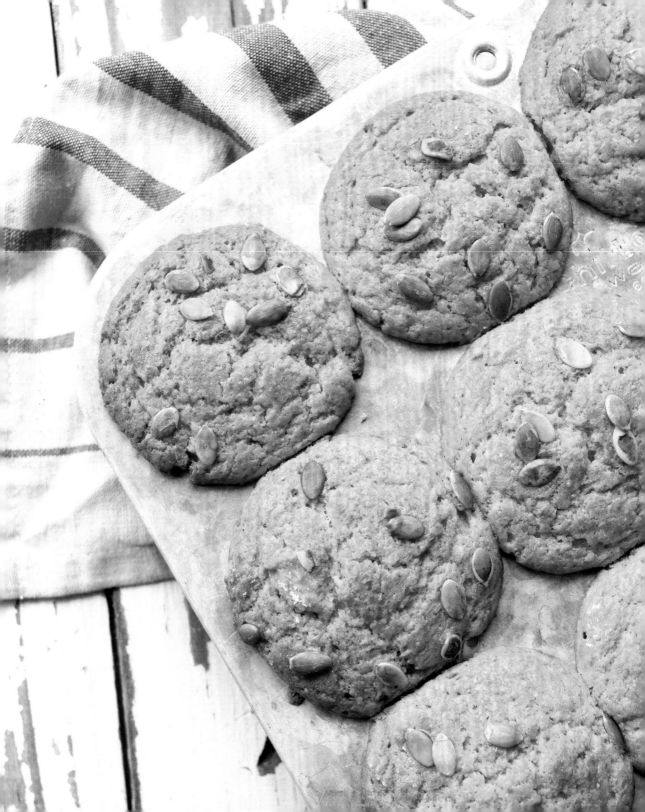

sweet potato corn muffins

Cornbread typically dries out quickly, but in this recipe, the baked sweet potato keeps the muffins moist while imparting vitamin-rich sweetness.

1 Preheat the oven to 375 degrees F. Lightly oil a muffin tin or line with paper muffin cups. Set aside.

2 In a large bowl, mix together the cornmeal, flour, baking powder, and salt and set aside. Mash the sweet potato, then, in a blender, put the sweet potato and water (there's your food for baby!) and blend until smooth. Add the butter, syrup, and eggs and pulse a few more times.

3 Combine the wet ingredients with the cornmeal mixture and incorporate with a minimum of strokes. Fill the muffin cups full with batter. Decorate the top of each muffin with a few pumpkin seeds. Bake for 25 to 30 minutes. The tops of the muffins will crack slightly when done.

FOR BABIES 6 MONTHS & OLDER: Reserve a portion of the baked sweet potato that has been pureed with water or mashed.

FOR BABIES 10 MONTHS & OLDER: Toast some pumpkin seeds in a dry skillet until they puff up and pop. Grind these to a meal and add about ½ teaspoon to baby's pureed sweet potato for extra nutrients.

PREPARATION TIME:

30 minutes

MAKES 12 MUFFINS

1½ cups cornmeal

1½ cups whole wheat pastry flour or barley flour

2 teaspoons nonaluminum baking powder

½ teaspoon sea salt

1 cup baked sweet potato

½ cup water or milk

½ cup (1 stick) unsalted butter, melted

½ cup maple syrup

2 eggs

2 tablespoons pumpkin seeds

fresh-baked bread & muffins

pumpkin pecan muffins

Baked sugar pie pumpkin or buttercup squash work beautifully in this recipe. These muffins make excellent snacks, breakfast food, or a nice accompaniment to Cannellini Kale Minestrone (page 183) and other savory soups.

PREPARATION TIME:

45 minutes

MAKES 12 MUFFINS

2 cups whole wheat
  pastry flour

1 cup unbleached white
  flour

½ cup unrefined cane sugar
  or brown sugar

1 tablespoon baking powder

1 teaspoon sea salt

1 teaspoon ground
  cinnamon

½ teaspoon ground cloves

½ teaspoon ground
  cardamom

½ cup (1 stick) unsalted
  butter

¼ cup molasses

¼ cup honey

1 cup mashed, cooked
  pumpkin or winter squash

½ cup milk or water

2 eggs

2 teaspoons vanilla extract

½ cup pecans, coarsely
  chopped

1 Preheat the oven to 375 degrees F. Lightly oil the muffin tin or line with paper muffin cups.

2 In a large bowl, mix together the flours, sugar, baking powder, salt, cinnamon, cloves, and cardamom and set aside.

3 In a small saucepan over low heat, melt the butter. Add the molasses and honey to the warm butter and stir to combine, then remove the pan from the heat.

4 In a blender, blend the cooked pumpkin and the butter-sweetener mixture and the milk until smooth. Add the eggs and vanilla and pulse to blend.

5 Add the wet ingredients to the flour mixture and fold together gently, using a minimum of strokes. Fold the pecans into the batter. Fill the muffin cups two-thirds full with batter. Bake until a knife inserted into the center of the muffin comes out clean, 25 to 30 minutes.

FOR BABIES 6 MONTHS & OLDER: Reserve some of the baked pumpkin or winter squash used in the muffins. Puree with a little breast milk or water.

cheese & green chili corn pudding

Here's my take on a favorite Puget Consumers Co-op deli item celebrating late summer with fresh corn and roasted poblano peppers (the mild kind). One ear of corn provides about one cup of kernels. Be sure to use corn flour (finely ground), not cornmeal, to make this recipe.

1 Preheat the oven to 350 degrees F. Butter or lightly oil an 8-inch springform pan or an 8-by-8-inch baking dish.

2 Roast the poblano by placing the pepper directly on the low flame of a gas burner, letting the skin char. Keep turning the pepper until skin is completely charred. Put the blackened pepper in a paper bag, allowing it to sweat and cool. Remove any black char under cool running water. Cut the pepper open, remove the seeds and stem, and dice it. In lieu of a gas oven, put the pepper in a shallow pan in the broiler to char the skin.

3 In a blender, puree 1 cup of the corn, the eggs, half-and-half, and yogurt. In a large bowl, put the flour, cheese, pepper, and salt. Add in the corn mixture and stir to incorporate. Pour the pudding into the prepared pan.

4 Bake the pudding until a knife inserted in the center comes out clean, 45 to 55 minutes. Turn the broiler on for 2 to 3 minutes to brown and bubble the top. Let the baked pudding rest for 10 minutes before slicing and serving.

FOR BABIES 6 MONTHS & OLDER: Blend the corn and water (without eggs) and snatch a few tablespoons of pureed corn for baby.

PREPARATION TIME:

70 minutes

MAKES 8 SERVINGS

1 (2-ounce) poblano pepper

2 cups fresh or frozen sweet corn, divided

3 eggs

½ cup half-and-half or milk

½ cup whole milk plain yogurt (not Greek yogurt)

1 cup corn flour

4 ounces jack cheese, grated

1¼ teaspoons sea salt

marilyn's best pizza dough

My dear friend and expert baker Marilyn McCormick shared this no-fail pizza dough recipe with me. It's easy to make, soft and chewy, and can be used for a variety of savory dishes—including pizza!

PREPARATION TIME:

15 minutes (for the dough); about 1 hour (for rising)

MAKES DOUGH FOR SIX 8-INCH PIZZAS

2 cups lukewarm water

2 teaspoons active dry yeast

1 tablespoon extra-virgin olive oil

3 cups whole wheat pastry flour

1 teaspoon sea salt

About 2 cups unbleached white bread flour, plus more for flouring

Sauce and toppings

1 In a large bowl, combine the water and yeast. Let it rest for 10 minutes while the yeast comes to life, then gently stir in the oil.

2 Gradually whisk in the pastry flour and salt. Beat for 1 to 2 minutes until it is stretchy and elastic. Begin gradually adding the bread flour to make soft dough. Let your hands sense when enough flour has been added. You want soft, bouncy dough that doesn't stick to your hands. Once it becomes difficult to stir, transfer the dough to a floured surface and knead it very briefly.

3 Clean, dry, and lightly oil the bowl. Place the dough in the bowl, cover, and let it rise in a warm place (75 to 80 degrees F is ideal) for 1 to 2 hours, until it has doubled in size.

4 Remove the dough from the bowl onto a surface lightly floured with white bread flour. Deflate the dough with the palms of your hands, then divide and shape the dough into six balls. Each ball will make an 8-inch pizza crust. At this point, all or half of the dough could be bagged, sealed, and frozen for later use, where it will keep for several months. If using now, cover the balls and let them rest 15 minutes to relax the dough.

5 Preheat the oven to 450 degrees F and place a pizza stone on the lowest rack of the oven.

6 On a floured surface, shape each ball into a flat round using your fingertips, making little tapping indentations rather than pulling or stretching the dough. Place the dough on an un-lipped baking sheet liberally dusted with cornmeal or rice flour or on a pizza peel. Top each pizza with your favorite sauce and toppings (see Veggie Lovers' Pizza Party, page 261, for ideas). Slide the pizza onto the stone from the baking sheet or peel. An 8-inch pizza will bake in about 6 minutes.

FOR BABIES 6 MONTHS & OLDER: If you use zucchini slices as a pizza topping, steam or puree some for baby.

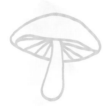

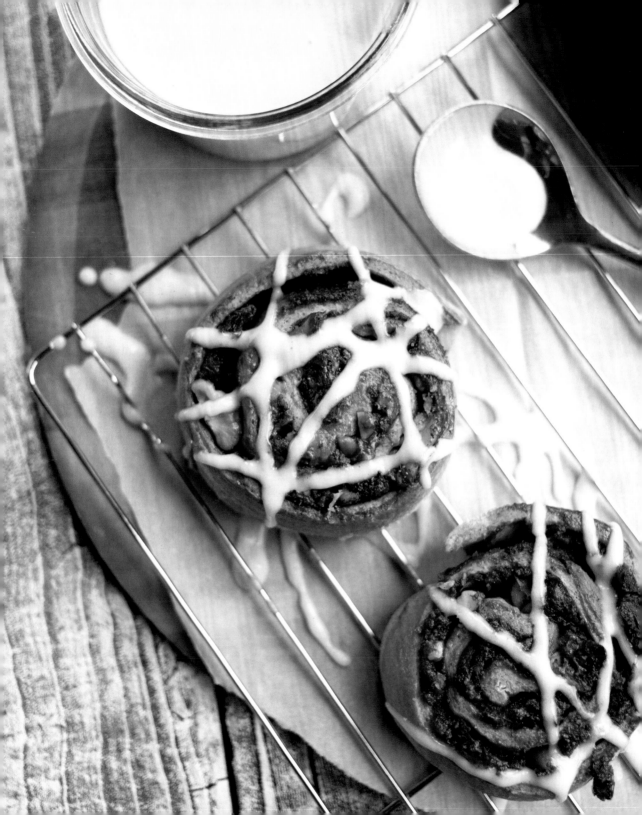

date & walnut cinnamon rolls

Did you know that dates have more fiber than prunes? They do! These cinnamon rolls provide a perfect snowy-day project. Young helpers will gobble up the outcome of their work. Share some with the neighbors!

1 In a small pan over low heat, warm ½ cup of the apple juice and the honey to lukewarm. Transfer the juice to a large bowl and add the yeast. Stir and set aside for 5 minutes until the mixture bubbles. In a medium bowl, combine the flours and set aside. To the juice mixture, add the eggs and enough of the flours to form a thin batter, about ¼ cup, and beat until smooth. Clean down the sides of bowl, cover with a damp cloth, and let it rise in a warm spot until doubled, about 30 minutes.

2 While the dough is rising, make the filling. In a small pan over low heat, place the dates and 1 cup of the apple juice. Heat the dates and juice to a simmer, cover, and cook until the liquid is absorbed, about 20 minutes. Let the dates cool, then puree them in a blender and set aside.

3 In a medium bowl, put the raisins and the remaining 2 cups apple juice. Let it sit for at least 15 minutes (or up to an hour) to soften and plump the raisins.

4 Return to the dough. Beat in the butter, zest, vanilla, and salt. Begin adding the remaining 2¾ cups of the flours to the dough. When it is too hard to stir, put the dough on a lightly floured surface and knead until smooth. Clean and lightly oil the bowl. Place the dough in the bowl, cover, and place in a warm place (around 80 degrees F) to rise until doubled, about 45 minutes.

5 Preheat the oven to 350 degrees F. Lightly oil a baking sheet or muffin tin. Set aside.

PREPARATION TIME:

2½ hours

MAKES 2 DOZEN CINNAMON ROLLS

3½ cups apple juice, divided

2 tablespoons honey

1 tablespoon dry active yeast

2 cups whole wheat pastry flour

1 cup unbleached white flour

2 eggs, beaten

1 cup pitted dates

2 to 3 cups raisins

½ cup (1 stick) unsalted butter, melted

1 tablespoon lemon zest (from 1 medium lemon)

1 teaspoon vanilla extract

½ teaspoon sea salt

⅔ cup walnuts, coarsely chopped

¼ cup unrefined cane sugar

1½ teaspoons ground cinnamon

For the icing:

½ cup sour cream

2 to 3 tablespoons honey

1 teaspoon vanilla extract

continued

6 On a lightly floured surface, roll out half of the dough to a rectangle about 10 by 16 inches. Strain the juice from the raisins. With the long end of the dough facing you, spread half of the date puree, strained raisins, and walnuts onto the dough. Sprinkle the dough with the sugar and cinnamon. Roll it up from the long side like a rug. An extra pair of hands helps! Cut the rolled dough into 1-inch slices and put them, cut side up, on the prepared baking sheet. Repeat with the other half of the dough. Bake the rolls until the edges of the rolls have turned golden, about 15 minutes.

7 While the rolls are baking, make the icing. In a small bowl, put the sour cream, honey, and vanilla and whisk together well. When the rolls have baked 15 minutes, spoon some of the icing on top of each roll and bake 10 to 15 more minutes. Let rolls cool to warm before serving.

FOR BABIES 10 MONTHS & OLDER: Add 1 teaspoon of softened date puree to baby's cereal.

---

cranberry, chestnut & sage thanksgiving dressing

My family begs me to make this dressing when November rolls around. Choose bread that is savory or neutral, not sweet. Ask a friend to help and make a lot—it is so good.

1 Preheat the oven to 400 degrees F.

2 Cut an *X* on the flat side of each chestnut. Place the nuts in a dry baking dish and bake until the shell comes away from the meat, about 20 minutes. Set aside to cool.

3 In a large skillet over medium heat, melt the butter. Add the onion and sauté until soft, 5 to 7 minutes.

4 Cut the bread into ½- to 1-inch cubes and put them in a large bowl. Add the celery, apple, and cranberries and toss to combine. Add the butter and onions and work the fat into the bread mixture.

5 In the skillet used for the butter and onion over medium heat, place ¼ to ½ cup water and heat the water to a simmer. Pour ¼ cup over bread mixture and work it in with your hands. If the mixture feels dry, add more water. It should feel moist but not soggy.

6 Peel the chestnuts, cut them into small pieces, and add them to the large bowl. Add all the herbs, salt, and pepper. Taste the mixture. Make sure the flavor pleases you. If desired, add more seasonings, especially salt or sage.

7 The stuffing is ready to be put into the turkey cavity or pressed into a 9-by-13-inch baking dish. If using a baking dish, cover and bake at 350 degrees F until baked throughout, about 45 minutes.

FOR BABIES 6 MONTHS & OLDER: Steam some apple slices until they are soft and puree them with applesauce.

PREPARATION TIME:

1½ hours

MAKES ABOUT 15 CUPS OF DRESSING

¾ cup toasted chestnuts

½ cup (1 stick) unsalted butter

1 medium onion, finely chopped

1 large (16-ounce) loaf whole grain or gluten-free bread

3 to 4 stalks celery, chopped

1 apple, chopped

1 cup fresh cranberries

Fresh sage, chopped

Fresh thyme

Fresh marjoram

Sea salt and freshly ground black pepper

FLOUR POWER

- - - - - - - - - - - - -

For more successful results, don't use just any flour you have for every baked good. Different varieties of wheat have different percentages of protein (gluten). Yeasted breads, which depend on gluten to form structure, require higher protein varieties of flour.

For yeasted breads, choose one of these whole grain flours:

- Hard red winter wheat
- Hard white spring wheat (a.k.a. whole white wheat flour)
- Unbleached white bread flour

All of these varieties have ample protein to yield the necessary amounts of gluten, the elastic component of dough that captures and holds carbon dioxide (the gas produced by yeast that raises your dough) for bread baking.

Whole white wheat flour is indeed a whole grain flour, complete with bran, germ, and endosperm, made from a type of whole grain wheat that doesn't have the genes that give it its bran color. Not only does it have a lighter color compared to hard red whole wheat but it also has a milder taste.

Less common whole grain gluten flours suitable for bread include:

- Triticale (cross of whole wheat and rye)
- Kamut (an ancient type of wheat)
- Spelt (an ancient type of wheat)

The high-protein flours, however, can make baked goods like cookies or piecrusts tough instead of tender!

For cookies, pastries, quick breads, and muffins, choose flours milled from low-protein soft wheat:

- Whole wheat pastry flour
- Soft whole white wheat flour
- Unbleached white all-purpose flour

Most reputable flour manufacturers give consumers clues on the package by labeling the flour "bread flour" or noting that the flour works well for muffins or pastries.

If choosing to use all-purpose or white flour, be sure to seek out a brand that doesn't bleach the flour (look for "unbleached" on the label).

And buy organic! Conventional wheat crops are sprayed with pesticides. Some theories blame glyphosates (a type of pesticide) for a whole host of health conditions.

For several good gluten-free formulas, see Have It Your Way: Flour, Fat, Milk, Sweetener, and Egg Substitutions (page 401). Remember that gluten-free flour mixes simply don't have the necessary components (gluten!) to stand in for the flour in yeasted breads. Most other flour-based products (muffins, cookies) are fine with a one-for-one swap.

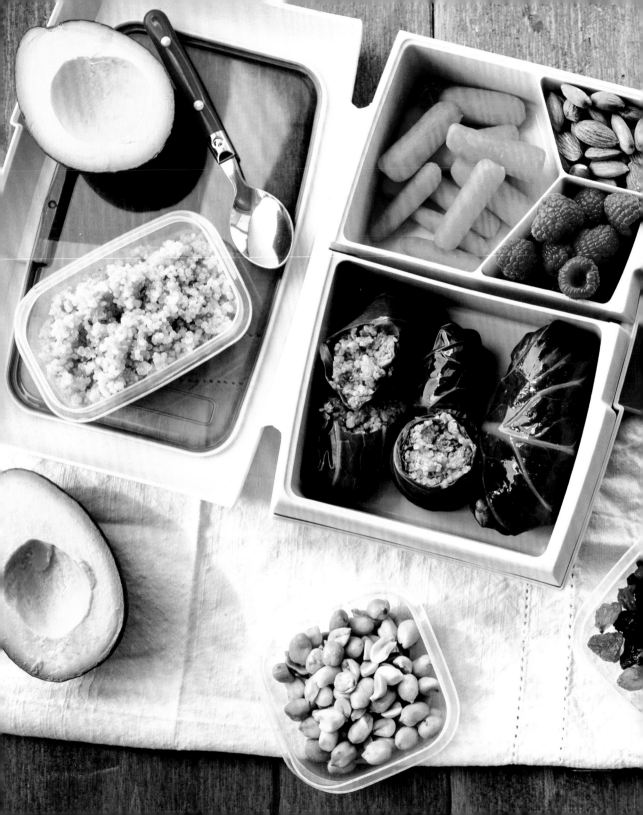

CHAPTER 6

lively
lunch boxes

When *Cookus Interruptus*, a web cooking show I cocreated, was launched in 2008, we immediately began looking for a way to support the site. Landing big advertisers required huge traffic numbers. Start-ups depended on each other to trade shout-outs and links to help build viewership.

One small web company we traded links with was Laptop Lunchboxes. The two women who started this company (now called Bentology) met in a new-moms group in 1995. As their babies grew into children and started school, they felt compelled to find a way to pack school lunches that would reduce food and packaging waste. Through extensive research, Amy and Tammy found that the bento-style lunch box system lent itself to well-balanced meals and set out to manufacture containers in an environmentally sustainable way. Their affordable lunch boxes were produced from plastic with no polyvinyl chloride (PVC) or bisphenol A (BPA). Sales skyrocketed.

The bento box is common in Japanese food culture. They are used for takeout or carefully home-packed meals. The box holds four or five smaller compartments so that several individual dishes can be included. The Japanese bento box typically includes one compartment with rice, one with fish, and two or three more holding vegetables and pickled vegetables.

Bento boxes are showing up as the latest trend in packing creative, healthy lunches for children. Those small inner compartments help promote variety and lend themselves to appropriately sized portions. As bento boxes become popular, so do the ideas to jazz things up by slicing and arranging food in the shape of cute animals and flowers. Creative ideas abound on Pinterest and food blogs.

We were always proud to highlight Amy and Tammy's products on *Cookus Interruptus*, and they were generous in linking to our videos. Helping each other out—can't overdo that.

creamy tahini sesame noodles

My daughter's godmother, Karen Brown, made these for our potlucks when we lived in New York, and they were the first entrée to disappear. Different nut and seed butters can be interchanged in this recipe to vary the flavor.

1 Fill an 8-quart pot with water and bring it to a boil over high heat. Add the noodles and salt and boil for the amount of time suggested on the package directions, usually 6 to 8 minutes.

2 Meanwhile, make the sauce. In a small bowl, put the tahini, vinegar, tamari, almond butter, syrup, oil, and coriander and stir well to blend. Add the warm water, a little at a time, to create a creamy, pourable consistency.

3 Rinse and drain the cooked noodles. Pour the sauce over noodles and toss to coat. Add the green onion and sesame seeds. Chill the noodles in the refrigerator for a minimum of 15 minutes before serving or packing.

FOR BABIES 10 MONTHS & OLDER: Omit the sauce. Cut plain noodles into bite-size pieces and serve.

VARIATION FOR CHILDREN: Try serving the sauce on the side and letting children dip the noodles in the sauce.

PREPARATION TIME:

15 minutes; 15 minutes (for chilling)

MAKES 4 SERVINGS

1 (8-ounces) soba or udon noodles

1 teaspoon sea salt

3 tablespoons tahini

2 tablespoons apple cider vinegar

2 tablespoons tamari (soy sauce)

1 tablespoon almond or cashew butter

1 tablespoon maple syrup

1 teaspoon toasted sesame oil

½ teaspoon ground coriander

2 to 4 tablespoons warm water

2 green onions, chopped, for garnish

1 tablespoon toasted sesame seeds (see below), for garnish

HOW TO TOAST SESAME SEEDS

In an 8-inch dry skillet over medium heat, put the sesame seeds. Keep the seeds moving until they give off a nutty aroma, pop, and begin to change color, 5 to 7 minutes. Remove the pan from the heat, and allow the sesame seeds to cool. The toasted sesame seeds will keep in an airtight container for several months.

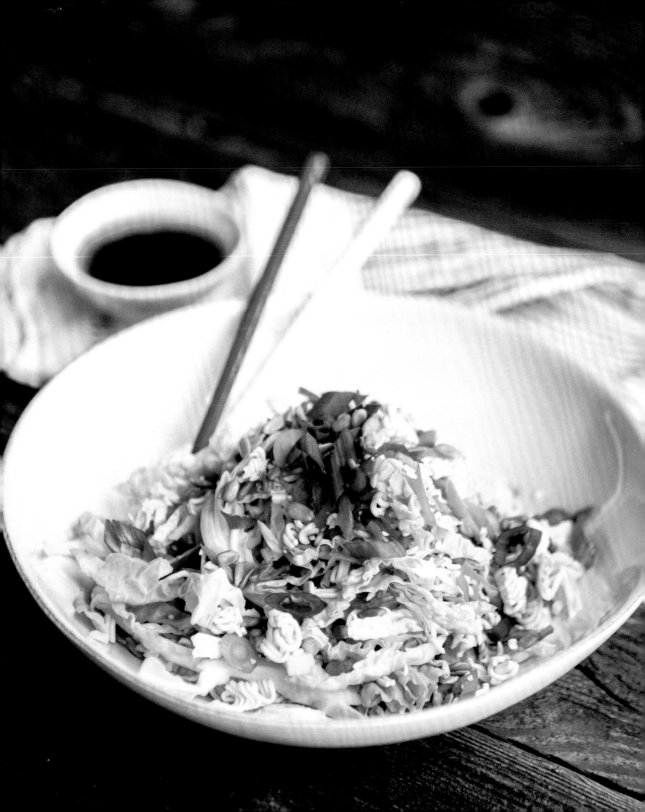

aunt cathy's
crunchy ramen coleslaw

Look for ramen made from whole grain flours. This slaw uses smashed dry noodles to give it the crunch factor.

1 To toast the sunflower seeds, in a small dry skillet over medium heat, put the seeds. Stir or shake the pan constantly until the seeds begin to emit a nutty aroma, about 5 minutes.

2 In a large bowl, combine the cabbage, green onions, carrot, and toasted seeds. Set aside. Put the ramen noodles on a cutting board. Using a rolling pin, roll over the uncooked noodles to break them into small pieces, then add them to the vegetables and toss.

3 In a small jar, combine the oil, vinegar, sugar, salt, and pepper. Shake to emulsify. Pour the dressing over the salad just before serving and toss again.

FOR BABIES 10 MONTHS & OLDER: Cook the unused half of the ramen noodles according to the directions on the package. Cut them into small pieces and serve plain.

PREPARATION TIME:

15 minutes

MAKES 6 SERVINGS

¼ cup sunflower seeds

3 cups finely shredded cabbage

3 green onions, finely sliced

1 small carrot, grated

½ (single serving) package brown rice ramen

¼ cup extra-virgin olive oil

3 tablespoons balsamic vinegar

1 teaspoon unrefined cane sugar

½ teaspoon sea salt

Freshly ground black pepper

lively lunch boxes

dilled brown rice & kidney beans

Summer cooks welcome this easy-to-make dish. Dill and red onion give the grain-and-bean combination its zip. Umeboshi plum vinegar, the leftover juice from the plum-pickling process, gives a unique salty-sour taste to food. Lemon juice and salt can be substituted for umeboshi *vinegar.*

PREPARATION TIME:

10 minutes

MAKES 4 SERVINGS

½ cup red onion, finely chopped

2 cups cooked brown rice

1½ cups cooked kidney beans

3 tablespoons extra-virgin olive oil

3 tablespoons rice vinegar

1 tablespoon *umeboshi* plum vinegar

2 tablespoons fresh dill, or 2 teaspoons dried dill

1 To take the sting out of raw onion, in a small bowl, put the onion, cover it with boiling water, and let it sit for 1 minute. Drain and put in a large bowl with the rice and beans.

2 In a small bowl, mix the oil, vinegars, and dill with whisk (or shake to combine in a small jar). Pour the dressing over the rice mixture and toss gently. If possible, let the dish set for 1 to 2 hours, as flavors integrate into starchy foods better with time.

FOR BABIES 6 MONTHS & OLDER: Reserve some of the cooked brown rice and blend it with water or breast milk.

FOR BABIES 10 MONTHS & OLDER: Reserve some plain cooked kidney beans and blend them with a pinch of dill to a smooth consistency, adding a little water if necessary.

santa fe black bean salad

Combine Southwestern ingredients for this "to-go" dish and serve with corn tortillas or Polenta Slices (page 253). Frozen corn can be thawed and used if fresh corn is unavailable.

1 To roast the peppers with a gas stove, put the pepper directly on the low flame of a gas burner, letting the skin char. Keep turning the pepper until skin is charred on all sides. To roast the peppers with an electric stove, put the pepper in a shallow pan and put in the oven under the broiler. Let the skin char. Turn the pepper every few minutes until skin is completely charred. Remove the pepper from the oven.

2 Place the blackened pepper in a paper bag, allowing it to sweat and cool for about 5 minutes. Remove any black char under cool running water. Cut the pepper open and remove the seeds and stem.

3 In a medium bowl, combine the roasted pepper, beans, corn, and cilantro and set aside. Put the garlic and salt on a cutting board and chop to a paste-like consistency. In a separate small bowl, mix together the garlic paste, oil, lime juice, cumin, and cayenne. Pour the dressing over the beans and vegetables and toss gently. Taste for salt and add more if needed.

FOR BABIES 10 MONTHS & OLDER: Blend fresh corn kernels into a puree before serving (or they will come out the other end whole!).

PREPARATION TIME:

30 minutes

MAKES 6 SERVINGS

1 red bell pepper

2 cups cooked black beans

1 cup fresh corn off the cob (about 1 ear)

⅓ cup chopped fresh cilantro

2 to 3 cloves garlic, minced

½ teaspoon sea salt

3 tablespoons extra-virgin olive oil

3 tablespoons freshly squeezed lime juice

½ teaspoon ground cumin

¼ teaspoon cayenne

lively lunch boxes

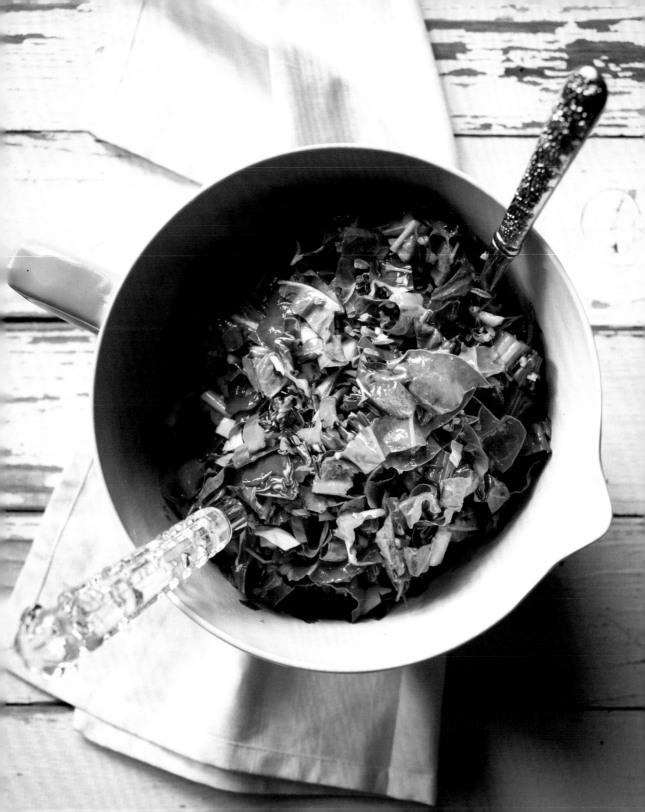

emerald city salad *with* wild rice, fennel & greens

This PCC deli salad is so popular that I have filled classes with the mere mention that I would be demonstrating how to make it.

1 In a 2-quart pan over high heat, bring the water and stock to a boil. Add ½ teaspoon of the salt, the butter, and rice. Bring the pan to boil again, cover, then reduce the heat to low and simmer until all water is absorbed, 55 to 60 minutes. If after 55 minutes the grain has opened up, but when tipped, there is still liquid in the pot, remove the lid and let the remaining water cook off.

2 In a large bowl, combine the lemon juice, garlic, and the remaining ½ teaspoon salt. Whisk in the oil to emulsify.

3 Place the fennel, bell pepper, cabbage, and parsley on top of the dressing. Remove the thick stems from the parsley and Swiss chard. Stack the chard leaves, roll up the pile (like a rug), and cut into ¼- to ½-inch ribbons. Pile the chopped greens on top of the other vegetables.

4 Once the rice is fully cooked, let it cool until it quits steaming but is still warm, and then lay it like a blanket on top of the raw greens to wilt them. When the rice cools to room temperature, fold it into vegetables and dressing. Taste the salad and adjust seasonings, adding addition salt or lemon if desired. Top with grated pecorino if desired.

FOR BABIES 6 MONTHS & OLDER: Add 1 teaspoon of fresh chopped parsley to baby's cereal.

FOR BABIES 10 MONTHS & OLDER: Offer baby 1 to 2 tablespoons of cooked wild rice grains. The flavor is strong. Stirring in a little baked sweet potato sweetens it.

PREPARATION TIME:

75 minutes

MAKES 6 TO 8 SERVINGS

1¼ cups water

1 cup Easy Vegetarian Stock (page 168), Simple Chicken Stock (page 165), or store-bought

1 teaspoon sea salt, divided, plus more for seasoning

1 teaspoon unsalted butter or extra-virgin olive oil

1 cup black wild rice (½ inch long)

¼ cup freshly squeezed lemon juice (from 2 small lemons)

1 clove garlic, minced

¼ cup extra-virgin olive oil

½ cup chopped fennel

½ red or yellow bell pepper, diced

½ cup chopped red cabbage

½ cup chopped fresh Italian parsley

6 to 7 Swiss chard leaves

Freshly ground black pepper

Pecorino cheese (optional)

tabbouleh salad *with* parsley & cherry tomatoes

Traditional tabbouleh salad makes splendid lunch box fare and packs well for a picnic or potluck. Serve the tabbouleh with Roasted Garlic Hummus (page 154) and Classic Greek Salad (page 208). Substitute three cups cooked quinoa for bulgur for a gluten-free tabbouleh.

PREPARATION TIME:

30 minutes

MAKES 4 SERVINGS

1 cup whole wheat bulgur

1 cup boiling water

⅓ cup finely chopped fresh Italian parsley

2 green onions, finely chopped

½ cup cucumber, chopped into small pieces

8 cherry tomatoes, halved or quartered

¼ cup chopped fresh mint

¼ cup freshly squeezed lemon juice (from 2 small lemons)

1 teaspoon sea salt

¼ cup extra-virgin olive oil

1 In a medium bowl, put the bulgur. Pour the boiling water over bulgur, cover, and let stand for 15 minutes. Make sure all the water has been absorbed, then fluff the bulgur with a fork.

2 When the grain has cooled to room temperature, add the parsley, green onions, cucumber, tomato, and mint to the cooled bulgur and toss gently.

3 To make the dressing, in a small bowl, blend lemon juice and salt with whisk. Drizzle in the oil slowly, while whisking, to emulsify. Pour the dressing over the bulgur and vegetables and toss again. Serve immediately or store in refrigerator in a covered container.

FOR BABIES 10 MONTHS & OLDER: Reserve some plain bulgur and serve it to baby as finger food with chopped cucumber and mint on the side.

VARIATION FOR CHILDREN: Keep the chopped vegetables separate from the bulgur and serve small piles of each on one plate.

lemon-basil potato salad

Consider growing basil in your yard or in a pot on the kitchen windowsill. Your child can learn about how food grows by assisting in the planting and harvesting.

1 Place a steamer basket in a large pot and fill it with about 2 inches of water. Bring the water to boil over high heat, then add the potatoes, cover the pot, and allow the potatoes to steam until a fork slides into the center of a potato easily, 15 to 20 minutes. Baby (1- to 1½-inch diameter) potatoes will take about 15 minutes, while larger (3-inch diameter) potatoes will take about 20 minutes.

2 Put the garlic, basil, zest, and salt on a cutting board. Chop the ingredients together to a paste-like consistency. In a small bowl, combine the paste with the oil.

3 When the steamed potatoes are warm but can be easily handled, slice the potatoes into a serving bowl and dress with the lemon juice. Add the basil paste and toss gently. Serve immediately or chill to serve later.

PREPARATION TIME:

30 minutes

MAKES 4 SERVINGS

1 pound (about 6 to 8) red potatoes, cut into chunks

3 to 4 cloves garlic

⅓ cup tightly packed fresh basil

1 tablespoon lemon zest (from 1 medium lemon)

1 teaspoon sea salt

¼ cup extra-virgin olive oil

¼ cup freshly squeezed lemon juice (from 2 small lemons)

FOR BABIES 6 MONTHS & OLDER: Reserve some steamed potato and mash with water or breast milk.

PACKING A WHOLESOME LUNCH BOX

Here are some suggestions for caretakers who pack lunch regularly for children:
• Include one item in the lunch box for each of the categories: vroom-vroom vegetables, giddy-up whole grain, power-on proteins, and fantastic fruits.

• Make a lunch box chart (sample chart follows). If your child is five or older, let them help plan and make the chart. Children are more likely to eat the food if they have helped plan the menu. Renew the chart as the seasons change. Post your chart where the less tall can view it.

• Though many food companies make convenient lunch foods wrapped in happy-looking packaging, remember to be discerning and read labels. Avoid foods with additives, preservatives, food coloring, cheap oils, and an excess of sweeteners.

• Rather than packing juice, tuck in a small container of fruity herbal tea if liquids need to be included. Juice does not signal a sense of fullness and metabolizes as quickly as table sugar.

• For an earth-friendly lunch box, use a cloth napkin and silverware instead of wasteful paper and plastic.

• On days where you feel like tucking in an extra treat, add a dried flower, poem, a special rock or crystal, a jingle bell, a cartoon, a finger puppet, or a love note from you instead of candy.

• If the staff and parents of your child's school are open to the idea, consider having "Hot Soup Fridays" where parents bring in enough hearty hot soup for the whole class on a rotating basis. This is especially appropriate during the winter months when warm food will be welcomed.

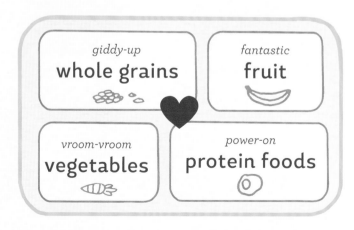

Let's Plan Your Lunch Box!

	VROOM-VROOM VEGETABLES	GIDDY-UP WHOLE GRAINS	POWER-ON PROTEINS	FANTASTIC FRUIT
MONDAY				
TUESDAY				
WEDNESDAY				
THURSDAY				
FRIDAY				

lively lunch boxes

asian noodle salad *with* broccoli & toasted sesame dressing

You can create an impressive summer meal by serving this with Nori-Wrapped Wasabi Salmon (page 288)—nutritionally impressive too!

PREPARATION TIME:

20 to 25 minutes

MAKES 4 TO 6 SERVINGS

1 (8-ounce) package soba noodles

3 tablespoons tamari (soy sauce)

3 tablespoons balsamic vinegar

2 tablespoons toasted sesame oil

1 tablespoon maple syrup

1 tablespoon hot pepper oil

2 cups Blanched Broccoli (page 191)

¼ cup toasted sesame seeds (see page 129 for toasting instructions)

¼ cup chopped cilantro leaves

1 Cook the noodles according to the directions on the package. Drain and rinse the noodles.

2 In a small bowl, combine the tamari, vinegar, sesame oil, syrup, and hot pepper oil and whisk together.

3 In a large bowl, put the noodles. Add the broccoli, sesame seeds, and cilantro. Drizzle in the dressing and toss gently.

FOR BABIES 10 MONTHS & OLDER: Reserve some of the blanched broccoli. Cut it up into tiny pieces.

VARIATION FOR CHILDREN: Omit the hot pepper oil. Some children may prefer plain noodles without any dressing and cut-up vegetables on the side.

---

feeding the whole family

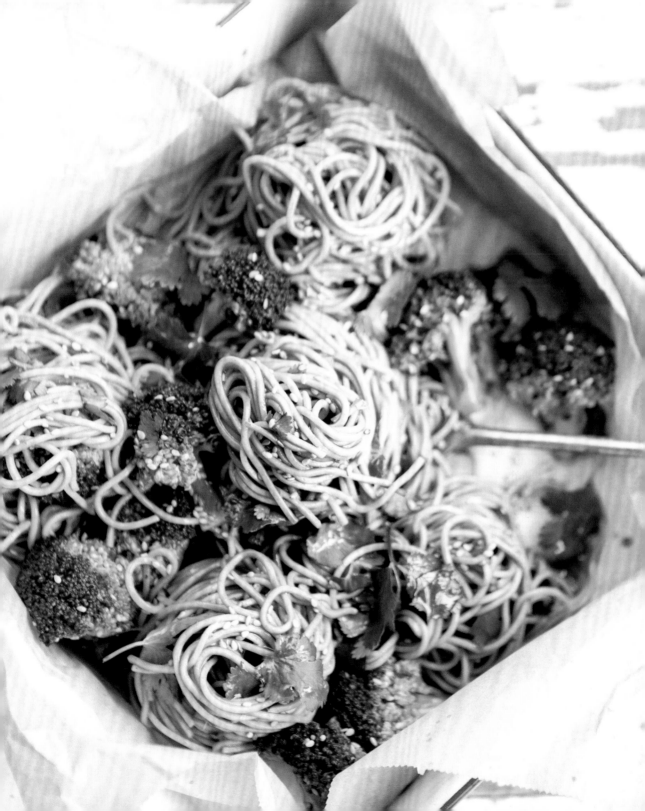

seared steak salad *with* cilantro-lime dressing

Choosing beef from healthfully raised cows is important nutritionally, ecologically, and politically. If you can't find grass-fed or humanely raised beef from a local farmer, ask at your food co-op or grocery store to find beef from cows that were not given antibiotics or hormones.

PREPARATION TIME:

1 to 12 hours (for marinating); 20 minutes (for preparing)

MAKES 4 SERVINGS

For the marinade:

⅓ cup lime juice (from 3 limes)

⅓ cup extra-virgin olive oil

¼ cup packed fresh cilantro, chopped

2 to 3 cloves garlic, minced

3 teaspoons honey or sugar

1 teaspoon hot pepper sesame oil

1 teaspoon sea salt

Freshly ground black pepper

1 pound (1 inch thick) sirloin or rib-eye steak

Sea salt and freshly ground black pepper

2 teaspoons high-heat vegetable oil, such as safflower or peanut

4 cups salad greens, torn

1 To make the marinade, in a small bowl, combine the lime juice, oil, cilantro, garlic, honey, hot pepper oil, salt, and pepper. Whisk together and set aside.

2 Season the meat with salt and pepper. Place the meat between two sheets of plastic wrap and, using a meat tenderizer mallet, pound the meat on both sides. (Alternately, you can massage the meat with your hands, breaking up the fibers.) Remove the plastic wrap and place the meat in a shallow pan. Pour half of the marinade over the meat. Cover the pan and let the meat marinate in the refrigerator for at least 1 hour or up to 12 hours.

3 When the meat is finished marinating, preheat the oven to 400 degrees F.

4 In a cast-iron or oven-safe skillet over medium-high heat, heat the oil. Place the marinated steak in the skillet and sear it for 1 minute on each side.

5 Transfer the steak to the oven then bake until the meat has browned and is firmer when pressed, 6 to 7 minutes if the cut is thicker, less if the steak is less than ¾ inch thick. Check the center for doneness (red for medium rare, pink for medium) or use an instant-read thermometer and aim for 130 to 135 degrees F. Remove the pan from oven when the meat is slightly

redder than you desire. Transfer the meat to a carving board and let it rest for 10 minutes before cutting it into thin slices on a diagonal, against the grain of the meat.

6 To assemble the salad, in a large serving bowl, toss the greens, onion, and cucumber with the remaining marinade and divide it among four plates. Top each plate with an equal portion of steak slices. If packing in a lunch box, consider replacing the salad greens with 2 cups of cooked noodles or keeping the dressing in a separate container, as lettuce leaves will not hold well after being dressed.

½ small red onion, cut into half moons

½ cucumber, peeled, seeded, and cut into half moons

FOR BABIES 10 MONTHS & OLDER: Cut a strip of cooked steak into tiny ¼-inch pieces or pulse it in a food processor before serving to baby.

VARIATION FOR CHILDREN: Instead of arranging this dish like a salad, keep the meat, noodles, and vegetables separate and serve a few tablespoons of the dressing on the side for dipping.

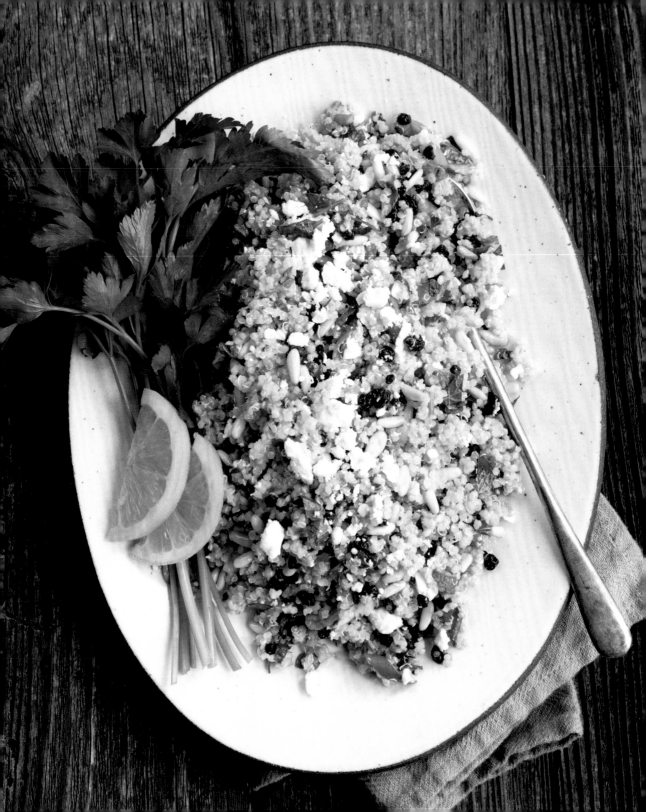

mediterranean quinoa salad
with feta, pine nuts & mint

Quinoa has high protein quality and is typically regarded as an adequate source of all essential amino acids, including lysine and isoleucine. This unique whole grain, which was a staple food of the Incas, also has appreciable amounts of manganese, a mineral associated with good bone formation.

1 In a 2-quart pot over high heat, put the water, quinoa, and salt, and bring it to a boil. Reduce the heat to low and simmer, covered, until all the water is absorbed, 15 to 20 minutes. Don't stir the quinoa while it is cooking. Remove the pot from the heat, remove the lid, and let the quinoa rest for 10 minutes.

2 While the quinoa is cooking, in a skillet over low to medium heat or a 300-degree-F oven, dry toast the pine nuts until they begin to change color and give off a nutty aroma, 5 to 7 minutes.

3 In a large salad bowl, put the lemon juice. Whisk in the oil a little at a time to incorporate. Add the currants. Using a fork, add the warm cooked quinoa a little at a time. Then add the toasted pine nuts, mint, parsley, and green onions; toss gently. Finish by crumbling the feta on top. Serve at room temperature.

PREPARATION TIME:

30 minutes

MAKES 4 SERVINGS

1¾ cups water

1 cup quinoa

1 teaspoon sea salt

¼ cup raw pine nuts

¼ cup freshly squeezed
   lemon juice (from
   2 small lemons)

¼ cup extra-virgin olive oil

¼ cup currants

3 tablespoons chopped
   fresh mint

3 tablespoons chopped
   fresh Italian parsley

2 green onions, chopped

⅓ cup crumbled feta cheese

FOR BABIES 6 MONTHS & OLDER: Puree a small amount of plain quinoa with water or breast milk.

tempeh avocado sushi rolls

Nori and other seaweed products are available at natural foods stores and Asian markets. These rolls travel well, making them perfect for the bento-style lunch box.

feeding the whole family

PREPARATION TIME:

30 minutes

MAKES 24 PIECES

2 tablespoons mirin

2 tablespoons brown rice syrup

2 tablespoons rice vinegar

4 cups cooked short-grain rice (see page 242 for cooking instructions)

2 tablespoons unrefined coconut oil

4 ounces tempeh, cut into 3-inch strips

4 sheets toasted nori

½ ripe avocado, cut into thin slices

1 carrot, cut lengthwise into long, thin strips

For the dipping sauce:

¼ cup tamari (soy sauce)

2 tablespoons water

1 tablespoon grated daikon (Japanese white radish)

¼ teaspoon prepared wasabi (optional)

1 In a small saucepan over low heat, heat the mirin, syrup, and vinegar until pourable, 1 to 2 minutes. In a large bowl, toss the mirin mixture with the rice to combine. It is best to season the rice while it is still warm.

2 In a skillet over medium-high heat, heat the oil. Add the tempeh, turning the strips until brown on all sides, about 1 minute on each side. Remove the tempeh to a paper towel.

3 Lay a sheet of nori shiny side down on a bamboo rolling mat or a clean dish towel. Spread a quarter of the rice mixture onto the nori, leaving ½ inch uncovered on the top and bottom of the nori sheet. Place a quarter of the tempeh, avocado, and carrot lengthwise in the middle of the rice. Lift the rolling mat or towel from the edge nearest you and begin to roll, tucking firmly into the center while lifting the mat up. Continue pulling in with your fingertips, tightening the ingredients, while rolling the nori. Gently squeeze the roll to make it even. With a sharp, wetted knife, using a back and forth sawing motion, cut the roll into 1-inch pieces. Repeat with the remaining three nori sheets.

4 To make the dipping sauce, in a small bowl, stir together the tamari, water, and daikon. Add the wasabi (not too much, if any, for young children). The sauce will hold well for several hours placed in a sealed container or wrapped in plastic wrap.

FOR BABIES 6 MONTHS & OLDER: Reserve some of the rice before dressing it. Puree the rice and a few bits of nori together with water or breast milk and serve. Mashed avocado is also an option.

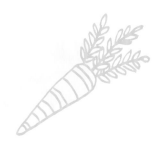

sticky rice balls rolled *in* sesame salt *with* ginger soy dipping sauce

During an after-school program, I led a cooking class and had children help make this simplest of snacks. To my surprise, they literally licked the plates.

PREPARATION TIME:

20 minutes

MAKES 12 TO 15 RICE BALLS

2½ to 3 cups pressure-cooked sweet and short-grain brown rice (see page 242 for cooking instructions)

1 cup brown sesame seeds

1 teaspoon sea salt

For the dipping sauce:

¼ cup water

¼ cup tamari (soy sauce)

1 teaspoon freshly grated gingerroot

1 Simmered or rice-cooker rice will not hold together to form balls. It is best to pressure-cook the rice and use a combination of ¼ cup sweet brown rice and ¾ cup short-grain brown rice. Allow the rice to cool to room temperature before making the rice balls.

2 Rinse the sesame seeds and drain them through a fine mesh strainer. In a medium dry skillet over medium heat, toast the seeds, stirring constantly, until the seeds begin to pop, change color slightly, and give off a toasty aroma, about 5 to 7 minutes. In a *suribachi* (a serrated ceramic mortar), put the toasted seeds and salt and grind with a pestle or pulse seeds and salt together. (Alternatively, you can grind the seeds and salt in a blender or food processor.) This condiment can be stored in a sealed container and used to flavor many foods (like on popcorn—yum).

3 To make the rice balls, on a plate or in a shallow baking dish, spread about ⅓ cup of the sesame salt. Moisten your hands with water and gather a small handful of cooked rice in your hand. Press your hands around the rice, packing it into small ball about the size of a ping-pong ball. Roll the ball in the sesame salt, covering all sides. Repeat until all the rice is used up or the desired amount is obtained. The rice balls will keep for 5 days in a covered container in the refrigerator.

4 To make the dipping sauce, in a small bowl, combine the water, tamari, and gingerroot.

FOR BABIES 10 MONTHS & OLDER: Pulverize a few tablespoons of the toasted sesame seeds before adding salt. Use this as a condiment on cereal or vegetables.

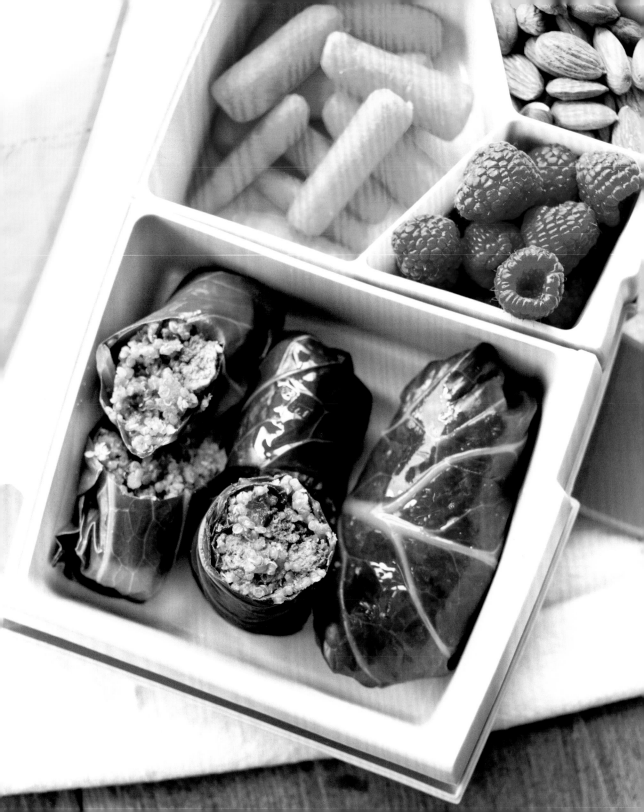

collard green wraps *with* spiced beef & quinoa filling

They sky is the limit as to what combination of grains, beans, nuts, and herbs you can use for the filling. Utilize leftovers! This fun use of collard greens works for lunch boxes, potlucks—and even makes a unique appetizer.

1 In a large skillet over medium heat, heat the oil. Add the onion and sauté until translucent, 5 to 7 minutes. Add the beef, 1 teaspoon of the salt, the cumin, paprika, cinnamon, and pepper. Break up the beef with a spatula until incorporated with the onion and spices and in small bits. When the beef is thoroughly cooked, about 5 minutes, fold in the cooked quinoa and remove the skillet from the heat.

2 Fill an 8-quart pot with water and bring it to a boil over high heat. Make a *V*-cut and remove the thickest part of the collards' center stems while leaving the leaves intact. Bisect the leaves lengthwise. You will have ten to twelve leaf halves, each approximately 5 inches wide. (If you are working with smaller leaves, remove the stem but keep the leaves whole.)

3 Put the leaves in the boiling water with the 1 remaining teaspoon salt. Don't stir but make sure the leaves are completely submerged. Allow them to boil until still bright green but limp, 2 to 3 minutes. Pour the contents of the pot through a large colander and rinse the leaves in cold water to stop the cooking.

4 Place each cooked leaf on a cutting board, stem end closest to you. Place 2 rounded tablespoons of the filling toward the bottom third of the leaf. Fold the edge closest to you over the filling and pull the filling in firmly. Fold

PREPARATION TIME:

40 minutes

MAKES 10 TO 12 ROLLS

2 teaspoons extra-virgin olive oil

1 medium onion, finely chopped

½ pound grass-fed ground beef

2 teaspoons sea salt, divided

½ teaspoon ground cumin

½ teaspoon ground paprika

¼ teaspoon ground cinnamon

Freshly ground black pepper

½ cup cooked quinoa (see page 242 for cooking instructions)

5 to 6 large (10-inch wide) collard leaves

Tzatziki Sauce (page 363) or store-bought

lively lunch boxes

continued

½ inch of each side toward the center and then roll the leaf closed—like you would roll a burrito. The rolls will be about 3 to 4 inches wide. Repeat the procedure until you have used all of your cooked leaves and stuffing.

5 Store the rolls in the refrigerator until ready to eat.

FOR BABIES 6 MONTHS & OLDER: Reserve some cooked quinoa and blend it with water or breast milk.

FOR BABIES 10 MONTHS & OLDER: Mix some of the beef and quinoa filling with a few bits of cooked collard greens.

VARIATION FOR VEGETARIANS

You'll need around 1½ cups of filling food to make these rolls.

- Scrambled Tofu and Pepper (page 97)

- Dilled Brown Rice and Kidney Beans (page 132)

- Mediterranean Quinoa Salad with Feta, Pine Nuts, and Mint (page 145)

- French Lentil Dijon Spread (page 159)

- Moroccan Rice and Lentils (page 257)

- Curried Cauliflower Dal (page 266)

- Lime and Chili Tempeh (page 267)

miso-tahini butter *with* carrot & pepper dippers

Tahini is a creamy paste made of crushed, hulled sesame seeds. Sesame is uniquely resistant to rancidity, which is perhaps why it has been enjoyed by many cultures for centuries. The miso adds a probiotic touch.

1 In small bowl, put the tahini and miso and mix well. Add the water, a few drops at a time, to get a creamier consistency. Stir in the green onions.

2 Serve as a dip for the carrots and pepper or any other fresh vegetables.

FOR BABIES 10 MONTHS & OLDER: Stir ½ teaspoon of the tahini into baby's warm whole grain cereal for added fat.

VARIATION FOR CHILDREN: For a sweeter flavor, omit the green onions and add 1 teaspoon of maple syrup to the dip.

PREPARATION TIME:

5 to 10 minutes

MAKES ⅔ CUP

½ cup tahini

1 tablespoon white or mellow miso

About 1 to 2 tablespoons warm water

2 to 3 green onions, finely chopped

2 carrots, cut into 3-inch sticks

1 red or yellow bell pepper, cut into thick strips

lively lunch boxes

roasted garlic hummus
with olive oil pool

This traditional Middle Eastern dish makes excellent vegetarian sandwiches, and it's a perfect dip for vegetables. The combination of chickpeas and tahini creates a high-protein spread. Roasting garlic (instead of adding it raw) softens the sharpness of the spread, which children may appreciate.

feeding the whole family

PREPARATION TIME:

35 minutes (for roasting);
10 minutes

MAKES ABOUT 3 CUPS

1 head garlic

4 to 5 teaspoons extra-virgin olive oil, divided

2 cups cooked chickpeas

5 tablespoons tahini

1 teaspoon sea salt, plus more if needed

⅓ cup freshly squeezed lemon juice (from 1½ to 2 medium lemons), plus more if needed

¼ teaspoon ground paprika

1 Preheat the oven to 400 degrees F.

2 Peel away some of the papery outer layers of the garlic bulb skin, leaving the skins of the individual cloves intact. Cut ¼ to ½ inch off of the stem side or top of the head, exposing the individual cloves of garlic.

3 Put the garlic head in a baking pan or a square of aluminum foil, then drizzle 1 to 2 teaspoons of oil over the open side, using your fingers to make sure the garlic head is well coated. Cover the baking pan or enclose the head in the aluminum foil. Bake until the cloves feel soft when pressed, 30 to 35 minutes.

4 Allow the garlic to cool enough so you can touch it without burning yourself. Use a small knife to lightly score the skin around each clove. Use a cocktail fork or your fingers to pull or squeeze the roasted garlic cloves out of their skins. Children like helping with this.

5 In a blender or food processor, blend the cooked chickpeas, tahini, salt, and lemon juice until smooth. Taste the garlic and decide if you want all of the roasted garlic or just some in the hummus. (The remainder can be saved and spread on toast or added to salad dressings.) Hummus presents an exercise in finding the right taste and texture. Add the roasted garlic a little at a time, tasting the mixture each step of the way. If a wee bit more salt or lemon is needed to please your palate, adjust those flavors as well.

6 If the mixture seems too thick, add some water, a tablespoon at a time. The hummus will thicken some as it cools. Place the hummus in a serving bowl, indent the top with the back of a spoon, and pool the remaining 1 tablespoon oil on top. Sprinkle the paprika around the perimeter.

7 This hummus stores well in the refrigerator for at least 1 week.

FOR BABIES 10 MONTHS & OLDER: Serve 1 teaspoon of soft hummus to baby.

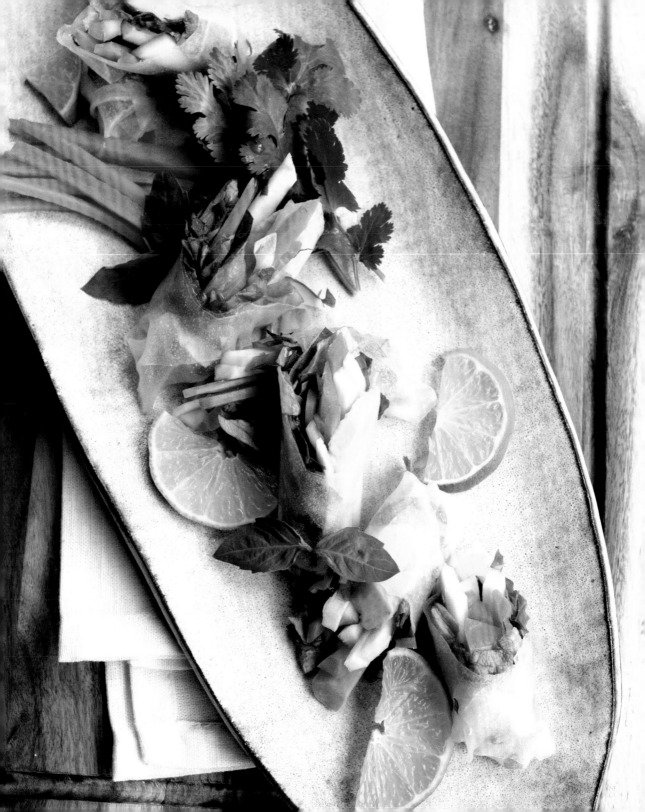

thai fresh vegetable rolls

These rolls are way yummy served with Coconut Peanut Sauce (page 361) as a dipping sauce. Rice wrappers are available in most Asian grocery stores.

1 Fill a large, round pie plate or cake pan with warm water. Soak the spring roll skins, one at a time, for about 15 seconds on each side, until soft but still firm to the touch. Remove the soft skin from the water and lay it flat on a hard surface—plastic or metal work best.

2 Build the rolls one at a time. Place a couple of avocado slices on the bottom third of the softened skin. Top with some of the lettuce, carrot, zucchini, and any other additions, forming a line. The key is not to add too many vegetables and overstuff the roll. Next, sprinkle some of the lime juice over the fillings.

3 Working quickly, fold the edge closest to you over the filling and drag the filling in toward you. Use a firm touch or the rolls won't hold together. Fold the sides toward the center and then roll it closed. Rolls should be about 4 inches long and 1½ inches wide. Repeat until you have made ten rolls.

4 Place the rolls in a sealed container and refrigerate until ready to serve.

FOR BABIES 10 MONTHS & OLDER: Any of the finely cut-up vegetables can be blended into baby's cereal or served as a finger food.

PREPARATION TIME:

30 minutes

MAKES 10 ROLLS

10 spring roll skins

1 medium ripe avocado, thinly sliced

2 lettuce leaves, thinly sliced (chiffonade)

1 medium carrot, cut into matchstick slices

1 medium zucchini, cut into matchstick slices

Fried tofu (optional)

Grilled chicken (optional)

Cooked shrimp (optional)

Fresh basil, mint, or cilantro leaves (optional)

2 tablespoons freshly squeezed lime juice

lively lunch boxes

smoked salmon & kraut reuben

Served with Cream of Tomato-Basil Soup (page 179), this sandwich dazzles. Be sure to buy the real-deal sauerkraut, which contains just cabbage and salt, and is found in the refrigerated section of the grocery store, or make your own (see page 223)!

PREPARATION TIME:

10 to 15 minutes

MAKES 2 SERVINGS

Avocado slices (optional)

Ketchup (optional)

Mayonnaise (optional)

Mustard (optional)

4 slices rye bread

½ pound smoked salmon, cut horizontally into ¼-inch pieces

2 slices Swiss cheese

¾ cup sauerkraut

2 teaspoons unsalted butter

1 To make each sandwich, spread avocado slices, ketchup, mayonnaise, mustard, or other preferred condiments on all four slices of bread. Place the salmon on two slices and the cheese on the other two. Put half of the sauerkraut on top of the salmon. Repeat for second sandwich.

2 In a large skillet over medium heat, heat the butter. Put the sandwiches together and place each sandwich in the skillet, salmon side down, to toast the bread. When the first side is toasted, 2 to 3 minutes, flip the sandwiches, cover the skillet with a lid, and toast the second side until the cheese melts, 2 to 3 more minutes. Cut each sandwich in half and serve.

FOR BABIES 6 MONTHS & OLDER: Mash up a few slices of avocado for baby.

FOR BABIES 10 MONTHS & OLDER: Break up some of the smoked salmon into tiny bits and serve with mashed vegetables or cereal.

french lentil dijon spread

French lentils are the tiny gray variety. This spread can replace the "B" in a "BLT" sandwich or be used as a dip for fresh vegetables. For basic lentil cooking instructions, see page 244.

1 In a food processor, pulverize the walnuts. Add the lentils, mushrooms, green onions, garlic, mustard, tamari, and pepper and blend until smooth. Add a little water if necessary to get the consistency you desire. This spread will keep in the refrigerator for several days.

FOR BABIES 10 MONTHS & OLDER: Reserve some plain cooked lentils and puree with a little water. Add baked sweet potato to puree for a nutritious combination.

PREPARATION TIME:

10 minutes

MAKES ABOUT 1 CUP

2 tablespoons raw walnuts

1 cup cooked French lentils

2 button or cremini
   mushrooms, sliced

1 green onion, sliced

1 clove garlic

1 tablespoon Dijon mustard

1 tablespoon tamari
   (soy sauce)

½ teaspoon freshly ground
   black pepper

apple miso almond butter sandwich

This sweet and nutty combo offers a fresh twist on the usual peanut butter and jelly.

PREPARATION TIME:

5 minutes

MAKES 4 SERVINGS

⅓ cup unsweetened apple butter

1 to 2 teaspoons white or mellow miso

8 slices Whole Grain Honey Oat Sandwich Bread (page 108) or store-bought

¼ cup smooth almond butter

1 In a small bowl, put the apple butter and stir the miso into it. Spread four slices of the bread with a light layer of almond butter and four slices of the bread the apple-miso butter. Put the slices together.

FOR BABIES 6 MONTHS & OLDER: Stir ½ teaspoon of apple butter into baby's whole grain cereal for a new flavor.

FOR BABIES 10 MONTHS & OLDER: Stir ½ teaspoon of almond butter into baby's warm whole grain cereal for added calories and other nutrients.

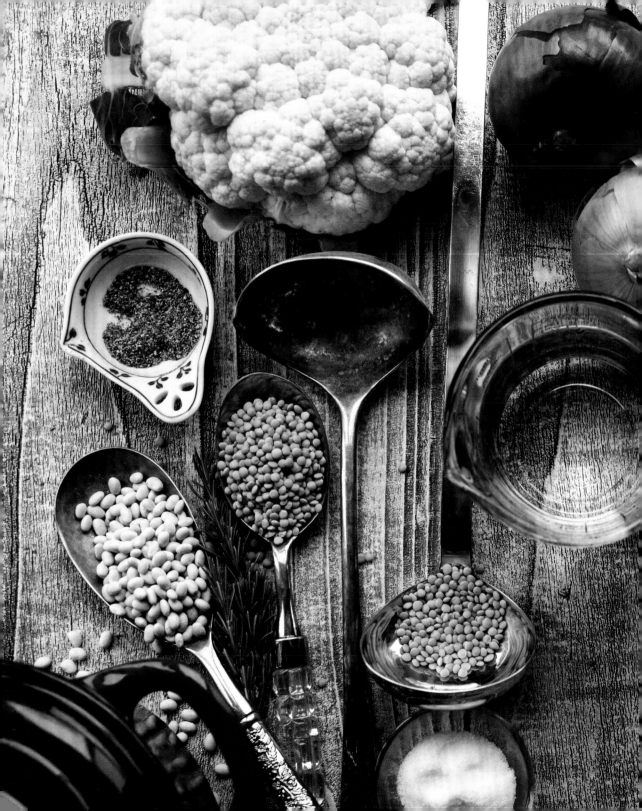

CHAPTER 7

- - - - - - - - -

soothing
soups

When a new baby arrives in the home, the senses of everyone in the family heighten. The primal instinct to protect an infant sharpens our abilities to see, smell, hear, touch, and taste. Schedules and sleep patterns may go awry during the adjustment. To honor the needs of all, food must be simple, available, and nourishing.

The use of broths and soups to nourish and heal is ancient and timeless. When bones, meat, vegetables, and other whole foods give up their vital energies to the liquid surrounding them, the result is a highly digestible meal full of nutrients. Soup is economical, costing only a few bucks to fill many tummies. You can construct soup with nearly anything you have on hand, substitute ingredients at will—the soup doesn't care but accepts what's offered and keeps on simmering.

Leave behind the stuffed animals and pastel booties. The perfect gift for a new family is a pot of homemade soup or a big jar of nourishing stock. Add a loaf of warm bread or muffins, and you'll never be forgotten. New moms can support each other by trading soup—it's just as easy to make a big pot as a small pot. The foods share their nutrients with the water; we share the soup with others.

Do you think of yourself as someone who's not a good cook? Making soups will help you shed that notion. Soups are supremely forgiving. Having a newborn child in the house can be daunting and overwhelming. Ladle up a bowl of warm forgiveness. To take it in, all you need is a spoon.

"Soup is a lot like a family. Each ingredient enhances the others; each batch has its own characteristics; and it needs time to simmer to reach full flavor."

—MARGE KENNEDY,
100 Things You Can Do to Keep Your Family Together

simple chicken stock

This nutritious stock can be used to cook rice, to simmer vegetables, to thin sauces, and to make super soups. By adding vinegar, some believe the minerals from the bones are extracted into the stock.

1 In a 4-quart soup pot over low to medium heat, heat the oil. Add the onion and salt and sauté until soft, 5 to 7 minutes. Add the water, bay leaves, chicken, and vinegar and bring to a boil. Reduce the heat to medium low and simmer for 30 to 45 minutes or longer. The stock flavors deepen with more time.

2 Taste it after 30 minutes to see if you are satisfied or want it to simmer longer. Add more salt if desired.

3 Allow the liquid to cool, remove the chicken and bay leaves, then strain the stock into glass jars and store it in the refrigerator until needed. Or parcel the stock into ziplock bags, ice cube trays, or sealable containers and store in the freezer. Stock will keep about 1 week in the refrigerator and several months in the freezer.

⁓

FOR BABIES 6 MONTHS & OLDER: Use stock to puree food for extra nourishment.

VARIATION FOR CHILDREN: Make a gentle and nourishing soup by stirring some cooked noodles into a cup of this stock.

⁓

* *Buying a whole chicken and using less desirable parts, such as the back and neck, while reserving the servable parts for other dishes, is economical and (for some) more respectful of the chicken. See How to Cut Up a Whole Chicken (page 166).*

PREPARATION TIME:

1 hour

MAKES 1 QUART

1 tablespoon extra-virgin olive oil

1 medium onion, roughly chopped

2 teaspoons sea salt, plus more if needed

4 cups water

2 bay leaves

½ pound chicken parts, bone-in*

1 tablespoon rice vinegar

HOW TO CUT UP
A WHOLE CHICKEN

– – – – – – – – – – – – – –

A sharp boning knife is best for this, but any sharp knife that you can handle comfortably will do. A pair of kitchen shears is also helpful.

If the chicken organs are stored in a packet in the cavity, remove those before beginning.

Start with the drumstick and thigh. Pull the leg and thigh away from the body and, with a small, sharp knife, cut through the skin between the breast and drumstick.

Pull the drumstick and thigh away from the bird and bend it back to pop the joint. Follow the line of where the thigh is attached to the breast and cut through the joint; repeat with the other leg.

Cut the drumstick and thigh into two pieces by cutting along the fat line that delineates the joint. Your knife should be able to go straight through at the joint here.

Next remove the wings. Pull the wing away from the body. Cut through skin to expose the joint. Cut through the joint and skin to separate the wing from body; repeat with the other wing.

Lift the chicken and snip along each side of the backbone between the rib joints with a kitchen shears, again following fat lines. Then use your knife to separate the back from the breast. The backbone can be saved in the freezer for stock.

Put the breast on a cutting board skin side down. Gently cut down through the center cartilage using a sawing motion. Follow the cut again, slicing through meat and skin to separate the breast into two even pieces.

Voila! You have eight pieces of chicken for your recipe and a backbone for stock.

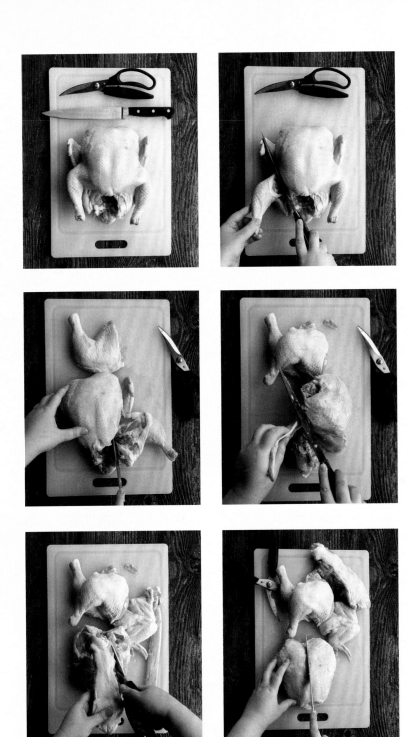

easy vegetarian stock

Kombu, a sea vegetable, serves to impart some of the same minerals the bones from animals might contribute.

PREPARATION TIME:

25 minutes

MAKES 1 QUART

1 medium yellow onion

1 tablespoon extra-virgin olive oil

1 carrot, cut into large chunks

1 rib of celery, cut into chunks

1 green onion or leek, cut into pieces

1 (3-inch) piece of kombu

1 bay leaf

1 teaspoon dried marjoram

1 teaspoon dried thyme

1 quart water

1 teaspoon sea salt

⅛ teaspoon freshly ground black pepper

1 Roughly chop the onion, reserving the skin. In a 4-quart soup pot over medium heat, heat the oil. Add the onion and sauté until soft, 5 to 7 minutes. Add the onion skin, carrot, celery, green onion, kombu, bay leaf, marjoram, thyme, and water and bring it to a boil. Add the salt and pepper. Reduce the heat to medium low and simmer for 20 minutes. Taste and adjust seasoning if desired.

2 Allow the liquid to cool, remove the vegetables and bay leaf, then strain the stock into glass jars and store it in the refrigerator until needed. Or parcel the stock into ziplock bags, ice cube trays, or sealable containers and store in the freezer. Stock will keep about 1 week in the refrigerator and several months in the freezer.

FOR BABIES 6 MONTHS & OLDER: Use the stock to puree food for extra nourishment.

VARIATION FOR CHILDREN: Make a gentle and nourishing broth by stirring a teaspoon of light miso into a cup of this stock.

dashi stock

Unlike a meat stock, dashi is light in body and adds a subtle, distinct oceanic flavor to any dish. Sea vegetables and bonito fish flakes distribute minerals and protein to the stock. Kombu and bonito flakes can be found in most international grocery stores or can be ordered online.

1 In a 4-quart pot, put the water. Add the kombu and let it soak in the water for at least 1 hour, or as long as 2 hours.

2 After soaking, bring the water to a boil over high heat. Just as it begins to simmer, add the bonito flakes and stir. Allow the liquid to come to a boil again and then simmer over low heat for 1 minute.

3 Remove the pot from the heat and allow the stock to steep for 10 minutes. Strain the stock through a fine mesh strainer over a large bowl. The stock can be stored in a jar in the refrigerator for about 1 week or several months in the freezer.

PREPARATION TIME:

1 to 2 hours (for soaking); 20 minutes (for cooking)

MAKES 1½ QUARTS

6 cups water

1 ounce kombu (about 20 inches)

1 ounce bonito flakes (3 to 4 loosely packed cups)

169

soothing soups

FOR BABIES 6 MONTHS & OLDER: Use the stock to puree cooked vegetables such as carrot or squash for added nutrients.

TAKE STOCK

Stock does not need to be fancy. In fact, it should be a utilitarian task. Unused raw chicken parts, an onion, a bay leaf, and a few vegetable scraps are really all you need. Alternately, you can begin with the carcass of your Thanksgiving turkey or the bone from the Easter ham. Cooked bones yield a stronger flavor and darker color than raw bones. Stock isn't on a schedule. So if you forget about it while you change a diaper and a nap or two later it is still simmering, don't worry. It's still good.

Concerned about babies and children getting enough vegetables in their diet? Make soup, baby cereal, rice, sandwich spreads, or beans for tacos with homemade stock to boost nutrient intake. Almost anything you cook that requires water can be replaced with stock!

There are many brands of organic stock that you can buy. They can't provide the love inherent in homemade stock but will definitely enhance flavor. Note that some of the prepackaged stocks, especially the vegetarian ones for some reason, are quite thick and heavy. Be sure to taste your stock before pouring it into a soup pot. Note the saltiness. It is better to use half stock and half water when the stock flavor is heavy or salty so that the stock doesn't overwhelm the other flavors of the soup.

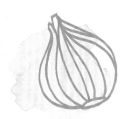

miso soup *with* tofu & bok choy ribbons

Wakame is a green, leafy sea vegetable high in calcium and other minerals. Beneficial bacteria are contributed to the dish from the miso (fermented soybean paste). When a family member feels fatigued or ill, serve this soup, which is brimming with highly digestible minerals, protein, and probiotics.

1 In a small bowl filled with cold water, put the wakame and soak it for 5 minutes to rehydrate. In a 4-quart pot over medium-high heat, add the stock, potato, and carrot and bring it to a simmer. Remove the wakame from the bowl, discard the thick spine, tear the leaf into pieces, and then add it to the broth. Cover and let the broth simmer until the vegetables are tender, 15 to 20 minutes.

2 Near the end of cooking time, roll up the bok choy leaves and make thin slices starting at one end. Add the bok choy ribbons and tofu cubes to the broth and let them simmer for 1 to 2 minutes.

3 Cooking miso at a high temperature can destroy its probiotic properties. Ladle ½ cup of the broth into each soup bowl. Dissolve 1 tablespoon of miso into the broth in each bowl. Add more broth with plenty of vegetables to each bowl and stir gently. Garnish each bowl with green onions.

PREPARATION TIME:

25 minutes

MAKES 4 SERVINGS

1 (3-inch) piece wakame

4 cups Dashi Stock (page 169)

1 small red potato, cut into ½-inch dice

1 small carrot, chopped

1 large or 3 baby bok choy leaves

¼ pound firm tofu, cut into small cubes

¼ cup white or mellow miso

2 green onions, thinly sliced, for garnish

FOR BABIES 6 MONTHS & OLDER: Remove some boiled potatoes or carrots from the soup after it simmers and puree or mash well.

FOR BABIES 10 MONTHS & OLDER: Babies with a few teeth who can handle soft things to chew will enjoy some pieces of cooked vegetables and tofu cubes from the soup along with some broth.

asparagus soup *with* lemon & dill

Rolled oats add extra whole grain nutrition and create a nondairy, fiber-rich, creamy texture. Serve this soup with Mediterranean Quinoa Salad (page 145) or Caribbean Lime Halibut (page 279) for a seasonal springtime meal.

PREPARATION TIME:

25 minutes

MAKES 4 TO 6 SERVINGS

2 tablespoons extra-virgin olive oil or unsalted butter

1 medium onion, finely chopped

1 stalk celery, chopped

1 teaspoon ground cumin

1 bunch asparagus, trimmed and cut into 2-inch pieces

2 cups Easy Vegetarian Stock (page 168), Simple Chicken Stock (page 165), or store-bought

2 to 3 cups water

1 bay leaf

½ cup rolled oats

1 teaspoon sea salt

1 tablespoon fresh dill, or 1 teaspoon dried dill

2 to 3 tablespoons freshly squeezed lemon juice

Sour cream, for garnish (optional)

1 In a 4-quart pot over medium heat, heat the oil. Add the onion and sauté until the onion is soft and beginning to caramelize. Stir in the celery and cumin.

2 Add the asparagus to the pot and sauté a few more minutes. Add the stock, water, bay leaf, oats, and salt and bring it to a boil. Lower heat to medium low and simmer until the oats are soft and asparagus is bright green, about 15 minutes. Let it cool slightly.

3 Remove the bay leaf. Transfer the contents of the pot to a blender or use an immersion blender. Add the dill and puree. If using a standing blender, cover the lid with a towel and start the blender on low to prevent splattering.

4 Reheat if necessary. Add the lemon juice, a little at a time, to taste. Top each serving of soup with 2 teaspoons of sour cream before serving. This soup can be served cold in warm weather.

FOR BABIES 10 MONTHS & OLDER: Use some of the rolled oats to make your baby a bowl of warm oatmeal. See page 84 for directions.

red lentil soup *with* east indian spices (masoor dal)

Red lentils are a small, flat, orange-colored legume, differing from the gray-green French lentil in flavor and appearance. A vegetarian Indian restaurant in Seattle called Silence-Heart-Nest used to serve this satisfying soup, whose proper name is Masoor Dal. *Ghee is clarified butter that is used frequently in Indian cooking. To learn more about ghee, see Homemade Ghee (page 383).*

1 In a 4-quart pot over medium heat, melt 1 tablespoon of the ghee. Sauté the onions and garlic until the onion caramelizes. Add the turmeric, cumin, and cayenne and stir until fragrant, 2 to 3 minutes. Add the tomatoes. Cook until they break down if using fresh tomatoes; if using canned, simply proceed.

2 Rinse and drain the lentils. Add the lentils, stock, and salt to pot. Bring the pot to a soft simmer and cook for 45 minutes, stirring often.

3 In a small skillet over medium-high heat, melt the remaining 1 teaspoon ghee and fry the seeds until they pop, 2 to 3 minutes. Stir the fried seeds, cilantro, and lemon juice into the finished soup. Taste and adjust salt and citrus to bring up the flavor.

FOR BABIES 10 MONTHS & OLDER: Use ¼ cup red lentils and simmer in a separate small pan with 1 cup water to make a simpler soup for baby. Or if baby is a fairly experienced eater, this soup is fine as is.

PREPARATION TIME:

1 hour

MAKES 6 SERVINGS

4 teaspoons Homemade Ghee (page 383) or unsalted butter, divided

1 medium onion, finely chopped

1 to 2 tablespoons minced garlic

1 teaspoon ground turmeric

1 teaspoon ground cumin

⅛ teaspoon cayenne

1 cup chopped tomatoes (from 1 large tomato)

1 cup dried red lentils

4 cups Easy Vegetarian Stock (page 168), Simple Chicken Stock (page 165), or water

2 teaspoons sea salt

1 teaspoon cumin

1 teaspoon mustard seeds

¼ cup chopped fresh cilantro

1 teaspoon freshly squeezed lemon juice or vinegar

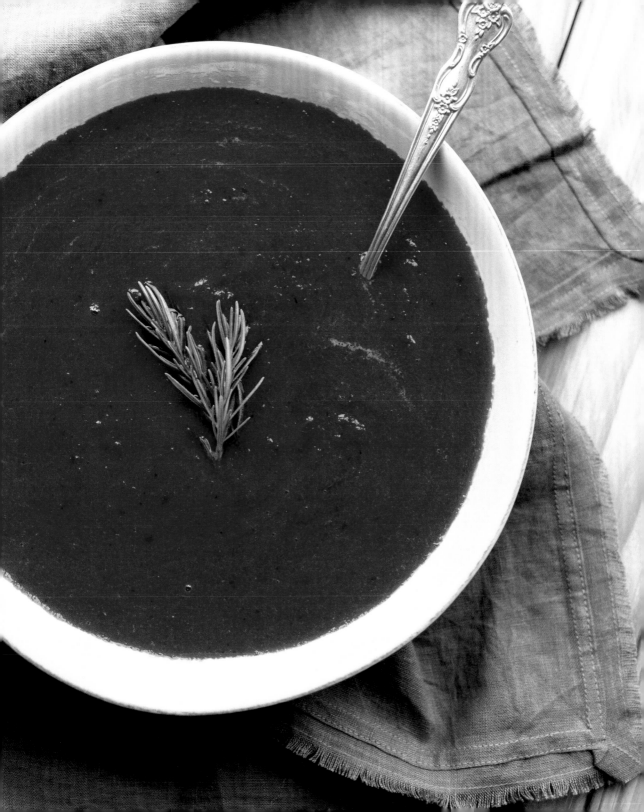

rosemary red soup

The gorgeous red color of this pureed soup has visual appeal. Pair the soup with Sweet Potato Corn Muffins (page 115) and Romaine and Blue Cheese Chop Salad with Basil Dressing (page 207).

1 Remove the leaves of the beets, if present, and the grainy top end where the stem comes out. Scrub and chop the carrots and beet and cut them into small chunks.

2 In a 4-quart pot over medium heat, heat the oil. Add the onion and sauté until soft, 5 to 7 minutes. Add the carrots and beet and sauté a few more minutes.

3 Rinse and drain the lentils. Add the lentils, rosemary, oregano, bay leaves, salt, and stock to the sautéed vegetables and bring the pot to a boil. Lower heat and simmer 40 minutes.

4 Remove the bay leaves. Let the soup cool slightly and puree it in small batches in a blender or use an immersion blender. In a small bowl, dissolve the miso in ½ cup water, and then stir it into the pureed soup. Gently reheat before serving.

FOR BABIES 6 MONTHS & OLDER: Steam a few carrot slices and puree with water.

VARIATION FOR CHILDREN: Make a face in the bowl with crackers!

PREPARATION TIME:

50 minutes

MAKES 6 TO 8 SERVINGS

1 medium or 2 small beets

3 medium carrots

1 tablespoon extra-virgin olive oil

1 large onion, diced

1 cup dried red lentils

1 (3-inch) sprig fresh rosemary, finely chopped, or 1 teaspoon dried rosemary

1 tablespoon fresh oregano, finely chopped, or 1 teaspoon ground oregano

2 bay leaves

1 teaspoon sea salt

6 cups Easy Vegetarian Stock (page 168), Simple Chicken Stock (page 165), or water

2 to 3 tablespoons light miso

split pea soup *with* fresh peas & potatoes

My daughter's second-grade class had a hot lunch program where parents took turns bringing hot soup to school lunch. This soup was a favorites. Leave out the ham bone to make this a vegetarian soup.

PREPARATION TIME:

4 to 6 hours (for soaking); 1 to 1½ hours (for cooking)

MAKES 4 SERVINGS

1 cup dried green split peas

2½ teaspoons sea salt, divided, plus more for seasoning

1 tablespoon unsalted butter or extra-virgin olive oil

1 medium onion, finely chopped

1 stalk celery, chopped

1 carrot, chopped

2 small red potatoes, cubed

1 teaspoon ground cumin

Freshly ground black pepper

4 cups Easy Vegetarian Stock (page 168), Simple Chicken Stock (page 165), or water

1 large bay leaf

1 small ham bone (optional)

2 teaspoons apple cider vinegar

½ cup fresh or frozen peas

1 tablespoon fresh dill, or 1 teaspoon dried dill

1 Soak the split peas for 4 to 6 hours in 5 cups of water and 1 teaspoon of the salt. This will help with digestibility, quicken the cooking time, and improve the texture of the soup.

2 In a pressure cooker or a 4-quart pot over medium heat, melt the butter. Add the onions and sauté until they begin to soften and caramelize, 5 to 10 minutes.

3 Add the celery, carrot, potatoes, cumin, and pepper and sauté for 3 to 4 minutes. Drain the split peas and discard the water. Add the split peas, then the stock, bay leaf, and the remaining 1½ teaspoons salt. Add the ham bone and vinegar to the pot.

4 If using a pressure cooker, bring up to the pressure on high heat, then reduce the heat and cook for 40 minutes. If using a pot, bring the contents to a boil over high heat, reduce the heat to low, and simmer for 1 hour and 15 minutes, or until the peas have melted.

5 Once the soup has become creamy, remove the ham bone and bay leaf. Cut off any meat, discard the skin and bone, and then dice the meat into small pieces and add them back to the soup. Toss in the peas and dill. Taste the soup; add more salt and pepper if desired. Continue cooking a few more minutes until the peas are tender and warm, and then serve.

FOR BABIES 6 MONTHS & OLDER: Reserve some fresh peas. Steam them until tender. Mash and serve.

golden mushroom–basil cashew cream soup

Friend and chef Jeff Basom showed me this inventive way of blending potatoes and cashew butter to create a creamy dairy-free soup base.

1 In a 4-quart pot over medium heat, heat 1 tablespoon of the oil. Add the onions and salt. Reduce the heat to low, cover, and simmer, stirring occasionally, until the onions cook down and caramelize, 15 to 20 minutes.

2 Add the potatoes, celery, carrot, and stock to the mixture, cover, and simmer until potatoes are soft, 15 to 20 minutes.

3 Let the soup cool slightly, then puree it in small batches in a blender with the cashew butter and tamari, blending until smooth. Return the soup to the pot. (Alternatively, you can add the cashew butter and tamari to the soup and puree it with an immersion blender.)

4 In a large skillet over medium heat, heat the remaining 1 tablespoon oil. Add the mushrooms and sauté until soft, 3 to 5 minutes. Stir the sautéed mushrooms, basil, and pepper into the blended soup. Taste and add vinegar and additional salt if needed to bring up the flavor.

FOR BABIES 6 MONTHS & OLDER: Remove some of the cooked potato from the soup and puree.

FOR BABIES 10 MONTHS & OLDER: Blend a portion of the soup before adding the tamari and sautéed mushrooms for baby.

PREPARATION TIME:

45 minutes

MAKES 6 SERVINGS

2 tablespoons extra-virgin olive oil, divided

2 large or 3 medium onions, diced

1 teaspoon sea salt

1 medium russet potato, diced

2 ribs celery, diced

1 large carrot, diced

4 cups Easy Vegetarian Stock (page 168), Simple Chicken Stock (page 165), or water

2 tablespoons cashew butter

2 tablespoons tamari (soy sauce)

¾ pound mushrooms, sliced

½ cup fresh basil leaves, finely chopped

Freshly ground black pepper

1 teaspoon apple cider vinegar

iron-replenishing cauliflower & dulse soup

A variation of Golden Mushroom–Basil Cashew Cream Soup (see previous page) is included for medicinal reasons. This soup utilizes iron-rich dulse, a sea vegetable with an impressive two milligrams of absorbable iron per teaspoon (breastfeeding moms require at least nine milligrams per day).

PREPARATION TIME:

45 minutes

MAKES 6 SERVINGS

1 tablespoons extra-virgin olive oil

2 large or 3 medium onions, diced

1 teaspoon sea salt

1 medium russet potato, diced

2 ribs celery, diced

1 large carrot, diced

4 cups Easy Vegetarian Stock (page 168), Simple Chicken Stock (page 165), or water

2 tablespoons cashew butter

2 tablespoons tamari (soy sauce)

1 small head cauliflower

⅓ cup dry dulse

Freshly ground black pepper

1 teaspoon apple cider vinegar

1 In a 4-quart pot over medium heat, heat the oil. Add the onions and salt. Reduce the heat to low, cover, and simmer, stirring occasionally, until the onions cook down and caramelize, 15 to 20 minutes.

2 Add the potatoes, celery, carrot, and stock to the pot, cover, and simmer until potatoes are soft, 15 to 20 minutes.

3 Let the soup cool slightly, then puree it in small batches in a blender with the cashew butter and tamari, blending until smooth. Return the soup to the pot. (Alternatively, add the cashew butter and tamari to the soup and puree it with an immersion blender.)

4 Remove the outer leaves of cauliflower and cut it into bite-size florets. Bring a 4-quart pot of water to boil over high heat and blanch the cauliflower pieces by submerging them in the water for about 5 minutes. Drain the cauliflower pieces and add them to the soup. Prepare the dulse by soaking it in a cup of cold water for 5 minutes to rehydrate it and then gently tearing into bite-size pieces. Add the dulse and pepper into the finished soup. Add the vinegar and taste to see if additional salt is needed to bring up the flavor.

FOR BABIES 6 MONTHS & OLDER: Steam some of cauliflower pieces until very soft, about 20 minutes. Puree the steamed cauliflower with a pinch of dulse and serve.

cream of tomato-basil soup

When I was a child, tomato soup was my main comfort food. The food company Muir Glen makes a "fire-roasted" canned tomato that adds another dimension of flavor to this recipe.

1 In a 4-quart pot over medium heat, heat the oil and butter. Add the onion, garlic, and salt and sauté until the onions are soft and translucent, 5 to 7 minutes. Add the stock, tomatoes, and honey, reduce the heat to low, and simmer for 10 to 15 minutes to marry the flavors.

2 Let the soup cool slightly, then put half of it into a blender with the sour cream and blend until smooth. Transfer the soup to another pot. Blend the other half of the soup and add to the pot. (Alternatively, add the sour cream to soup and puree with an immersion blender.) Reheat the blended soup. Add the pepper and stir in the basil just before serving.

FOR BABIES 6 MONTHS & OLDER: Serve this soup with steamed broccoli on the side. Puree some steamed broccoli with water for baby.

PREPARATION TIME:

25 to 30 minutes

MAKES 4 SERVINGS

2 tablespoons extra-virgin olive oil

1 tablespoon unsalted butter

1 medium onion, finely chopped

2 to 3 cloves garlic, minced

1 teaspoon sea salt

2 cups Easy Vegetarian Stock (page 168), Simple Chicken Stock (page 165), or store-bought

1 (14.5-ounce) can chopped tomatoes

1 tablespoon honey

¼ cup cultured sour cream or crème fraîche

Freshly ground black pepper

¼ cup finely chopped fresh basil

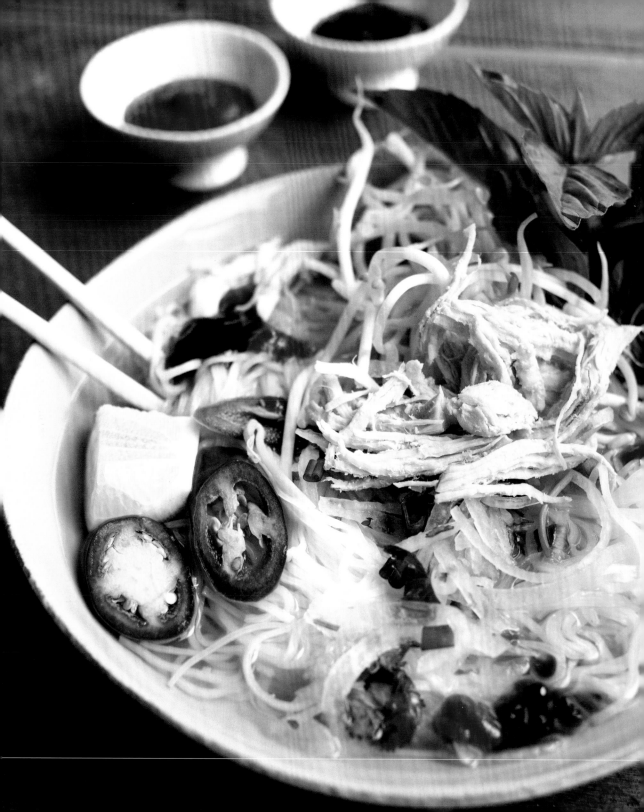

vietnamese pho ga soup

My-Duyen Huynh taught me the authentic way of making Pho Ga. The "pick and choose" aspect of adding condiments satisfies the young child's desire to express independence. Put the stock together and watch a movie or play a board game while it simmers.

1 To make the stock, in an 8-quart pot over medium-high heat, bring the water to a simmer. Wash the chicken thoroughly. If starting with a whole chicken, cut it into pieces (see How to Cut Up a Whole Chicken, page 166). Remove any excess fat and skin. As soon as water is simmering, add the back, neck, and/or legs. (Don't include the breast, which will be added later.)

2 Preheat the oven to broil. In a baking dish, put the ginger and shallots and broil until slightly charred on the edges, 8 to 10 minutes.

3 Add the ginger, shallots, cloves, cardamom, star anise, cinnamon, salt, and sugar to the pot. Bring it to a simmer. If the temperature is too high, the broth will be cloudy, not clear. Skim any fat that rises to the surface off the top of the broth. Let the stock simmer, covered, for 2 hours. If the chicken breast is one large piece, bisect it lengthwise. Add the chicken breast during the last 15 minutes of cooking.

4 Taste the broth. Add additional salt if desired. Remove the chicken breast, allow it to cool, and then remove the skin and bones. Cut the meat into thin slices and set aside.

5 Prepare the rice noodles according to the directions on the package. The threadlike vermicelli noodles will cook through in just a few minutes. Thicker flat rice noodles will take around 10 minutes. Pay attention and

PREPARATION TIME:

2 hours and 20 minutes

MAKES 4 TO 6 SERVINGS

For the stock:

3 quarts water

1 pound bone-in, skin-on chicken parts (back, neck, legs)

1 (3-inch) piece fresh ginger-root, thinly sliced

2 shallots, thinly sliced

6 to 8 whole cloves

3 to 4 whole cardamom pods

1 star anise

½ cinnamon stick

5 teaspoons sea salt

1 tablespoon sugar

1 pound bone-in, skin-on chicken breast

1 (8-ounce) package rice noodles

Sesame oil

½ bunch cilantro, chopped (about 1 cup)

4 green onions, chopped

Freshly ground black pepper

soothing soups

continued

For garnish:

3 limes, cut into wedges

1 cup bean sprouts

½ cup chopped Thai basil

2 jalapeños, sliced

3 tablespoons hoisin sauce

2 tablespoons sriracha
   sauce

test the noodles frequently, as they'll become mushy if overcooked. Once the noodles are tender, drain them and run them under cool water to stop the cooking. Toss them with a few drops of sesame oil to keep the noodles from sticking.

6 Put a small handful of noodles in each bowl. Top with a few slices of chicken breast, some of the cilantro, green onion, and black pepper. Pour the hot stock over the top of each bowl.

7 Arrange the garnishes, each in a small bowl, on a tray or platter. Diners can add the condiments of their choice to their soup.

FOR BABIES 6 MONTHS & OLDER: Use the magical aromatic broth to blend cooked vegetables into purees.

cannellini kale minestrone
with grated pecorino

This recipe was inspired by one of my favorite cookbooks, Sundays at Moosewood Restaurant *by the Moosewood Collective. The kale adds energy-boosting vitamins and minerals, while the beans provide a simple protein base.*

1 In a small bowl of cold water, place the kale and set aside.

2 In a 4-quart pot over low to medium heat, heat the oil. Add the garlic and sauté, making sure it sizzles but doesn't burn, 1 to 2 minutes.

3 Reserve 1 cup of the beans. Add the remaining 2 cups of beans and 1½ cups of the stock to the pot and stir. In a blender, put the reserved 1 cup beans, the remaining 1 cup stock, the tomato paste, and the sage and puree. Stir the pureed bean mixture into the soup, creating a creamy base. Add salt and pepper to taste.

4 Mix the kale into the simmering soup and cook until the kale wilts, about 5 minutes. Add the lemon juice and enough water to make the soup a desirable consistency. Taste for salt and pepper and adjust seasonings as desired. Serve the soup topped with the pecorino.

FOR BABIES 10 MONTHS & OLDER: Reserve several tablespoons of the pureed bean mixture before adding it to the soup and serve it to baby.

PREPARATION TIME:

30 minutes

MAKES 3 TO 4 SERVINGS

½ bunch (about 12 to 15 leaves) lacinato kale, thinly sliced (chiffonade)

1 tablespoon extra-virgin olive oil

2 large cloves garlic

3 cups cooked cannellini beans (see page 244 for cooking instructions), or 2 (15-ounce) cans cannellini beans, drained

2½ cups Easy Vegetarian Stock (page 168), Simple Chicken Stock (page 165), or store-bought

1 tablespoon tomato paste

4 fresh sage leaves

1 teaspoon sea salt

Freshly ground black pepper

1 tablespoon freshly squeezed lemon juice

Freshly grated pecorino cheese

soothing soups

smoky navy bean soup
with bacon & apple

Using animal foods, like bacon, in small amounts as a flavoring demonstrates frugality and places these food in the right ratio in a mostly plant-based diet. Be sure to seek animal products from producers using humane practices. Serve this soup with Romaine and Blue Cheese Chop Salad with Basil Dressing (page 207) for a satisfying meal.

PREPARATION TIME:

8 to 10 hours (for soaking), 75 minutes (for cooking)

MAKES 4 SERVINGS

1 cup dried navy beans

2 teaspoons sea salt, divided, plus more if needed

3 strips bacon

1 medium onion, diced

1 medium apple, diced

4 cups Easy Vegetarian Stock (page 168), Simple Chicken Stock (page 165), or water

1 chipotle chile

½ teaspoon ground paprika

¼ teaspoon ground allspice

2 teaspoons apple cider vinegar

Freshly ground black pepper

1 tablespoon heavy cream (optional)

1 In a large bowl, put the dry beans with 5 cups of water and 1 teaspoon of the salt. Allow them to soak for 8 to 10 hours.

2 In a pressure cooker or a 4-quart pot over medium-high heat, add the bacon strips. Fry the bacon, turning occasionally, until crisp. Drain the bacon on a paper towel and set aside. Leave the bacon fat in the soup pot.

3 Add the onion to the bacon fat and sauté until soft, 4 to 5 minutes. Add the apple to the onion, and sauté 3 more minutes. Next add the drained beans, stock, chile, paprika, allspice, and the remaining 1 teaspoon salt. Increase the heat to high to establish a simmer and cover or, if using a pressure cooker, bring up to pressure, then reduce heat to low, while keeping the pressure steady. Cook until beans are soft, 1 hour in pot or 45 minutes in a pressure cooker.

4 Remove the chili pod. Add another ½ teaspoon of salt if desired, the vinegar, and pepper. Stir to incorporate. Using and immersion blender, blend the soup until textured but creamy, or puree the soup in a blender, then add it back to the pot. If the heat from the chile seems too much, add the cream to tame the flame before serving. Serve soup garnished with crumbled bacon.

FOR BABIES 10 MONTHS & OLDER: Omit the chilies. A small portion of this soup pureed is fine for an older baby.

VEGETARIAN VARIATION

Omit the bacon and sauté the onion in 1 tablespoon of extra-virgin olive oil or butter. Use smoked paprika instead of regular paprika to enhance the smoky flavor.

curried lentil & potato stew

This hearty stew transforms economical ingredients into big flavor. The tiny French lentils are wonderful, but if you can't find them, substitute regular brown lentils. You can replace all the individual spices in this recipe with one heaping tablespoon of Homemade Curry Paste (page 382).

PREPARATION TIME:

70 minutes

MAKES 6 SERVINGS

1 tablespoon Homemade Ghee (page 383) or extra-virgin olive oil

1 medium onion, finely chopped

1 teaspoon ground cumin

1 teaspoon ground coriander

1 teaspoon freshly grated gingerroot

1 teaspoon ground turmeric

¼ teaspoon ground allspice

¼ teaspoon cayenne

¼ teaspoon ground cinnamon

⅛ teaspoon freshly ground black pepper

2 red potatoes, cut into cubes

1 parsnip, sliced

1 stalk celery, diced

1 carrot, chopped

4 cups Easy Vegetarian Stock (page 168), Simple Chicken Stock (page 165), or water

1 cup French lentils

1½ teaspoons sea salt

Yogurt Cucumber Topping (page 364) or sour cream, for garnish

1 In a pressure cooker or a 4-quart soup pot over medium heat, melt the ghee. Add the onion and sauté until the onion is soft and beginning to caramelize. Add the cumin, coriander, ginger, turmeric, allspice, cayenne, cinnamon, and pepper and sauté until fragrant, 2 to 3 minutes.

2 Add the potatoes, parsnip, celery, carrot, stock, lentils, and salt, then bring the heat up to high to take the stew to a boil. Reduce the heat to low and simmer, covered, until the potatoes are tender and the lentils are creamy, 50 to 60 minutes. If using a pressure cooker, bring up to pressure over high heat, then reduce the heat and cook until the lentils become creamy, about 40 minutes.

3 Garnish the hot stew with the yogurt topping just before serving.

FOR BABIES 10 MONTHS & OLDER: A small portion of this pureed soup should be fine for the older baby.

---

thai coconut chicken soup

Otherwise known as Tom Ka Gai, this traditional Thai soup uses coconut milk, lemongrass, and fish sauce to form its flavorful base. For a vegetarian version, use tofu cubes instead of chicken and omit the fish sauce (you will need to add additional salt to compensate for this).

1 In a 4-quart soup pot over medium heat, warm the oil. Stir in the onion, garlic, and salt and sauté until the onion is translucent. Add the ginger, coriander, cumin, and red pepper flakes and cook until fragrant, 2 to 3 minutes.

2 Bisect the lemongrass stalk lengthwise. You will see a small core at the bottom. Cut out the core and then chop about ½ inch off each stalk half where it is tender (tender means you can easily insert a fingernail). Add the chopped lemongrass to the other spices and reserve a piece of the stalk.

3 Tenderize the chicken breast with a meat pounder on both sides and then cut it diagonally into thin strips. Add the chicken to the onion and spices and cook, stirring constantly, until the chicken is white on the outside.

4 Add the water, coconut milk, fish sauce, and lemongrass stalk and simmer until the chicken is thoroughly cooked and the flavors are well blended, 5 to 10 minutes, depending on the size of the strips. Add the bok choy and simmer for 3 more minutes. Remove the lemongrass stalk before serving. Stir in the cilantro and lime to finish.

FOR BABIES 10 MONTHS & OLDER: Remove ¼ cup of the spiced coconut broth. Tame the intensity by blending it with cooked carrot or sweet potato.

PREPARATION TIME:

1 hour

MAKES 4 SERVINGS

2 tablespoons extra-virgin olive oil or unrefined coconut oil

1 medium onion, thinly cut into half moons

2 to 3 cloves garlic, minced

1 teaspoon sea salt

2 tablespoons freshly grated gingerroot

1 teaspoon ground coriander

1 teaspoon ground cumin

½ teaspoon red pepper flakes

1 (6- to 8-inch) stalk lemongrass

½ pound boneless, skinless chicken breasts

2 to 3 cups water

1 (14-ounce) can coconut milk

3 to 4 tablespoons fish sauce

1 large baby bok choy, thinly sliced

¼ cup chopped fresh cilantro

1 tablespoon freshly squeezed lime juice from ½ lime)

soothing soups

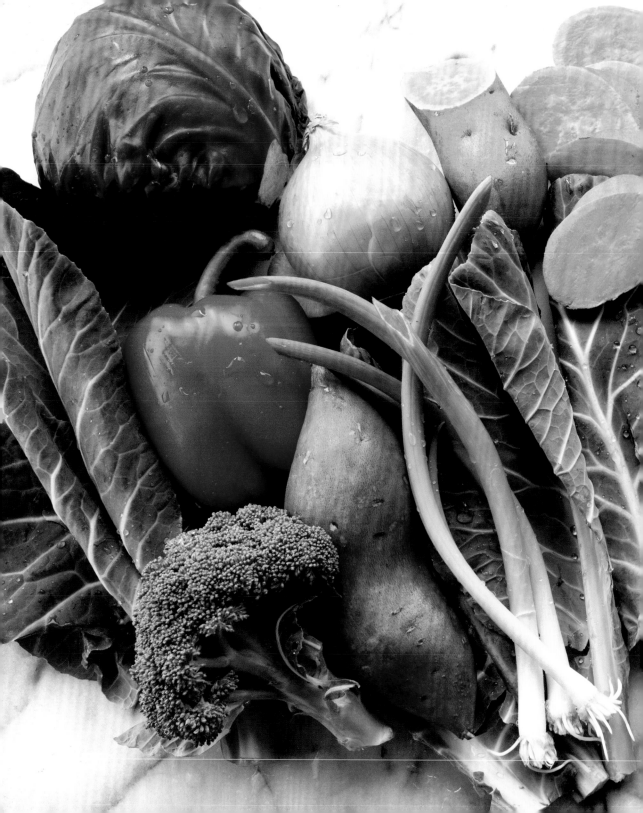

CHAPTER 8

vivacious vegetables

One drizzly Seattle evening, in a school parking lot, I was pulling books from my car for a PTA talk about family eating. Out of the dark, a small woman approached me. With grave anxiety, she let it all spill out: how her child wouldn't eat vegetables and she was at her wit's end. "I tell him every night that he has to eat them. He needs the vitamins. He won't grow without them. But he refuses even one bite. What should I do?"

I asked her if I might address her questions during the lecture, as this is a common issue for parents. "How old is he?" I asked, walking toward the school door. "He's four," she answered. My intuition told me that ideas for tasty spinach recipes would be of no use here. She was in a state of fear, and it sounded like the fear was landing on her young son.

This happened many years ago. What stays with me is the distressed look on her face. Though I regularly talk, write, and teach about feeding children good food and believe what I say with all my heart, there are more important things to give your children than broccoli.

Always ask yourself, is he growing? Does he have energy and like to play? Is his mind curious, his smile frequent? If you got mostly yeses, relax about how many servings of vegetables go in the pie hole. Make salads and squashes and veggies you like and enjoy them. Let him pick up the joy vibe. Don't use words, just your fork. Wait for him to ask for a bite.

one-trick vegetables

The flavor of a single vegetable can really shine if the right cooking technique is applied. Blanching brings out the flavor of broccoli—maybe better than steaming, definitely superior to raw! Beets turn silky in the pressure cooker. And, of course, the single cooked vegetable makes outstanding food for baby.

blanched broccoli

1 Bring a 4-quart pot of water and salt to a boil over high heat.

2 Fill a large bowl or sink with ice-cold water.

3 Drop the broccoli into the boiling water. Let the vegetables boil until they are bright green and tender, less than 1 minute. Drain the water off and immediately plunge the vegetables into the ice bath until they are cool. This keeps the broccoli in a tender but crunchy state.

4 Remove the broccoli from the ice bath. Let it dry on a clean dish towel, then serve immediately or store it in a sealed container in the refrigerator.

PREPARATION TIME:

10 minutes

MAKES 4 TO 6 SERVINGS

1 teaspoon sea salt

1 large bunch broccoli, florets cut into uniform-size pieces

sautéed green beans

1 Trim the ends of the green beans. Rinse and drain.

2 In a 12-inch skillet over medium heat, heat the butter; don't let it burn. Add the green beans—they should sizzle—and keep them moving until they turn bright green, 3 to 4 minutes. Test one! You're aiming for a tender crunch. Remove the skillet from the heat and sprinkle the green beans with a little salt and a squeeze of lemon before serving.

PREPARATION TIME:

10 minutes

MAKES 4 TO 6 SERVINGS

½ pound green beans

2 teaspoons unsalted butter

Sea salt

Lemon

continued

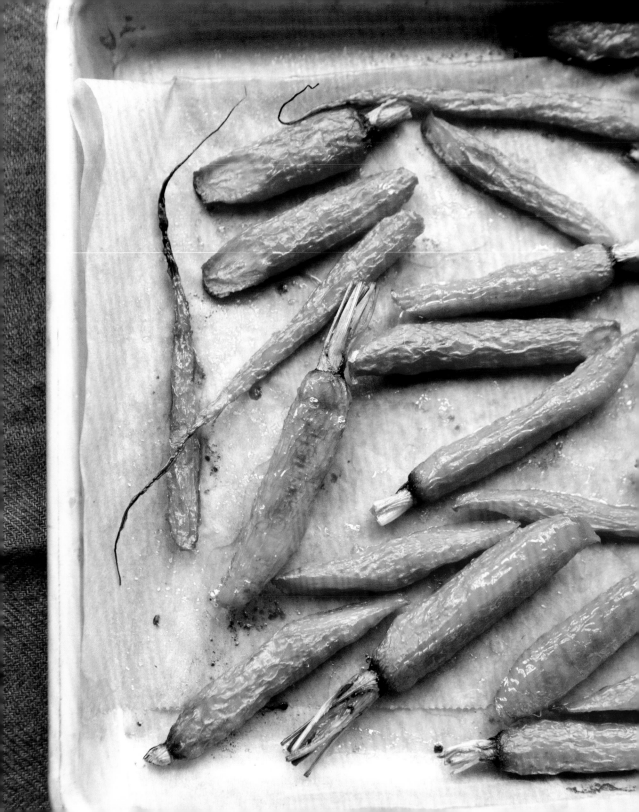

pressure-cooked beets

1 Remove the leafy tops from the beets and wash the beets to remove any dirt. Do not cut off the root or the nubby crown. If you do, the beets will "bleed" into the water they are cooked in and lose flavor and nutrition. In a pressure cooker filled with enough water to cover the bottom half of the beets, put the whole beets and secure the lid. Bring the heat to high. When cooker has reached pressure, reduce the heat to medium low and cook for 20 to 25 minutes.

2 Remove the cooker from the heat and let the pressure come down naturally. The beets should be quite tender when pierced with a fork. When cool enough to handle, slip the skins off the beets under cool running water. Trim the ends if needed.

3 Slice the beets, dress them with a bit of butter and vinegar, and serve.

PREPARATION TIME:

30 minutes

MAKES 4 SERVINGS

4 large beets

Unsalted butter or extra-virgin olive oil (optional)

Balsamic vinegar (optional)

roasted carrots

1 Preheat the oven to 400 degrees F.

2 Place the carrot slices in a baking dish. Brush each carrot with oil and sprinkle it with salt. Roast the carrots until they are tender when pierced with a fork, about 10 to 15 minutes, depending on size.

PREPARATION TIME:

20 minutes

MAKES 4 SERVINGS

4 to 5 carrots, cut into 2-inch-long angled slices (at least ¼ inch thick)

1 tablespoon extra-virgin olive oil

½ teaspoon sea salt

continued

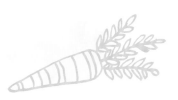

baked winter squash

PREPARATION TIME:

40 minutes to 1½ hours

MAKES 4 SERVINGS

1 (2- to 3-pound) winter
    squash
Unsalted butter
Sea salt

1 Preheat the oven to 350 degrees F and lightly oil a baking dish.

2 Using a utility knife with a serrated edge, begin by cutting off the stem and root end of the squash so you have flat surfaces on either end of the gourd. Bisect the squash by placing one of the flat ends on the cutting board and sawing straight down the middle. Scoop out the pith and seeds.

3 Rub butter on the face of the squash, sprinkle it with a few grains of salt, and lay it facedown on the prepared baking dish. Cover the dish and bake until tender. Test the squash for doneness by inserting a fork; it should slide in easily and feel soft. Small squashes, such as delicate, will only take 35 to 45 minutes to bake, while a squash weighing 3 pounds may take up to 90 minutes.

FOR BABIES 6 MONTHS & OLDER: One-Trick Vegetables make perfect food for babies. Puree the cooked vegetable with a little breast milk or formula and serve. Serve minimal amounts of cooked beets to baby (only 1 teaspoon). The fiber in beets moves through the bowels quickly—an action most babies don't need help with!

---

quick-boiled collard greens
with apple cider vinegar

Assertive greens like collards can be bitter and tough, requiring heat and water to become tame and sweet. Vitamin A, vitamin C, folic acid, calcium, iron, and even protein are a part of most dark leafy greens. These powerful vegetables should be a daily part of the diet, especially for nursing mothers.

1 Remove the collard leaves from the thick central stem, keeping the leaves whole. Rinse the greens carefully. An easy way to do this is to fill a sink with cold water and submerge the greens. If the water has sediment, drain the sink and repeat.

2 In a 6- or 8-quart pot over high heat, bring 2 quarts of water and salt to a boil. Submerge the whole leaves. Timing is everything—if you remove the collards too soon they will be bitter; if you let them cook too long they will lose nutrients and have a flat taste. Tougher, more mature leaves will take 4 to 5 minutes to cook, while smaller, younger leaves may only require about 2 minutes. Remove a piece and test it every minute or so. You are looking for a slightly wilted leaf that still has a bright-green color and (most importantly) a succulent, sweet flavor.

3 Pour the cooked collards into a colander in the sink. Let them cool. Squeeze out any excess water with your hands, pressing the cooked leaves into a tight ball. Chop the ball into bite-size pieces. Toss the chopped collards with a dot of butter and a sprinkle of vinegar.

PREPARATION TIME:

10 minutes

MAKES 4 SERVINGS

1 large bunch collard greens
2 teaspoons sea salt
Unsalted butter, for garnish
Apple cider vinegar,
    for garnish

195

FOR BABIES 10 MONTHS & OLDER: Take 1 teaspoon of plain cooked collards and puree it with whatever grains or starchy vegetables baby is eating.

GREEN GOODNESS

When people think of greens, they often assume "salad." Explore the wide variety of greens and the many ways to prepare them. Green vegetables are rich in vitamins A and C, folic acid, calcium, and iron. The darker the color, the more nutrients present. Remember, though, that nutrients like vitamin A and calcium are better absorbed if there is fat present, so don't be shy about using butter or olive oil in any greens dish!

ARUGULA is also known as roquette. This leaf has a peppery flavor and is very popular to add to "wild greens" mixes. Buy fresh-looking leaves. Arugula adds a spicy dimension to lettuce-based salads.

BEET GREENS are the tops of the beet plant. Often you can purchase beets with the tops still attached. Only use them if the leaves are turgid and vibrant, not wilted.

BOK CHOY is a curvy vegetable with a crunchy white base that melds into dark-green leaves. You can chop up the whole plant and use it; however, the white part will require a bit more cooking time than the leaves. Bok choy is delicious sautéed in butter and garlic with a tiny splash of vinegar.

BROCCOLI sports a beautiful treelike structure that is often fascinating to children. Blanching the florets, then providing a sauce or a dip, is an easy way to add appeal for children.

CHINESE CABBAGE (napa or nappa) looks like green cabbage with a perm. It has a curly edge to its leaves and a more delicate flavor than common cabbage. Napa can be used in place of green cabbage in any recipe.

COLLARD GREENS are big, broad oval-shaped dark-green leaves that need cooking time to bring out their goodness—braising or quick boiling work well. They are easy to grow and over-winter nicely in temperate climates.

DANDELION GREENS are the most bitter of all of the greens. Some folks yearn for that strong bitter flavor, as it stimulates the digestive juices in the mouth.

ENDIVE, the most common variety being Belgian endive, is a small cream to pale-green cigar-shaped plant. It only needs a brief whisper of heat or can be served raw in salad.

ESCAROLE is a variety of endive whose leaves are broader and less bitter than other members of the endive family. It is most often used as a leafy green in salads but can be cooked briefly or added to soups near the end of cooking time.

GREEN CABBAGE, also known as common cabbage, is really not common at all. Slice a head in half and stare at that pattern! The way the leaves are tightly woven is amazing. Cabbage is wonderful lightly cooked, raw in slaws, or used as a wrapper. Also, it is a must for making sauerkraut.

KALE, a member of the cabbage family, comes in a number of shapes, sizes, and types. There is curly-leafed kale, red kale, dinosaur (lacinato) kale, and more. All kales have an assertive flavor and benefit from cooking. Kale is rich in vitamins, minerals, and bioflavonoids.

MUSTARD GREENS are another member of the kale family. These leaves have a strong, peppery flavor. Mizuna is a type of mustard green that is milder than some.

SWISS CHARD has big majestic-looking leaves with white, yellow, pink, or red stems—a beautiful looking plant. Cook it as you would collards or kale but with much less cooking time.

WATERCRESS likes to grow near running water. It has small round leaves and a bright, sharp taste. Use it like a fresh herb to finish soup or grain or bean dishes, or add it raw to salads for a fresh spark.

There's more that are not listed here. Please forgive me. Many of my favorite fresh herbs, like basil, oregano, sage, cilantro, and parsley, are nutrition-packed dark leafy greens too. Let's graze!

butter-braised kale *with* onion

Braising is an excellent cooking method for sturdy greens, as it fully tenderizes the leaf while adding flavor. All varieties of kale benefit from this cooking method; however, pay attention to the leaves you have chosen to cook. Lacinato or dinosaur kale has a more tender leaf and a milder flavor and so will require less cooking time, while curly-leaf kale benefits from more cooking time.

feeding the whole family

PREPARATION TIME:

15 to 20 minutes

MAKES 4 SERVINGS

2 tablespoons unsalted butter

½ medium onion, cut into crescents

1 large bunch kale, de-stemmed and cut into bite-size pieces

2 tablespoons water

1 tablespoon tamar (soy sauce)

1 tablespoon mirin

Rice or sherry vinegar

1 In a large 12-inch skillet over medium heat, add the butter and onion. Sauté the onion, stirring occasionally, until translucent and soft, about 3 to 5 minutes.

2 Add the kale and toss to coat it with the butter. Using tongs, keep turning the leaves so they continuously contact the heat, begin to turn brilliant green, and wilt down.

3 In a small bowl, mix together the water, tamari, and mirin. Pour the mixture over the greens. Cover the skillet tightly. Cook until the leaves are tender, about 3 to 5 minutes. Taste to check for doneness; the greens should be tasty, not bitter and still green, not gray. After removing the kale from the skillet, sprinkle it with a few drops of vinegar and serve.

FOR BABIES 10 MONTHS & OLDER: Blend 1 to 2 teaspoons of cooked kale with cereal or sweet potato.

garlic sautéed
rainbow swiss chard

Rainbow chard, with its beautiful red, pink, yellow, and white stems, warrants a moment of admiration before cooking.

1 Pull the Swiss chard leaves off of the central stem. Rinse the chard carefully. Shake off any excess water, pile the leaves one on top of the other, and chop them into 1-inch strips.

2 In a 12-inch skillet over medium heat, heat the oil. Get the heat high enough that after 1 minute you can feel heat when you place your hand above the oil but low enough that the oil doesn't smoke. Add the garlic and sauté until fragrant, taking care not to burn the garlic, about 1 minute.

3 Add the chopped leaves and keep them moving in the skillet. Turn the skillet frequently so that all the chard reaches the heat. Remove a piece and test it every 30 seconds or so. You are looking for a slightly wilted leaf that still has a bright-green color and (most importantly) a succulent, sweet flavor.

4 When all the greens have turned bright green and begun to wilt, remove them from the skillet. Sprinkle the cooked chard with salt and a few drops of vinegar and toss. Taste and adjust the amount of vinegar and salt to your liking.

PREPARATION TIME:

15 minutes

MAKES 4 SERVINGS

1 large bunch rainbow Swiss chard

2 tablespoons extra-virgin olive oil

4 cloves garlic, minced or pressed

Sea salt, for garnish

Apple cider vinegar, for garnish

199

vivacious vegetables

FOR BABIES 10 MONTHS & OLDER: Before adding the vinegar, take 1 to 2 tablespoons of the cooked Swiss chard and puree it with cooked quinoa or Baked Winter Squash (page 194).

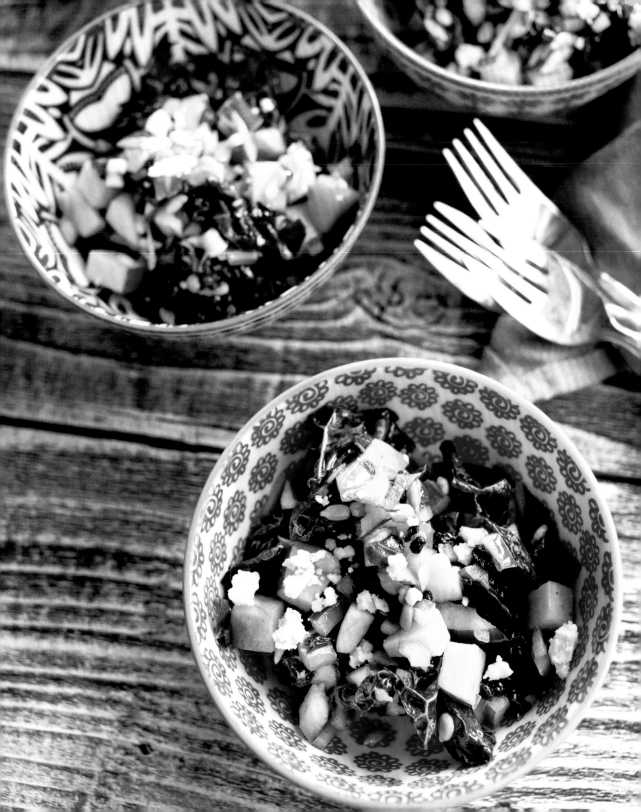

massaged kale & apple salad
with currants & gorgonzola

Friend and colleague Jennifer Adler, MS, CN, contributed this recipe. This salad keeps well in the refrigerator. Make a big batch to ensure that dark leafy greens are ready on busy days.

1 In a large bowl, put the kale and salt. Massage the salt into the kale with your hands for 2 minutes. The volume will reduce by almost half as the kale leaves wilt. In a clean bowl, put the massaged kale and discard the liquid extracted from massaging.

2 To toast the seeds, in a dry skillet over low to medium heat, put the seeds and stir constantly for a few minutes until they change color and give off a nutty aroma, about 3 to 4 minutes.

3 Add the apple, currants, onion, and toasted seeds to the kale and toss to combine. Add the oil and vinegar and toss again. Taste for salt and vinegar, adding more if necessary. Toss in or sprinkle on the cheese.

FOR BABIES 10 MONTHS & OLDER: Simmer slices from remaining ½ apple in water until soft. Puree it into a sauce for baby.

PREPARATION TIME:

15 minutes

MAKES 4 TO 6 SERVINGS

1 large bunch (about ¾ pound) kale, de-stemmed and thinly sliced (chiffonade)

1 teaspoon sea salt

⅓ cup sunflower seeds

½ large apple, diced (about ¾ cup)

⅓ cup currants

¼ cup diced red onion

¼ cup extra-virgin olive oil

2 tablespoons unfiltered apple cider vinegar

⅓ cup Gorgonzola cheese, crumbled

wilted sesame spinach

These greens make a tasty and impressive side dish for any Asian-influenced meal. It's particularly yummy served with Sticky Szechwan Tempeh (page 275).

PREPARATION TIME:

15 minutes

MAKES 4 SERVINGS

2 medium bunches spinach (about 1 pound)

1 teaspoon maple syrup

1 to 2 teaspoons rice vinegar

1 teaspoon toasted sesame oil

1 teaspoon hot pepper oil

½ teaspoon sea salt

2 tablespoons toasted sesame seeds (see page 129 for toasting instructions)

1 Remove the stems from the spinach and wash the leaves. Rest the leaves on a clean dish towel to absorb excess water.

2 In a 12-inch skillet over low or medium heat, add half of the moist spinach leaves. The water on the leaves will begin the wilting process. Turn the leaves constantly with tongs, bringing those from the bottom of the skillet to the top. They will wilt within 15 to 30 seconds. Add the remaining half of the leaves and repeat the process. Remove the spinach to a serving dish.

3 Dry any remaining water from the skillet with tongs and a paper towel. With the heat on low, add the maple syrup, vinegar, oils, and salt. Whisk together briefly until the flavors meld. Pour the dressing over the spinach, then add the toasted seeds and toss well. Serve warm, cold, or at room temperature.

FOR BABIES 6 MONTHS & OLDER: Wilted spinach is quick to make and a mild-tasting beginner green for baby. Remove 1 tablespoon before adding the dressing and puree.

---

feeding the whole family

cashew curry swimming greens

You have to have some of the Homemade Curry Paste (page 382) on hand to make this dish, and if you haven't made it routine to have the paste in your refrigerator, here is another excuse to start.

1 In a medium serving bowl, put the cooked collards.

2 In a saucepan over low heat, whisk together the cashew butter, curry paste, tamari, and water. Once the mixture is creamy smooth and warm, about 3 to 4 minutes, pour it over the cooked greens.

3 Top with cashews and serve immediately.

FOR BABIES 10 MONTHS & OLDER: Stir ½ teaspoon of cashew butter into baby's warm cereal for added calories.

PREPARATION TIME:

15 minutes

MAKES 4 SERVINGS

2 cups Quick-Boiled Collard Greens (page 195), without the added butter or vinegar

¼ cup cashew butter

1 tablespoon Homemade Curry Paste (page 382) or store-bought

1 tablespoon tamari (soy sauce)

¾ cup water

¼ to ⅓ cup whole roasted cashews

vivacious vegetables

spinach, peach & maple bacon salad

Be conscientious when shopping for bacon and other pork products. Select pork from ranchers who allow the pigs to live outdoors. Pigs don't sweat to keep clean. They eat dirt (along with other food, and the carbon in the dirt passes through their system, collecting unneeded particles along the way).

PREPARATION TIME:
15 to 20 minutes

MAKES 4 SERVINGS

4 strips bacon

1 tablespoon maple syrup

2 medium peaches, sliced

1 teaspoon unrefined cane or brown sugar

5 to 6 cups baby spinach leaves

1 to 2 tablespoons champagne or white wine vinegar

Sea salt and freshly ground black pepper

1 In a 12-inch skillet over medium heat, fry bacon. Once the bottom side is crisp, turn the bacon over and drizzle the top of each piece with the maple syrup. Remove the fried bacon to a plate (the maple syrup will make it stick to a paper towel). Once cool, chop the bacon into ½- to 1-inch pieces.

2 Pour the bacon grease into a small container and clean the skillet. Heat the skillet to medium heat, then add 2 teaspoons of the reserved bacon grease. Add the peaches. Increase the heat slightly and cook until the peaches sizzle and begin to caramelize, about 2 to 3 minutes. Turn each slice, sprinkle the sugar over the top of the peaches, and cook until the other side shows the browning of caramelization, 2 to 3 more minutes.

3 Add the spinach. Begin to gently turn the spinach and peaches until all of the spinach is slightly wilted. Place the spinach and peaches into a salad bowl.

4 Add the bacon pieces to the salad. Just before serving, dress the salad with 1 tablespoon of the vinegar. Taste the salad and add more vinegar if desired. Sprinkle the salad with a pinch of salt and pepper and serve immediately. This one doesn't keep well.

FOR BABIES 6 MONTHS & OLDER: Pureed peaches! Awesome.

feeding the whole family

arugula salad *with* tofu goddess dressing

The sharp taste of calcium-rich arugula greens works well with an easy-going tofu dressing. Mizuna mustard greens can be used in place of arugula, and the creamy pale-green dressing doubles as a sauce for pasta or grains.

1 Wash the arugula and lettuce by placing the leaves in a sink full of cold water. Drain and repeat. Spin or pat dry. Tear the greens into bite-size pieces and put them in a large salad bowl with the radishes and sprouts on top. Set aside.

2 To make the dressing, in a blender, put the tofu, oil, lemon juice, parsley, dill, water, garlic, salt, and sugar and blend until smooth and creamy. (An immersion blender will also work.) Add some extra drops of water if a thinner consistency is preferred; the dressing should be pourable. Taste and add more salt, lemon, or sugar if desired.

3 Toss the salad with the dressing just before serving. Any leftover dressing will keep in the refrigerator for about 1 week.

FOR BABIES 10 MONTHS & OLDER: Reserve some of the tofu. Cut it into small cubes. Steam and serve warm.

PREPARATION TIME:

10 minutes

MAKES 4 TO 6 SERVINGS

½ bunch arugula greens

¼ head green leaf lettuce

4 red radishes, sliced

1 handful alfalfa sprouts

For the dressing:

¼ pound tofu

2 tablespoons extra-virgin olive oil

2 tablespoons freshly squeezed lemon juice, plus more if needed

2 tablespoons chopped fresh Italian parsley

1 tablespoon fresh dill, or 1 teaspoon dried dill

1 tablespoon water

1 small clove garlic

½ teaspoon sea salt, plus more if needed

Pinch sugar, plus more if needed

vivacious vegetables

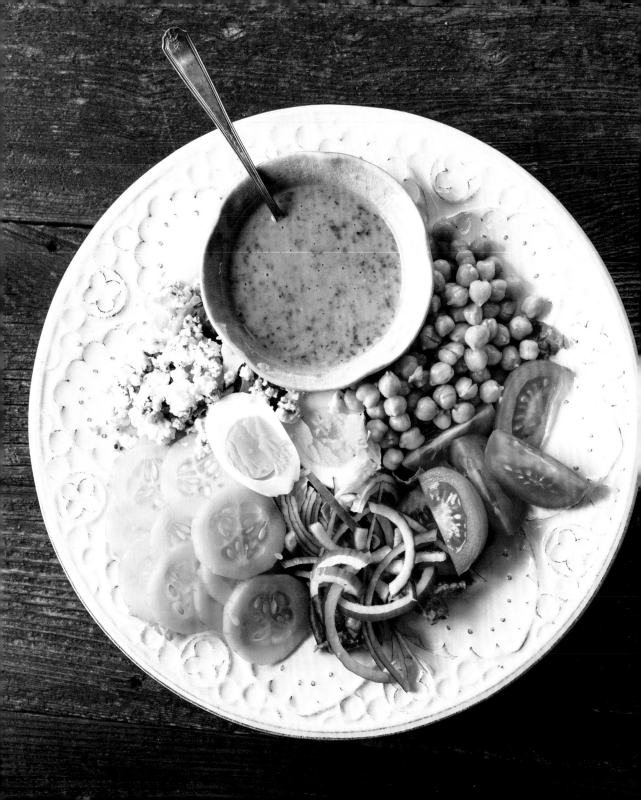

romaine & blue cheese chop salad *with* basil dressing

Chopping ingredients into a similar size gives the salad an even look and integrated flavor. Served with whole grain bread and butter, it makes a fine summer meal.

1 To make the dressing, in a blender, put the garlic, vinegar, mustard, and honey and blend well. With the blender running, slowly pour in the oil drop by drop. Once the oil is incorporated, add the basil and pulse a few times to combine.

2 In a 1-quart pan filled with cold water, place the egg. Bring the pan to a boil over high heat. As soon as it is boiling rapidly, turn off the heat, cover, and set a timer for 10 minutes. When the timer goes off, drain the water from pan and refill it with cold water repeatedly until the egg is cool. Peel the egg.

3 Break apart clean lettuce leaves. Stack the leaves on top of each other. Bisect the stack with a knife, then begin chopping the lettuce into approximately 1-inch squares. Place the chopped lettuce in a salad spinner and spin dry, then add it to a large salad bowl.

4 Dice the cucumber, red onion, tomato, and peeled egg into ½-inch pieces and add them to the salad bowl. Add the chickpeas and blue cheese. Pour the dressing over the salad and toss well. Serve immediately.

FOR BABIES 10 MONTHS & OLDER: Mash some of the cooked chickpeas with a leaf or two of chopped basil or puree them in the blender with a little water.

PREPARATION TIME:

15 minutes

MAKES 4 SERVINGS

For the dressing:

2 cloves garlic

3 tablespoons rice vinegar

1 teaspoon Dijon mustard

1 teaspoon honey

¼ cup extra-virgin olive oil

⅓ cup fresh basil

1 egg

½ large head romaine lettuce

½ cucumber

⅓ cup chopped red onion

1 large or 2 small ripe tomatoes

½ cup cooked chickpeas

⅓ cup crumbled blue cheese

classic greek salad
with pickled red onions

Create a Greek feast by serving this salad with Roasted Garlic Hummus (page 154), Tabbouleh Salad (page 136), and Middle Eastern Chickpea Falafel (page 268). Warm whole wheat pita on the side completes the meal. The bright pink pickled red onions perk up sandwiches, bagels and cream cheese, and even make a great hostess gift.

feeding the whole family

PREPARATION TIME:

1 hour (for pickling); 10 minutes (for preparation)

MAKES 4 SERVINGS

For the pickled onions:

½ medium red onion, cut
    into thin half moons

1 cup very hot water
    (not boiling)

¼ cup rice or white wine
    vinegar

½ cup cold water

1 tablespoon unbleached
    sugar

¼ teaspoon sea salt

2 peppercorns

1 dried red chili pepper

For the dressing:

1 tablespoon rice vinegar

1 teaspoon honey or sugar

Sea salt and freshly ground
    black pepper

3 tablespoons extra-virgin
    olive oil

1 To make the pickled onions, in a medium bowl, put the onions. Add the hot water and let it sit for 1 minute.

2 Drain the water from the onions. Add the vinegar, cold water, sugar, salt, peppercorns, and pepper, and stir to dissolve the sugar. Cover and chill for at least 1 hour. These onions will keep in a sealed container in the refrigerator for several weeks.

3 To make the dressing, in a large salad bowl, whisk together the vinegar, honey, and the salt and pepper to taste. Add the oil drop by drop, whisking vigorously, to emulsify.

4 To assemble the salad, add the olives, cucumber, tomato, and pickled onions to the dressing bowl and toss everything gently, bringing the dressing up from the bottom. Add the feta and gently fold it in or leave it on top.

10 (about ⅓ cup) pitted kalamata olives, halved

½ cucumber, peeled, halved
lengthwise, deseeded,
and diced into half moons

1 plum tomato, cut into
bite-size wedges

¼ pound feta, cut into cubes

FOR BABIES 10 MONTHS & OLDER: Serve this salad with
hummus or falafel and reserve some of the plain cooked
chickpeas to mash up for baby.

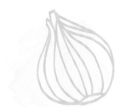

spinach salad *with* caramelized onions & maple-glazed nuts

This hearty salad goes with just about any main dish you could dream up. Leftover vinaigrette works well on grain or bean salads for lunch boxes.

PREPARATION TIME:

30 minutes

MAKES 6 SERVINGS

1 to 2 tablespoons unsalted butter or extra-virgin olive oil

1 medium onion, cut into half moons

Pinch of sea salt

1 bunch spinach, stems removed

⅓ cup Maple-Glazed Walnuts (page 371)

For the dressing:

2 tablespoons balsamic vinegar

1 teaspoon maple syrup

¾ teaspoon Dijon mustard

¼ teaspoon sea salt

¼ teaspoon freshly ground black pepper

3 to 4 tablespoons extra-virgin olive oil

1 In a 12-inch skillet over medium heat, heat the butter until it starts to sizzle but not burn, for just a minute or less. Add the onions and salt and move them around until the onions are coated. Lower the heat slightly and let the onions slowly cook down, decreasing in volume. Continue stirring and watch as the onions' color become more and more golden. If you feel that the onions are sticking to the bottom of the pan too much, add a very small amount of water and stir vigorously; this is called "deglazing."

2 To make the dressing, in a large salad bowl, place the vinegar, maple syrup, mustard, salt, and pepper and stir to mix. Add the oil a drop at a time, whisking it into the other ingredients to emulsify.

3 Tear the spinach into bite-size pieces and put them in the bowl, then add the caramelized onions and glazed nuts. Toss the salad with dressing just before serving.

FOR BABIES 6 MONTHS & OLDER: This salad makes a completely satisfying meal served with a thick soup or stew. Serve it with The Three Sisters Stew (page 265). Remove some of the cooked squash from the stew, puree, and serve to baby.

creamy lemon coleslaw

This has the familiar look and taste of traditional coleslaw but is not so mayonnaise-sloppy. The lemon gives it a fresher taste. Serve it with Sloppeh Tempeh Joes (page 269) for a new twist on traditional fare. Or go classic and serve with Mom's Meatloaf Muffins (page 305).

1 In a large salad bowl, combine the cabbages, carrot, and green onion. Toss together and set aside.

2 To make the dressing, in a small bowl, combine the mayonnaise, lemon juice, maple syrup, salt, and pepper to taste and whisk until mixed well. Pour the dressing over vegetables and toss again.

FOR BABIES 6 MONTHS & OLDER: Steam or bake an extra carrot and puree it for baby.

VARIATION FOR CHILDREN: Serve separate little piles of the grated or shredded vegetables before adding dressing.

PREPARATION TIME:

10 minutes

MAKES 6 SERVINGS

3 cups shredded green cabbage (from about ¼ of a large head)

1 cup shredded red cabbage

1 carrot, grated

1 green onion, chopped finely

For the dressing:

3 tablespoons mayonnaise

2 tablespoons freshly squeezed lemon juice

1 teaspoon maple syrup

½ teaspoon sea salt

Freshly ground black pepper

vivacious vegetables

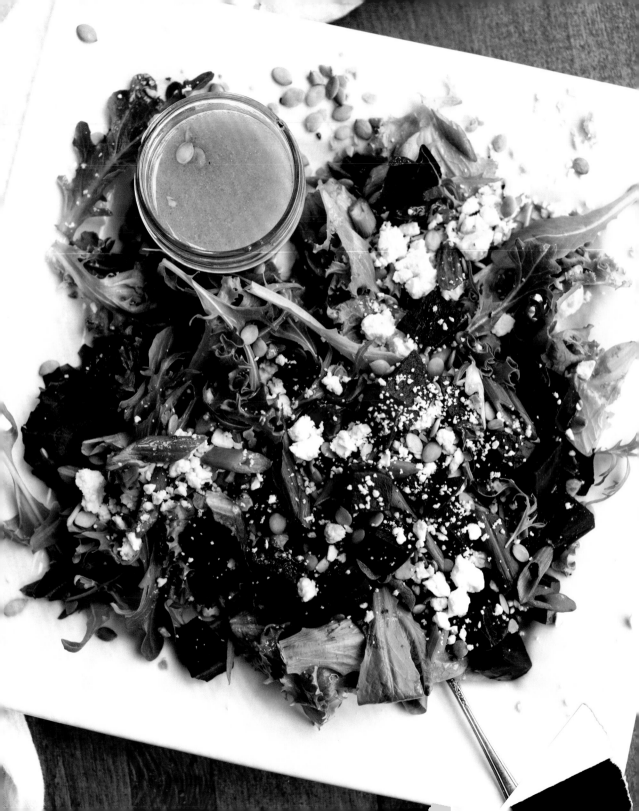

luscious beet salad *with* toasted pumpkin seeds

The key to making beets taste good is cooking them until they are fully tender. This recipe works well using golden beets, or would look stunning (color!) with a combination of both red and golden beets.

1 To make the dressing, in a ½-pint jar, put the oil, vinegar, basil, mustard, salt, and pepper and shake well to emulsify. Set aside.

2 Remove the greens from the beets and set aside. Wash the beets and put them in a 4-quart pot covered with water, then bring the water to a boil over high heat. Reduce the heat to low and simmer until the beets are fork-tender all the way to the center of the beet, about 1 hour. You can hasten this step by pressure-cooking the beets (see Pressure-Cooked Beets, page 193). Set aside to cool.

3 In a dry skillet over medium heat, put the pumpkin seeds. Moving the skillet back and forth over the heat with one hand, stir the seeds using a wooden spoon with the other hand. This will toast the seeds evenly and prevent burning. The seeds are ready once they begin to puff up and give off a nutty aroma, about 2 to 3 minutes. Remove the seeds from the skillet and set aside.

4 If your beet greens are vibrant, not wilted, follow the directions for Quick-Boiled Collard Greens (page 195) to cook them. Squeeze any excess water out of the cooked beet greens and chop into bite-size pieces. There will not be much volume. (If the greens look poor, substitute 1 to 2 cups of raw salad greens.)

PREPARATION TIME:

1 hour (for cooking); 15 to 20 minutes (for assembly)

MAKES 6 SERVINGS

For the dressing:

3 tablespoons extra-virgin olive oil

2 tablespoons balsamic vinegar

1 tablespoon finely chopped fresh basil

¾ teaspoon Dijon mustard

¼ teaspoon sea salt

¼ teaspoon freshly ground black pepper

4 large beets with greens

¼ cup pumpkin seeds

4 cups mixed salad greens

2 green onions, finely chopped

¼ pound feta cheese

continued

5 Peel the beets by holding them under a trickle of cold water and pushing the skins off with your fingers. Cut them into small cubes. In a large salad bowl, put the cubed beets, beet greens, pumpkin seeds, salad greens, and green onion. Pour the dressing over the salad just before serving and toss gently. Crumble the feta cheese on top.

FOR BABIES 10 MONTHS & OLDER: Reserve a teaspoon of the toasted pumpkin seeds, grind them to a fine powder, and stir them into baby's cereal or pureed vegetables for extra calories and other nutrients.

VARIATION FOR CHILDREN: Separate the different salad ingredients into piles and let them pick and choose.

watercress salad *with* amazing ginger dressing

The dressing for this salad may seem a bit fussy (lots of ingredients), but trust me, it is worth the effort. The recipe originated from a peaceful Indian restaurant in Seattle called Silence-Heart-Nest. Watercress is rich in minerals and is usually free of pesticides, as it grows easily and abundantly.

1 Wash the watercress and lettuce by placing the leaves in a sink full of cold water. Drain and repeat. Spin or pat dry. Tear the greens into bite-size pieces and put them in a large salad bowl. Add the cucumber and set aside.

2 To make the dressing, in a blender, put the oil, sesame seeds, ginger, celery, maple syrup, ketchup, pepper, and celery seeds and blend until thoroughly combined. Add the tamari, vinegar, and water and blend again until creamy. Before serving, toss the salad with the dressing.

FOR BABIES 10 MONTHS & OLDER: Add a few leaves of watercress to baby's cereal before blending. Offer a raw leaf or two as finger food as well.

PREPARATION TIME:

10 minutes

MAKES 4 SERVINGS

1 bunch watercress, tough stems removed

½ head red leaf lettuce

1 cucumber, thinly sliced

For the dressing:

3 tablespoons extra-virgin olive oil

1½ tablespoons toasted sesame seeds (see page 129 for toasting instructions)

1 tablespoon peeled, chopped gingerroot

1 teaspoon chopped celery

½ teaspoon maple syrup

½ teaspoon Kitchen Ketchup (page 377) or store-bought

⅛ teaspoon white pepper

⅛ teaspoon celery seeds

2 tablespoons tamari (soy sauce)

2 tablespoons rice vinegar

1 tablespoon water

napa cabbage slaw
with lime & roasted almonds

Napa or nappa cabbage is referred to as "Chinese cabbage" in much of the world. With only thirteen calories per cup, it is surprisingly filling.

PREPARATION TIME:

25 to 30 minutes

MAKES 4 SERVINGS

⅓ cup raw almonds

For the dressing:

2 tablespoons freshly
squeezed lime juice

2 tablespoons rice vinegar

1 teaspoon tamari
(soy sauce)

1 tablespoon sugar

½ teaspoon sea salt

3 tablespoons extra-virgin
olive oil

2 teaspoons toasted
sesame oil

½ head of napa cabbage,
shredded or thinly sliced
(about 4 cups)

2 green onions, finely
chopped

¼ cup chopped fresh
cilantro

1 Preheat the oven to 325 degrees F.

2 On a dry baking sheet, roast the almonds until the color begins to darken and they give off a nutty aroma, about 20 minutes. Turn the oven off and keep the almonds inside as it cools; this will crisp the nuts.

3 To make the dressing, in a large salad bowl, combine the lime juice, vinegar, tamari, sugar, and salt and stir to incorporate. Whisk in the oils a few drops at a time to create an emulsification, then whisk the rest in more rapidly.

4 Place the cabbage, green onions, and cilantro on top of the dressing. Toss the salad from the bottom up, coating the slaw with dressing. Taste for salt and add more if necessary. Chop the toasted almonds into chunks and sprinkle them on top before serving.

FOR BABIES 10 MONTHS & OLDER: Pulverize a few toasted almonds to a fine powder. Add ¼ teaspoon to yogurt or mashed avocado for baby.

feeding the whole family

succulent fall supper salad *with* apples, chickpeas & pumpkin seeds

Legumes and fruit transport this salad from side dish to meal.

1 Wash the lettuce, spinach, and arugula by placing leaves in a sink full of cold water. Drain and repeat. Spin or pat dry. Tear the greens into bite-size pieces and then put them in a large salad bowl.

2 Add the cabbage, apple, avocado, raisins, seeds, green onions, tomatoes, and chickpeas to the greens and toss gently.

3 To make the dressing, in a small bowl, put the vinegar, mustard, syrup, salt, paprika, and garlic. Whisk in the oil a few drops at a time to create an emulsification, then whisk the rest in more rapidly. Dress the salad just before serving and toss well.

FOR BABIES 6 MONTHS & OLDER: Reserve a slice or two of avocado, mash or blend, and serve.

FOR BABIES 10 MONTHS & OLDER: Mash cooked chickpeas with avocado for a creamy meal.

VARIATION FOR CHILDREN: Serve the salad in separate piles of raisins, apples, pumpkin seeds, avocado, and greens.

PREPARATION TIME:

20 minutes

MAKES 8 SERVINGS

½ head romaine lettuce

1 small bunch spinach (about 3 cups)

½ bunch arugula (about 2 cups)

1 cup chopped red cabbage

1 tart apple, cut into bite-size pieces

1 ripe avocado, cut into bite-size pieces

¼ cup raisins

¼ cup toasted pumpkin seeds

3 green onions, finely sliced

1 large or 2 small fresh tomatoes, cut into wedges

⅔ cup cooked chickpeas

For the dressing:

3 tablespoons balsamic vinegar

2 teaspoons Dijon mustard

2 teaspoons maple syrup

¼ teaspoon sea salt

⅛ teaspoon ground paprika

1 clove garlic, minced

¼ cup extra-virgin olive oil

vivacious vegetables

A+ avocado arame almond salad

Adding sea vegetables, like arame, is the perfect way to boost minerals in your diet. Pairing arame with the creaminess of avocado and the crunch of toasted almonds gives this salad a variety of delightful textures.

PREPARATION TIME:

20 to 25 minutes

MAKES 4 SERVINGS

¼ cup raw almonds

For the dressing:

3 tablespoons rice vinegar

2 tablespoons honey

2 teaspoons Dijon mustard

2 teaspoons poppy seeds

½ teaspoon sea salt

2 tablespoons toasted
    sesame oil

1 tablespoon extra-virgin
    olive or sesame oil

4 cups salad greens

⅛ cup dry arame

1 ripe avocado, cut into long
    strips

1 Preheat the oven to 350 degrees F.

2 On a dry baking sheet, roast the almonds until aromatic, 12 to 15 minutes. Turn the oven off and keep the almonds inside as it cools; this will crisp the nuts.

3 While the almonds are toasting, make the dressing. In a large salad bowl, combine the vinegar, honey, mustard, poppy seeds, and salt, and whisk to incorporate. Slowly add in the oils drop by drop to emulsify.

4 Wash the salad greens in a sink full of cold water. Spin or pat dry. Place the greens on top of the dressing in the salad bowl. Soak the arame for 5 to 10 minutes in 1 cup of water until softened, then drain and add it to the greens. Once cooled enough to touch, coarsely chop the almonds.

5 Gently fold the avocado into the salad. Toss to combine just before serving and garnish with the almonds.

FOR BABIES 6 MONTHS & OLDER: This one's easy—some mashed ripe avocado is just right for baby.

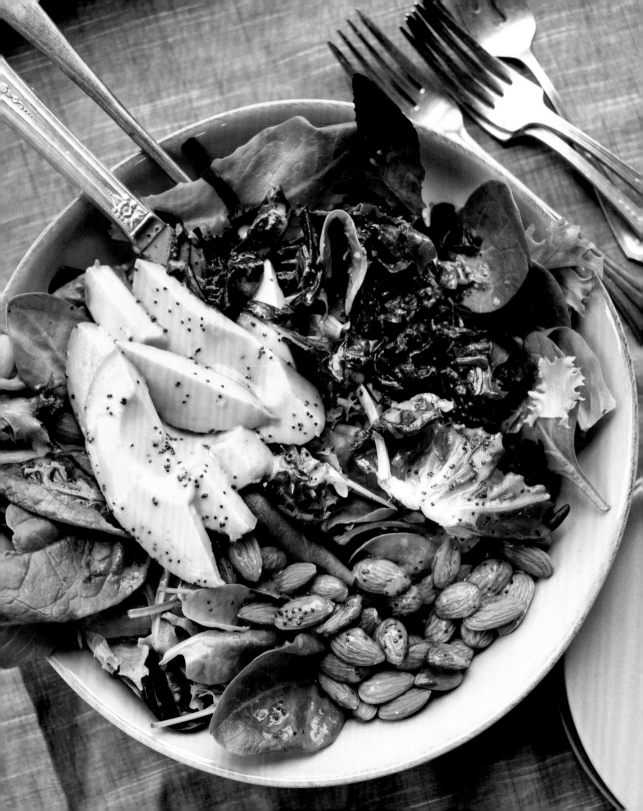

grilled vegetable salad *with* sweet poppy seed dressing

Grilled vegetables are satisfying whether served over rice, in a pocket pita, or in this incredible salad.

PREPARATION TIME:

30 minutes

MAKES 8 SERVINGS

1 medium eggplant, cut into ½-inch rounds

1 medium red bell pepper, cut into large wedges

1 medium onion, cut into large wedges

1 medium zucchini, cut into long, fat strips

1 portabella mushroom, cut into long, fat strips

3 tablespoons extra-virgin olive oil

8 cups salad greens

2 ounces feta cheese, crumbled

For the dressing:

¼ cup maple syrup

1 tablespoon Dijon mustard

1 tablespoon fresh dill, or 1 teaspoon dried dill

2 teaspoons poppy seeds

¼ cup extra-virgin olive oil

1 Heat up your grill (a small hibachi works fine).

2 While the grill is heating, brush both sides of each eggplant, pepper, onion, zucchini, and mushroom piece with a light coat of the oil. Place the vegetables on the hot grill and cook until the vegetables just start to brown, a few minutes on each side. Set aside.

3 Wash the salad greens by placing leaves in a sink full of cold water. Drain and repeat. Spin or pat the greens dry. Tear the greens into bite-size pieces and place them in a large salad bowl. Cut the grilled vegetables into bite-size pieces and add them to the salad greens.

4 To make the dressing, in a small bowl, whisk together the maple syrup, mustard, dill, and poppy seeds. Add the oil a few drops at a time to create an emulsification, then whisk the rest in more rapidly. Pour the dressing onto the salad and toss before serving. Crumble the feta on top.

FOR BABIES 6 MONTHS & OLDER: Reserve some slices of zucchini pieces and steam them until soft. Puree or mash them for baby.

VARIATION FOR CHILDREN: Skewer the oiled vegetables and grill them. Serve the shish kebab with dressing on the side.

iron woman salad

Struggling to add iron to your diet? Search no more. Nursing moms require at least nine milligrams of iron per day. Dulse tallies over eight milligrams in just two tablespoons.

1 Soak the dulse in cold water for 5 minutes to rehydrate it. To reduce the "bite" of the raw onion, cover the slices with boiling water for 1 minute, drain, and then cover them in cold water. Clean the soaked dulse well, removing any small pebbles. Pat the dulse dry. In a medium bowl, combine the dulse, onion, celery, vinegar, and salt and refrigerate for about 1 hour.

2 To make the dressing, in a blender, combine the tahini, water, oil, lemon juice, tamari, and garlic and blend until smooth. Serve the marinated dulse on a bed of lettuce leaves with the dressing on top. Extra dressing can be stores in the refrigerator, where it will keep for 7 to 10 days.

FOR BABIES 6 MONTHS & OLDER: Toast the dry dulse in a 250-degree oven for 12 to 15 minutes. Crumble the toasted dulse into flakes and store it in a sealed jar. Sprinkle some flakes into baby's cereal or other foods to make them iron fortified.

PREPARATION TIME:

1 hour (for marinating);
15 minutes (for assembly)

MAKES 4 SERVINGS

¼ cup dry dulse

1 red onion, cut in thin half moons

1 to 2 stalks celery, cut into bite-size pieces

1 tablespoon rice vinegar

Pinch of sea salt

For the dressing:

3 tablespoons tahini

3 tablespoons water

2 tablespoons extra-virgin olive oil

1½ to 2 tablespoons freshly squeezed lemon juice

1 teaspoon tamari (soy sauce)

1 clove garlic

1 small head of butter lettuce

braised brussels sprouts
with carrots & raisins

Braising these tiny cabbages lessens the bitter flavor that repels some children, and carrots and raisins sweeten the dish.

PREPARATION TIME:

10 to 15 minutes

MAKES 4 TO 5 SERVINGS

1 pound brussels sprouts

2 tablespoons unsalted
   butter or extra-virgin
   olive oil

1 large carrot, cut into
   matchsticks

1½ cups Easy Vegetarian
   Stock (page 168), Simple
   Chicken Stock (page 165),
   or store-bought

⅓ cup raisins

1 teaspoon chopped fresh
   thyme

Sea salt and freshly ground
   black pepper

1 Clean and trim the brussels sprouts by removing any browned outer leaves and trimming off the hard end. Split each one in half, or in thirds if they are large.

2 In an 8-inch skillet over medium-low heat, heat the butter until it slightly sizzles but doesn't brown, just 1 or 2 minutes. Add the sprouts and carrots and sauté until the vegetables begin to caramelize on the face and edges.

3 Add the stock, raisins, and thyme and simmer, covered, until tender (test one!), 4 to 5 minutes.

4 Add salt and pepper and taste. Don't be afraid to add a little more salt; it will bring out the sweetness. Remove the vegetables with a slotted spoon into a serving dish.

FOR BABIES 6 MONTHS & OLDER: Nab a few cooked, soft carrot slices before completing the dish. Mash well with a fork or blend with a touch of breast milk or water.

---

apple-fennel sauerkraut

Make homemade kraut to nourish your friendly gut microbes and enjoy a tangy condiment to add to rice, eggs, sandwiches, and more. Children can help with the massaging and pressing part of the process.

1 Weigh the head of the cabbage at the store or at home and note the amount.

2 Begin by halving the cabbage north to south, so you are cutting through the core. Notice the thick, white, *V*-shaped core. Follow the outside of the *V* with your blade and cut away the core from each half. Then cut each half lengthwise so you have four wedges. Take one wedge and remove enough of the inside section so that you can flatten the outer section with your hand. Hold it down with curved fingers, aim your knife perpendicular to the triangle-shaped stack of leaves, and. starting at the apex, cut it into ⅛-inch ribbons. Repeat this with the internal section of the wedge, then with all of the wedges, creating a cutting board full of confetti cabbage. Put all the cabbage ribbons into a large bowl.

3 You will use 1 teaspoon of salt per ½ pound of whole cabbage weight. Adjust the salt according to this ratio if your cabbage weighs more or less than 2 pounds. Sprinkle the salt over the shredded cabbage.

4 Remove the stems from the fennel bulb. Bisect the bulb, cut away the core from each half, and then cut each half into thin strips. Grate the apple slices on the large holes of a box grater. In a separate medium bowl, put the onion, fennel, apple, and thyme.

PREPARATION TIME:

15 minutes; 7-plus days (for fermenting)

MAKES 5 TO 6 CUPS

1 (2-pound) head green cabbage

4 teaspoons kosher salt

1 (8- to 10-ounce) head fennel

1 large or 2 small apples, cored and sliced

1 medium white onion, cut into thick half moons

1 tablespoon fresh thyme, finely chopped

2 teaspoons dried thyme

223

vivacious vegetables

continued

5 The salting will have given the cabbage a chance to begin releasing water. With clean hands, begin massaging the cabbage, pressing the salt into the strands to release more liquid and reduce the size of the chopped cabbage. Massage for a minimum of 3 minutes.

6 Add the fennel-apple mixture to the massaged cabbage and toss together with your hands.

7 In a fermentation vessel (two widemouthed quart jars or a large ceramic crock work well), put the mixed vegetables. Use your fist to compress the vegetables into the bottom of the vessel. Add the vegetables gradually, pushing down hard after each handful. You can't hurt the vegetables with the forceful pressing. In fact, it will help them release more liquid.

8 The goal is to submerge the vegetables in their own brine by applying even more compression to the top of the mixture. If using a ceramic crock, you can place a small plate directly on top of the vegetables and then add a weight on top of the plate (a 1-quart jar filled with water works as a weight; so does a clean rock!). If using widemouthed quart jars, place a sealed ½-pint jar filled with water on top of the vegetables to create more compression. Cover the crock or jars with a clean dish cloth to keep out dust.

9 Make sure the crock or jars are on a counter or table that is part of your normal walking path through the house. Pay the vegetables several visits during the next 24 hours. Push down on the weight to keep the vegetables submerged. Within 8 to 10 hours, there should be enough extracted liquid in the container to cover the veggies completely. After that, they'll only need a daily peek and a push to make sure the vegetables stay submerged.

10 After 7 days, lift up the weight and have a taste. This is very young kraut. It will likely still taste fresh with a mild tang. Want it tangier, krautier? Let it sit longer. Like it the way it is? Remove the weight, seal the jar, and refrigerate. Fido jars—a jar with metal hinge and rubber gasket—work best. The kraut will continue to ferment and change flavor but at a much slower rate in the refrigerator.

FOR BABIES 6 MONTHS & OLDER: Steam the apple slices. Puree or mash for baby.

DISCOVER SQUASH

The autumn harvest brings pumpkins and sweet potatoes and a wide variety of winter squashes, each with its own unique look and flavor. These vegetables not only score high on taste but are rich in vitamin A, vitamin C, fiber, and trace minerals. Look for squash that has clear skin and no mold or rotting on the stem end. Here is a description of some of the varieties to shop for.

ACORN SQUASH is shaped like a large acorn with prominent ridges and comes in dark-green, yellow, or orange; it has sweet, light-yellow flesh.

BUTTERCUP SQUASH is shaped like a pumpkin but smaller, with green or gold skin; the meat is dark orange, moist, and creamy.

BUTTERNUT SQUASH is gourd-shaped, with a neck and a bulbous base, buff-colored skin, and firm orange flesh.

DELICATA SQUASH has a small oblong shape, yellow skin with green stripes, and particularly sweet golden-colored flesh.

GOLDEN TURBAN is like a double-decker pumpkin with its distinctive turban shape, and comes in hues of green, gold, orange, and red; it has a mild, pleasant flavor.

HUBBARD SQUASH is large, smooth-skinned squash with a gray-green color and classic orange flesh.

KABOCHA SQUASH is pumpkin-shaped with dark-green skin that sports gray-brown nubs; it has dark orange flesh inside.

SPAGHETTI SQUASH is a large oval-shaped squash with yellow skin; the insides become long, thin golden strands when cooked.

SUGAR PIE PUMPKINS are small, dark-orange pumpkins, perfect for pie making.

SWEET POTATOES have beige or brown skins and are shaped like a potato with pointed ends. The meat is gold or dark orange. Some varieties of sweet potatoes are called yams. However, botanically they are all still sweet potatoes. True.

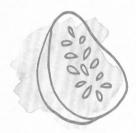

savory maple roasted butternut squash

Combining salty (tamari) and sweet (maple syrup) delights most palates.

PREPARATION TIME:

1 hour

MAKES 4 TO 6 SERVINGS

1 to 2 tablespoons unsalted butter, divided

1 (2- to 3-pound) butternut squash

½ teaspoon sea salt

1 tablespoon maple syrup

1 teaspoon tamari (soy sauce)

1 Preheat the oven to 400 degrees F and lightly butter a baking dish.

2 Using a utility knife with a serrated edge, cut off the stem and root end of the squash so you have two flat surfaces. Then halve the squash, cutting between the neck and the bulb. Bisect both pieces by placing one of the flat ends on the cutting board and sawing straight down the middle. Remove the pith and seeds from the two bulb-end pieces. You should have four squash pieces.

3 Rub 1 to 2 teaspoons of butter on the surface of each squash piece, sprinkle the salt over the butter, and place all four face pieces cut side down in the prepared baking dish. Roast until fork-tender, about 50 minutes.

4 In a small bowl, combine the maple syrup and tamari. Remove the squash from the oven, turn each piece over, and drizzle them with the maple syrup–tamari mixture. Return the dish to the oven and bake until the squash surfaces are brown, about 5 more minutes. Serve the squash warm.

FOR BABIES 6 MONTHS & OLDER: Puree or mash the roasted squash before adding maple syrup and tamari to make food for baby.

feeding the whole family

steamed cauliflower
in cheddar cheese sauce

It's true; folks of all ages dive into vegetables bathed in creamy cheese sauce. Homemade sauce is a snap to make, plus you can choose which cheese you prefer. Cheddar is used here, but Swiss or Gruyère are also options.

1 Remove the outer leaves and core from the cauliflower head, then cut or break it into small florets.

2 Fill a 4-quart pot with 1 to 2 inches of water and place a steamer basket in the water. Put the cauliflower into the basket and bring the water to a boil over high heat. Cover the pot and steam the cauliflower until tender, 8 to 10 minutes. Remove the cauliflower from the basket to a serving bowl.

3 Meanwhile, in a 2-quart saucepan over low heat, melt the butter. Add the flour and stir with a whisk until it becomes a thick paste, 1 to 2 minutes. Slowly add the milk, stirring constantly. Continue stirring until sauce has thickened, 3 to 4 minutes. When the sauce is smooth, add the cheese, salt, and pepper. Stir until cheese is melted. Thin the sauce with more milk if needed.

4 Pour the cheese sauce over the steamed cauliflower and mix gently. Serve immediately.

PREPARATION TIME:

10 minutes

MAKES 4 SERVINGS

1 (2½- to 3-pound) head cauliflower

2 tablespoons unsalted butter

1 to 2 tablespoons whole wheat pastry flour

1 cup whole milk

4 ounces grated cheddar cheese

½ teaspoon sea salt

Freshly ground black pepper

FOR BABIES 6 MONTHS & OLDER: Reserve a few pieces of soft steamed cauliflower and puree for baby.

VARIATION FOR CHILDREN: Serve the cheese sauce as a dip.

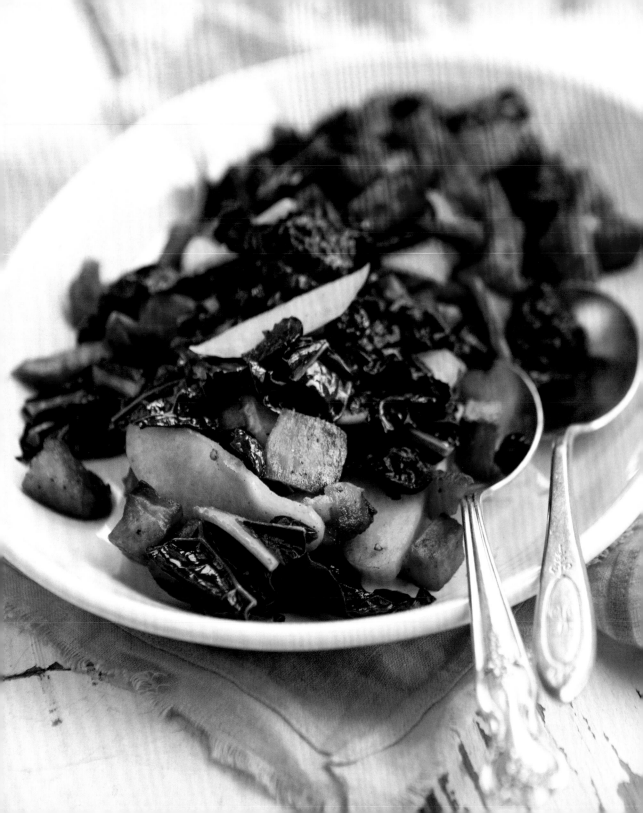

roasted sweet potatoes
with braised apples & kale

With its vibrant fall colors and natural sweetness, this is a welcome side dish for the holiday season.

1 Preheat the oven to 375 degrees F.

2 In a 9-by-13-inch baking dish, put the sweet potatoes. In a small bowl, mix together the oil, cumin, cinnamon, salt, and cayenne and drizzle it over the sweet potatoes. Turn the sweet potatoes with a large spoon so they are evenly coated. Cover the pan with aluminum foil and bake until fork-tender, 30 to 35 minutes.

3 While sweet potatoes are roasting, prepare the other vegetables. In a large skillet over medium heat, heat 1 tablespoon of the butter until it begins to sizzle. Add the apples and sauté, stirring frequently, for 1 to 2 minutes. Add the sugar, allowing it to melt on the apples, then add the remaining 1 tablespoon butter. When the second tablespoon of butter has melted, add the cranberries and kale. Allow the kale to be coated by the fat by folding it into the apples and butter with tongs. When the kale is shiny and beginning to get limp, about 3 minutes, add the juice. Cover the skillet and allow fruits and vegetables to braise until the kale is still green but wilted, 3 to 5 minutes.

4 In a large serving bowl, place the sweet potatoes, then add the braised apple-cranberry-kale mixture. Toss together gently. Drizzle 1 teaspoon of the vinegar on top and fold it in. Taste the composition. Add more vinegar or salt if desired. Serve warm or at room temperature. Leftovers will keep well in the refrigerator for several days.

PREPARATION TIME:

1 hour

MAKES 4 SERVINGS

2 sweet potatoes, scrubbed and cut into 1-inch chunks

2 tablespoons extra-virgin olive oil

1 teaspoon ground cumin

½ teaspoon ground cinnamon

½ teaspoon sea salt

Pinch of cayenne

2 tablespoons unsalted butter, divided

½ apple, cut into thin slices

1 tablespoon unrefined cane sugar or brown sugar

⅓ cup dried cranberries

6 to 8 kale leaves, cut into thin strips

¼ cup apple juice

1 to 2 teaspoons balsamic vinegar

vivacious vegetables

FOR BABIES 6 MONTHS & OLDER: Mash a few pieces of roasted sweet potato, void of oil and spices, for baby.

edamame succotash
with lemon herb butter

Succotash (named from a stew made by the Narragansett Indian Tribe of Rhode Island called msíckquatash, *"boiled corn kernels") is a dish consisting primarily of corn and lima beans or other shell beans.*

PREPARATION TIME:

10 minutes

MAKES 4 SERVINGS

1½ cups shelled edamame

1 cup corn kernels

1 large carrot, cut into
¼-inch dice

1 teaspoon lemon zest

2 tablespoons unsalted
butter, divided

1 medium red bell pepper,
cut into ¼-inch dice

2 tablespoons chopped
fresh herbs (basil, marjoram, and/or thyme)

½ teaspoon sea salt

1 tablespoon freshly
squeezed lemon juice

Freshly ground black pepper

1 Bring a 4-quart pot of water to boil over high heat. Add the edamame, corn, and carrot and boil for 2 to 3 minutes. Pour the vegetables through a large strainer and then plunge them into cold water for 2 to 3 minutes, then strain the vegetables.

2 In a large skillet over medium heat, add the zest and 1 tablespoon of the butter. When the butter sizzles, add the bell pepper and sauté for 1 minute, until more tender and less turgid.

3 Add the remaining 1 tablespoon butter, the cooked edamame, corn, and carrots, and the fresh herbs and salt. Toss until thoroughly warmed. Add the lemon juice and pepper to taste and serve immediately.

FOR BABIES 10 MONTHS & OLDER: Awesome finger food for little ones!

---

feeding the whole family

rosemary & garlic roasted potatoes

At breakfast, lunch, dinner, snack, or lunch box time, roasted potatoes are proven winners. Roast a pan while doing other chores. They take care of themselves.

1 Preheat the oven to 375 degrees F.

2 Wash the potatoes, scrubbing off any dirt and removing any eyes, and then cut them into halves or quarters, depending on the size. Put the potatoes in a 9-by-13-inch baking dish.

3 In a small bowl, mix the oil, garlic, and rosemary. Drizzle the oil mixture over the potatoes and shake pan to coat. Sprinkle the salt and a few grinds of pepper over the top. Roast the potatoes until they are tender inside and browned on the outside, 40 to 50 minutes.

4 Turn the oven off, leaving the pan of potatoes inside, and let them finish in the oven as it cools off. This gives the potatoes a crisper surface.

***

FOR BABIES 10 MONTHS & OLDER: Smash a few potatoes with a fork and serve!

PREPARATION TIME:

1 hour

MAKES 4 SERVINGS

12 small red potatoes, halved or quartered

3 tablespoons extra-virgin olive oil

5 to 6 cloves garlic, minced

2 tablespoons fresh rosemary leaves, minced

1 teaspoon sea salt

Freshly ground black pepper

vivacious vegetables

ruby-red pickled beets

You can either boil or pressure-cook beets to ready them for pickling. Dark-red, nutrient-rich beets are enhanced and preserved by this quick-pickle method.

PREPARATION TIME:

1 hour

MAKES 2 TO 3 CUPS

2 pounds whole red beets

4 to 5 whole cloves

1 cinnamon stick

1 teaspoon whole allspice

1 cup apple cider vinegar

1 cup water

½ cup unbleached white sugar

2 tablespoons unrefined cane sugar or brown sugar

1 Remove the leafy tops from the beets and wash the beets to remove any dirt. Do not cut off the root or the nubby crown; if you do, the beets will "bleed" into the water they are cooked in and lose flavor and nutrition.

2 To pressure-cook the beets, in a pressure cooker with enough water to cover the bottom half of the beets, put the beets. Secure lid and bring the heat to high. When cooker has reached pressure, reduce the heat to medium low and cook for 20 to 25 minutes. Remove the cooker from the heat and let the pressure come down naturally.

3 To cook the beets on the stovetop, fill a 4-quart pot with water and bring it to a boil over high heat. Add the beets, cover, and simmer until fork-tender, about 1 hour.

4 Meanwhile, in a coffee or spice grinder, pulse the cloves, cinnamon, and allspice for a few seconds. Place the roughly ground spices in a piece of cheesecloth and secure it with a string to make a bag. In a 4-quart pot over medium heat, put the vinegar, water, sugars, and spice bag and heat until the mixture simmers and the sugar dissolves, 2 to 3 minutes.

5 When the beets are cool enough to handle, slip the skins off each beet under cool running water. Trim the ends and slice the beets. Add the beets to the simmering liquid and cook to infuse the beets with the spices, about 5 minutes more.

6 Pack the beets into clean glass jars and cover them with the spiced liquid. If eaten within 1 to 2 weeks, the beets will store nicely in the refrigerator. If you want to keep the beets for months, process the jars as you would other canned vegetables.

FOR BABIES 10 MONTHS & OLDER: Cooked beets are a natural remedy for constipation. If your baby or child is suffering from this malady, try some mashed, well-cooked beets (before pickling)—no more than 1 tablespoon!

whipped adobe sweet potatoes

The candy sweetness of the baked sweet potato, cream, and butter merged with a little smoky heat will make you swoon, I promise. Regular sweet potatoes or Oriental yams (both have light-yellow flesh) are preferable to the orange-fleshed sweet potatoes.

PREPARATION TIME:

70 minutes

MAKES 4 TO 6 SERVINGS

3 small sweet potatoes
(1¾ to 2 pounds)

2 tablespoons unsalted
butter

¼ cup heavy cream

½ teaspoon sea salt

About 1 teaspoon chipotle
chili in adobe sauce

1 Preheat the oven to 400 degrees F.

2 In a baking dish, put the sweet potatoes and pierce each one a few times with a fork to create steam holes. Bake the sweet potatoes until they are fork-tender in the center, about 1 hour.

3 When the sweet potatoes are cool enough to handle, remove the skin and cut away any dark spots or eyes. In a food processor, put the sweet potato flesh with the butter, cream, and the salt and puree until smooth. Taste and add more salt if necessary. Add the chili a little at a time to get the heat and smokiness desired. The whipping can also be accomplished with an electric hand mixer.

FOR BABIES 6 MONTHS & OLDER: Puree or mash the sweet potato for baby before adding the butter, cream, and chili.

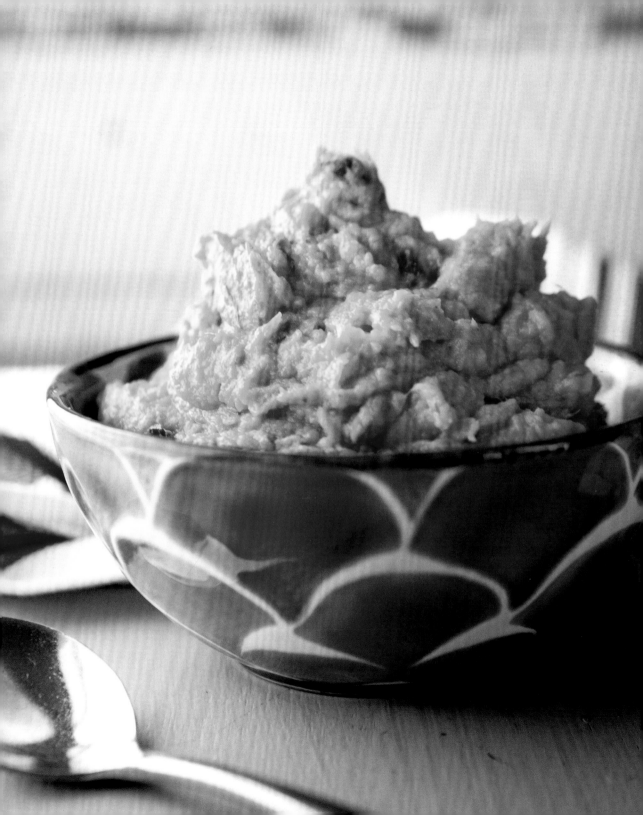

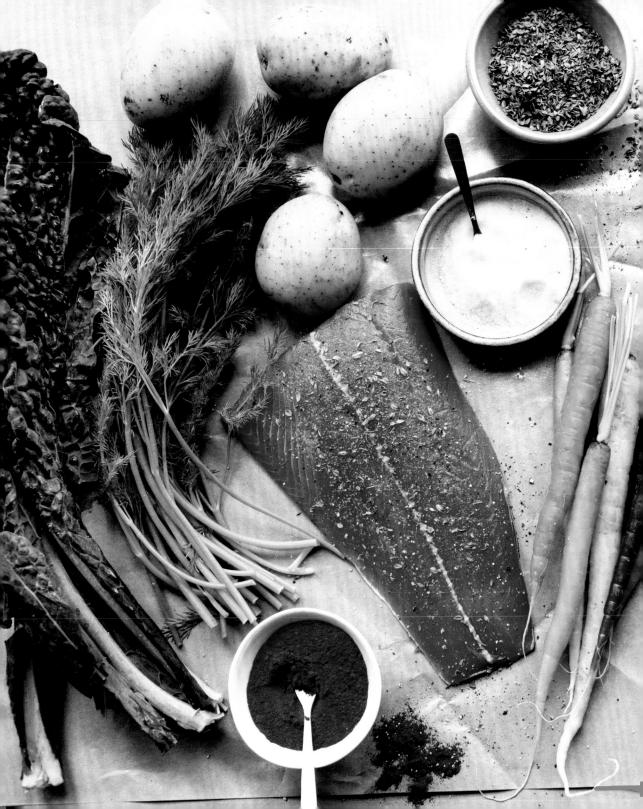

CHAPTER 9

substantial suppers

My daughter wants to be a vegetarian!"

I heard this often when I first began teaching cooking classes. Meat-and-potatoes parents wanted to learn how to make grain-and-bean entrées, which was my specialty. I had stretched my regime to include fish but stayed intent on the "mostly plants" diet, despite being raised in Kansas where dinner wasn't dinner unless steak was involved.

As my teaching expanded to the university level, I began to learn more about how the meat we eat is produced, while continuing to lean in the vegetarian direction. Feeling unprepared to cover the topic of meat production in a lecture, I invited guest speakers to share their knowledge. Oregon ranchers Connie and Doc Hatfield spoke to my class and taught us that there's a way to produce meat that's good for both people and the environment. Paradigm shifted. Later Eiko and George Vojkovich of Skagit River Ranch became regular guest speakers in my classes. Their cows were fed and cared for better than most people I know. Mind blown.

I was still a mostly vegetarian mom when my eight-year-old daughter pulled a switcheroo. I had lugged in the grocery bags from the car. She enjoyed helping me put things away. I had bought some beef stew meat to delight our two Jack Russell terriers, and the plastic-wrapped package was perched on top. She snatched it and asked, "Can I eat this?"

I paused, shrugged, and said, "Sure," suggesting that we cook it first.

The wok was pulled out and stir-frying began. The first six seared-beef chunks weren't enough. We cooked up the whole pound of beef. She ate all of it, ravenously. Her quick metabolism and early penchant for participating in sports made demands on her body. Lesson learned. Thankfully, it is possible to purchase meat, poultry, and eggs from conscientious ranchers. The price tag will be higher, reflecting the true cost. My advice: pony up.

We're not all the same. Even within one family. That's why this section straddles the fence.

"The farmer and the cowman should be friends,
Oh, the farmer and the cowman should be friends.
One man likes to push a plough,
the other likes to chase a cow,
But that's no reason why they cain't be friends."

—RODGERS and HAMMERSTEIN,
Oklahoma!

whole grains *from* scratch

Often cooks encounter the Goldilocks syndrome when preparing whole grains from scratch. The end product is too mushy or too hard, and never "just right." Follow these instructions to the letter and a pot of successful whole grains are less than an hour away.

feeding the whole family

PREPARATION TIME:

55 minutes

MAKES 2½ TO 3 CUPS

1 cup whole grains (such as quinoa, brown rice, or millet)

½ teaspoon sea salt

1¾ to 2 cups water

1 Rinsing: The best way to rinse grains is to place the grains in the pan with a generous amount of water. Swirl the grains in the water with your hand. As you touch the grain, remember your gratefulness to the farmers, soil, sun, and water for providing this food. Pour off the water through a fine mesh strainer. Repeat this process again until the water you pour off is clear.

2 Toasting (optional): Put the rinsed grains in a dry 2-quart pan. Bring the heat up to medium and stir the grains until they are dry and begin to give off a slightly nutty aroma, about 5 minutes. Toasting the grain before cooking increases the separateness of the final product, making it a worthwhile step for grains that will eventually become salads.

3 Cooking: In the 2-quart pan, add the salt and water to the grains. Sea salt brings out the sweetness in grains and helps the grain open up. Grains cooked without salt will taste very flat.

4 Over high heat, bring the water and grain up to a bubbling boil. Make sure it is a full boil and make sure that you don't leave the grain at the boiling stage for more than a few seconds. Lower the heat immediately, cover the pan, turn the heat to low, and establish a gentle simmer. Peek inside and make sure there is movement but no bubbling. If the heat on your stovetop is not flexible using a "flame-tamer" or heat diffuser, a perforated metal plate with a handle, placed between the pan and the heat source, can be helpful. When grains turn out too stiff and separate, usually it's because the grain was cooked at a high temperature for too long. If the grain turns out soggy or clumped together, the heat may not have been high enough or you may have used too much water.

5 *Don't stir cooking grains.* Whole grains create their own steam holes from the bottom of the pan to the top so that they cook thoroughly. Stirring them disturbs the tiny tunnels. Whole grains that have been ground or cereals are another matter. They can be stirred.

6 To test for doneness without disturbing the steam holes, remove the lid and gently tip the pan to one side. If even a tiny bit of liquid pools, replace the lid and return grains to heat. You want all of the liquid to be absorbed get a properly cooked grain.

7 **Resting:** The step is essential for "just right" grains. Remove the lid of the fully cooked grain and let it sit for 10 minutes before serving. The grain will lose any remaining liquid through steam and become fluffier.

beans *from* scratch

The personality of the unpretentious bean shares similarities with your friend or relative who simply does not like to be rushed. Trying to hurry up the cooking of the humble bean will not give you good results. "Low and slow" is the motto for cooking beans. Keep the temperature at a low simmer and give the beans plenty of time to change and open up, just like your friend.

PREPARATION TIME:

8 hours (for brining); 40 to 60 minutes (for cooking)

MAKES 6 CUPS COOKED BEANS

2 cups dried beans

14 cups water, divided

4 teaspoons sea salt, divided

1 Selecting: Buy dried beans at a store that has a rapid turnover, store them in an airtight container, and use them within a few months. If your beans are older than six months, they will take longer to become tender (or may never get tender!). You can tell if dried beans are aged by their appearance; the color will be faded, not rich, and the outside of the bean dull instead of shiny. Sort through beans bought in bulk and pick out any stones or bits before brining or soaking.

2 Brining: Place beans in a large bowl. Add 10 cups of the water and 2 teaspoons of the salt to the beans. Let stand for 8 hours or overnight. Brining works best as the salt speeds up the process of opening up the bean. If you brine beans for less than 8 hours, you will need to adjust the cooking time and the amount of water, adding more time and water. If the beans were brined for longer than 8 hours, less water and less time can be used during cooking.

3 Simmering or Pressure-Cooking (choose one): To simmer: Drain off the brine. In a 4-quart pot, place the beans, the remaining 4 cups fresh water, and the remaining 2 teaspoons salt. Over high heat, bring the beans and water to a full boil. Reduce heat, cover, and simmer until beans are quite tender, 55 to 60 minutes.

feeding the whole family

4 A well-cooked bean can be easily mashed on the roof of your mouth with your tongue. If extra water is needed, you may have the beans simmering on too high of heat. Remember "low and slow" works best for beans.

5 Cook until all of the water is absorbed, or if you are satisfied with the texture and there is still water present, uncover the pot and let the extra water escape through steam rather than draining the beans.

6 To pressure-cook: Pressure-cooking beans renders the most tender bean outcome. Less time is needed and the beans carry more flavor. Today's pressure cookers are safe and "explode-proof." Drain the brine off of the beans. In a 6- or 8-quart pressure cooker, put the beans, the remaining 4 cups fresh water, and remaining 2 teaspoons salt. Lock the lid in place, then turn the heat to high until the pressure gauge rises up. Once the gauge is firmly up, lower the heat to low and begin timing for 40 to 45 minutes. Keep the heat at a temperature where you can hear a steady but soft hissing sound coming from the cooker. This may take a few minor heat adjustments until you get it just right.

7 At the end of the cooking time, remove the cooker from the heat and allow the pressure and gauge to come down. As the pot cools this will happen naturally or you can speed up the process by running a small stream of cold water over the edge of the cooker. Test the beans. If they are tender and some liquid remains in the pot, cook off the liquid with the lid off to preserve flavor.

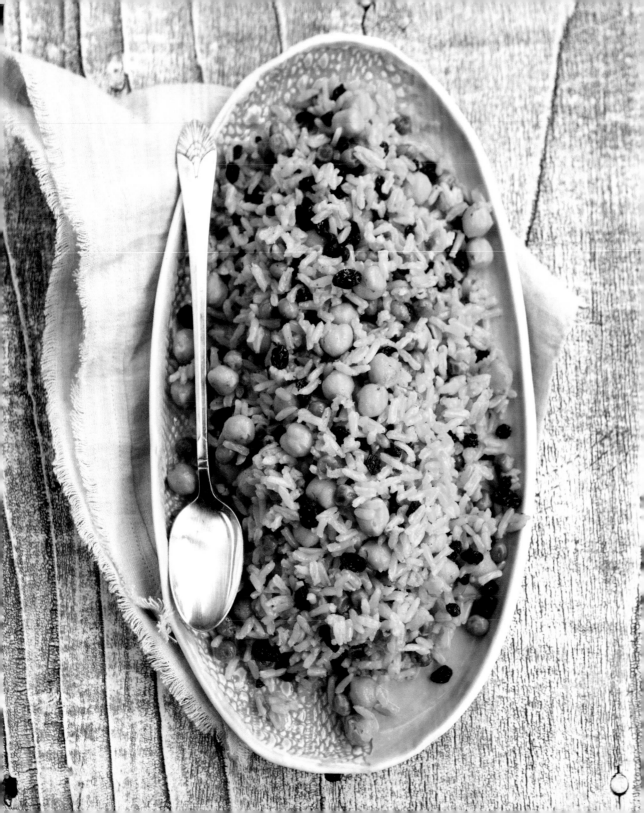

golden spice rice *with* chickpeas

Sautéing rice before cooking it results in a more separate finished grain. By adding a few simple spices, fragrance and a lovely golden color are imbued into the rice. Cooked chickpeas bring balance to the dish by combining the whole grain with a legume.

1 In a 2-quart pan over low to medium heat, heat 1 teaspoon of the ghee until melted. Rinse and drain the rice well. Put the rice in the pan and sauté it until well coated. Add the turmeric and stir again. Add the water, cardamom, and salt. Bring the pan to a full boil over high heat. Reduce the heat to low, establishing a light simmer. Cover the pan and let the rice simmer until all the water is absorbed, 45 to 50 minutes. Don't stir the rice while it is cooking.

2 Allow the rice to rest, uncovered, for 10 minutes.

3 In a large skillet over low to medium heat, heat the remaining 1 tablespoon of ghee. Add the chickpeas, green peas, and currants and stir until the peas are tender, 2 to 3 minutes. Fold in the cooked rice gradually. Serve while warm.

PREPARATION TIME:

55 minutes

MAKES 4 SERVINGS

4 teaspoons Homemade Ghee (page 383) or extra-virgin olive oil, divided

1 cup basmati brown rice

¼ teaspoon ground turmeric

1¾ cups water

2 green whole cardamom pods

½ teaspoon sea salt

1 cup cooked chickpeas

½ cup frozen green peas

¼ cup currants

FOR BABIES 10 MONTHS & OLDER: Either pureed golden rice or mashed cooked chickpeas from this dish are an easy offering for baby.

deep-fried millet croquettes *with* tamari ginger sauce

Properly done, deep-frying is actually quite low in calories. Keeping oil at the correct temperature is the key. Compare the amount of oil you're using before and after cooking—only a few teaspoons should be missing! Serve Millet Croquettes with Cannellini Kale Minestrone (page 183) for a whole grain, bean, green combo.

PREPARATION TIME:

45 to 50 minutes

MAKES 8 TO 10 CROQUETTES

1 cup millet

2½ cups water

½ teaspoon sea salt

1 carrot, grated

2 green onions, finely chopped

1 quart expeller-pressed high-heat vegetable oil, such as safflower or peanut (the pan you use to deep-fry should be ⅔ full)

For the sauce:

1 heaping tablespoon kudzu, or 2 teaspoons arrowroot

1 cup water

1 teaspoon freshly grated gingerroot

3 tablespoons tamari (soy sauce)

Lemon wedges, for garnish

1 Rinse and drain the millet two or three times. In a 2-quart pot over high heat, add the millet, water, and salt and bring it to a boil. Reduce the heat to low, cover, and let it simmer until all the water is absorbed, 25 to 30 minutes. Remove the pot from the heat and let it rest for 10 minutes.

2 In a large bowl, put the cooked millet, carrot, and green onions and mix well. With moist hands, form the mixture into croquettes about the size of a golf ball, packing tightly.

3 In a deep stainless-steel pot or wok, heat the oil to 375 degrees F. Use an instant-read thermometer to make sure the temperature is correct. If the temperature is too high, it will burn the outside of the croquettes and leave the inside raw. If the temperature is too low, it will result in soggy croquettes. When the temperature is correct, there will be dancing ripples on the bottom of the pan. Spread a brown paper bag or paper towel on a baking sheet for draining the fried croquettes.

4 With a slotted spoon, lower three or four croquettes into the hot oil. The croquettes should drop to the bottom and then quickly rise to the top. Fry until the croquettes are golden on the outside, 1 to 2 minutes, then, using a slotted spoon, remove them to the prepared lined baking sheet.

5 To make the sauce, in a small pan, dissolve the kudzu in the water. Add the ginger. Bring the mixture to simmer over medium heat, stirring constantly. When the mixture becomes clear and thick, about 5 minutes, remove the pan from the heat. Stir in the tamari. Squeeze the lemon wedges over the croquettes, then top them with the sauce or serve the sauce on the side.

FOR BABIES 6 MONTHS & OLDER: Reserve some cooked millet and puree it with water or breast milk and serve.

FOR BABIES 10 MONTHS & OLDER: Reserve some cooked millet and puree it with an extra carrot that has been sliced and steamed.

mexican brown rice

Need to spark up the rice you serve next to tacos or enchiladas? Adding a bit of this and that to rice as it cooks pumps up the flavor. This rice pairs perfectly with pinto beans.

PREPARATION TIME:

1 hour

MAKES 4 SERVINGS

1 cup long-grain brown rice

1 teaspoon extra-virgin olive oil or unsalted butter

1 teaspoon ground cumin

1 teaspoon chili powder

½ onion, finely diced

½ teaspoon sea salt

1¾ to 2 cups water

1 tablespoon tomato paste or sauce

1 Rinse and drain the rice and set aside. In a 2-quart pot over medium heat, heat the oil. Add the cumin and chili powder and sauté for a few seconds. Add the onion and salt and continue cooking until the onion is golden and soft, about 3 to 5 minutes.

2 Add the rice and stir well, coating the rice. Add the water and tomato paste, raise the heat to high, and bring it to a boil. Reduce heat to low and simmer, covered, until all of the water is absorbed, about 40 minutes. Remove the pot from the heat, and let the cooked rice rest, uncovered, for 10 minutes.

FOR BABIES 6 MONTHS & OLDER: Serve this rice with fresh avocado slices on top and mash part of the avocado for baby.

bok choy & buckwheat noodles *in* seasoned broth (yakisoba)

This traditional Japanese dish is a favorite in my home. From kindergarten to college, my daughter smiled when yakisoba was served. Pan-frying the tofu cubes before adding them adds a crispy texture, but the dish is equally good if the tofu is added raw.

1 Cook the noodles according to the directions on the package. Set aside.

2 In a 4-quart soup pot over medium heat, heat the oil. Add the onion and garlic and sauté until onion begins to soften, about 3 minutes. Add the carrot and mushroom pieces and sauté 2 to 3 more minutes. Add the water, tamari, tofu, and ginger. Increase the heat to medium high until the mixture begins to simmer. Reduce the heat to low, cover, and simmer for 10 more minutes.

3 Add the bok choy to the pot and simmer until the leaves are bright green, 1 to 2 minutes. Serve this dish by placing a handful of noodles in each bowl. Ladle the broth and vegetables over the noodles. Garnish with the green onions.

FOR BABIES 6 MONTHS & OLDER: Retrieve some cooked carrots and bok choy from the broth. Puree with some water and serve.

FOR BABIES 10 MONTHS & OLDER: Serve cubes of cooked tofu and/or cooked soba noodles cut into small pieces.

PREPARATION TIME:

30 minutes

MAKES 4 SERVINGS

1 (8-ounce) package soba noodles

2 tablespoons toasted sesame oil

1 medium onion, cut into thin half moons

2 to 3 cloves garlic, minced

1 carrot, cut into matchsticks

5 shiitake mushrooms, cut into bite-size pieces

4 cups water

⅓ cup tamari (soy sauce)

½ pound firm tofu, cut into ½-inch cubes

1 tablespoon freshly grated gingerroot

1 small head baby bok choy, cut into thin ribbons

2 green onions, thinly sliced, for garnish

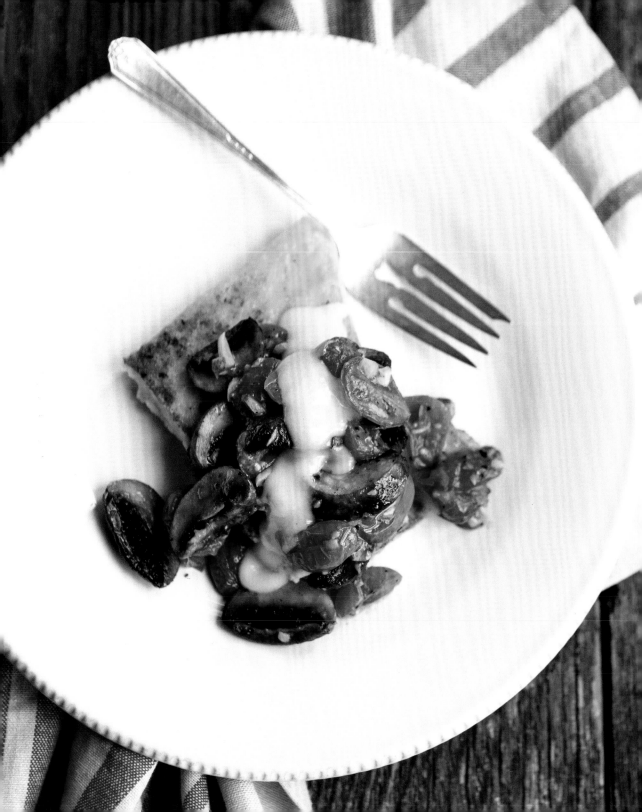

roasted mushrooms
& tomatoes *on* polenta slices

The combination of polenta and mushrooms simply rocks. Dazzle your vegetarian self and/or friends. These heavenly mushrooms also work served on cooked lentils or baked chicken. The polenta can be prepared ahead of time, even the day before.

1 To make the polenta slices, lightly oil a pie plate or an 8-by-8-inch pan (for squares). Set aside.

2 In a 4-quart (or larger) pot over high heat, bring the water and stock to a rapid boil. Add the butter and salt and stir to incorporate. Slowly add the polenta, stirring continuously with a whisk or wooden spoon.

3 Reduce the heat to low and continue stirring in a clockwise motion, making sure that the heat is at a temperature where the polenta puckers but does not boil. Normally the heat will need to be adjusted several times over the course of stirring to maintain the soft pucker.

4 Stir slowly and continuously for about 25 minutes, then stir in the Parmesan. Stir for 5 more minutes, until the grains become less individualized and the mixture is thick and creamy.

5 Pour the polenta into the prepared pan and smooth the top. Let it cool to room temperature, and cut into eight slices.

6 Preheat the oven to 425 degrees F.

7 Wipe any dirt off of the mushrooms with a damp towel. Remove any hardened stem ends. Cut the mushrooms into ¼-inch-thick slices.

PREPARATION TIME:

65 minutes

MAKES 4 SERVINGS

For the polenta slices

4 cups water

1 cup Simple Chicken Stock (page 165) or store-bought

2 teaspoons unsalted butter or extra-virgin olive oil

½ teaspoon sea salt

1 cup polenta or corn grits

¼ cup grated Parmesan or Asiago cheese (optional)

1 pound cremini mushrooms

½ pound cherry tomatoes, halved

3 to 4 green onions, diced

3 cloves garlic, minced

¼ cup extra-virgin olive oil

1½ teaspoons sea salt

Freshly ground black pepper

½ teaspoon dried thyme

½ teaspoon dried oregano

substantial suppers

continued

1 tablespoon balsamic
    vinegar

½ cup cooked gigante (large
    white) beans (optional)

1 tablespoon unsalted
    butter

1 tablespoon flour

¼ cup half-and-half

¼ cup white wine

8 In a large bowl, place the mushrooms, tomatoes, green onions, garlic, oil, salt, pepper, thyme, and oregano and toss to coat. In a 9-by-13-inch baking dish, put the mushroom mixture and roast them for about 10 minutes. Stir the mushroom mixture and continue roasting them until the mushrooms are soft and juicy, 5 to 10 more minutes. Remove the baking dish from the oven from oven, add the vinegar and beans, and toss again.

9 In a large skillet over medium heat, melt the butter. Once the butter is sizzling, add the flour, reduce the heat to low, and whisk or stir constantly to make a thick paste (roux). Slowly add the half-and-half, a little at a time, continuing to whisk as the liquid combines with the roux to make a thick sauce. Whisk in the wine to establish a smooth cream sauce. Add the roasted mushrooms mixture to the skillet. Be sure to include all of the juices from the baking dish. Stir gently to coat.

10 Put two polenta slices in each of four bowls and divide the mushroom sauce on top of the polenta.

FOR BABIES 10 MONTHS & OLDER: Reserve some of the soft polenta—the perfect texture for baby.

sweet rice timbales
with black sesame sprinkles

Serving rice formed into pleasing shapes offers visual appeal. Pressure-cooking yields sticky rice that is easy to mold. Lovely served next to grilled fish or Sticky Szechwan Tempeh (page 275) and A+ Avocado Arame Almond Salad (page 218).

1 Rinse and drain the brown and sweet brown rice. In a pressure cooker, put the rice, salt, and water. Lock the cooker, place it on high heat, and bring up to pressure. When the pressure gauge rises and is firm, you will hear a gentle, steady hissing sound. Reduce the heat and cook for 35 to 40 minutes. Remove the cooker from the heat and allow the pressure to come down naturally or by drizzling cold water over the edge of the lid. Allow the rice to cool slightly, until just warm. (Alternatively, the rice can also be simmered in a heavy pot. Simmering takes 45 to 50 minutes.)

2 While rice is cooking, in a small saucepan over low heat, put the mirin, honey, and vinegar and cook until the honey melts and the mixture is warm. Pour the mirin mixture over the warm rice and stir to combine.

3 To serve, oil a small ramekin or cup. Pack the rice into the cup as densely as possible, keeping the top surface level. Place a serving plate on top of the ramekin and invert the ramekin. Garnish the top of the rice with some of the toasted seeds. Repeat with the remaining rice.

FOR BABIES 6 MONTHS & OLDER: Blend some of the cooked brown rice with breast milk or formula to make fresh-cooked cereal for baby!

PREPARATION TIME:

55 minutes

MAKES 6 TO 8 TIMBALES

1½ cups brown rice

½ cup sweet brown rice

½ teaspoon sea salt

3 cups water

2 tablespoons mirin

2 tablespoons honey

2 tablespoons rice vinegar

2 teaspoons toasted brown or black sesame seeds (see page 129 for toasting instructions)

substantial suppers

red bean & quinoa chili

Nutritious quinoa provides the bulk that ground beef would typically add to chili. Give this vegetarian version a whirl some chilly evening.

PREPARATION TIME:

30 minutes

MAKES 6 TO 8 SERVINGS

1 tablespoon extra-virgin olive oil

1 medium onion, finely chopped

2 teaspoons sea salt, divided

2 cloves garlic, minced

1 large green bell pepper, chopped

1 teaspoon ground cumin

1 teaspoon dried oregano

¼ teaspoon ground cinnamon

⅛ teaspoon cayenne

⅔ cup quinoa

1 cup fresh or frozen corn

1 to 2 cups tomato sauce

1 cup water

3 cups cooked kidney beans (see page 244 for cooking instructions), or 2 (15-ounce) cans kidney beans, drained

Grated jack or cheddar cheese (optional), for serving

1 In 4-quart pot over medium heat, heat the oil. Add the onion and sauté until the onion becomes soft and golden, 5 to 7 minutes. Add 1 teaspoon of the salt, the garlic, pepper, cumin, oregano, cinnamon, and cayenne. Sauté until aromatic, 2 to 3 minutes.

2 Rinse and drain the quinoa and then stir it into the pot. Add the corn, tomato sauce, and water. Increase the heat to high to establish a simmer, then reduce the heat to low, cover, and simmer until the quinoa has opened and become tender, about 20 minutes. Add the kidney beans and the remaining 1 teaspoon salt and simmer for 10 more minutes.

3 Top each serving with grated cheese.

FOR BABIES 10 MONTHS & OLDER: Serve cooked, mashed beans or puree some extra cooked corn. Or both!

moroccan rice & lentils *with* caramelized onions (mojadra)

Inexpensive and filling, this recipe takes rice and beans to a higher plane. Garlic Sautéed Rainbow Swiss Chard (page 199) makes an ideal side dish.

1 In a 4-quart pot over low heat, heat 1 tablespoon of the ghee. Add the rice and lentils and sauté until evenly coated, about 2 minutes. Add the garlic, 2 teaspoons of the salt, the cumin, coriander, turmeric, allspice, cinnamon, and cayenne and sauté, stirring constantly, until fragrance fills the air, about 2 more minutes. Add the water. Bring the rice and lentils to a bubbling boil, then reduce the heat to low, and simmer, covered, until all the water has been absorbed, about 40 minutes. Remove the pot from the heat, remove the lid, and allow the mixture to rest for a minimum of 10 minutes before serving.

2 In a 12-inch skillet over medium-low heat, melt the remaining 1 tablespoon ghee until it starts to sizzle but not burn. Add the onions and the remaining 1 teaspoon salt and move them around until the onions are coated. Reduce the heat to low and let the onions slowly cook down, stirring frequently, until the onions are golden, about 30 minutes.

3 If you feel that the onions are sticking to the bottom of the pan too much, add a small amount of the water (or white wine) to the pan and stir to deglaze them.

4 In a small bowl, combine the yogurt and dill. Serve the rice and lentils with the caramelized onions piled on top and a spoonful of yogurt dip on top of that!

PREPARATION TIME:

50 minutes

MAKES 6 SERVINGS

2 tablespoons Homemade Ghee (page 383) or unsalted butter, divided

1 cup basmati brown rice

1 cup dried brown or green lentils

2 cloves garlic, minced

3 teaspoons sea salt, divided

2 teaspoons ground cumin

1½ teaspoons ground coriander

1 teaspoon ground turmeric

1 teaspoon ground allspice

½ teaspoon ground cinnamon

⅛ teaspoon cayenne

3¾ cups water

2 large onions, thinly sliced into half moons

¼ cup water or white wine

1 cup plain whole milk yogurt, for serving

1 tablespoon fresh dill, or 1 teaspoon dried dill, for serving

substantial suppers

FOR BABIES 10 MONTHS & OLDER: Puree some of the lentil-rice mixture.

pan-fried tofu & greens *with* almond-ginger drizzle (bathing rama)

The traditional way to make the Thai dish Bathing Rama features tofu served on a bed of cooked spinach. For a new twist on this classic, this recipe replaces spinach with collards and swaps out white rice with soba noodles. Creamy cashew butter can be subbed in for the almond butter, or, another slightly richer option, Coconut Peanut Sauce (page 361) works well too.

PREPARATION TIME:

8 hours (for marinating);
30 minutes

MAKES 4 SERVINGS

For the marinade:

3 cloves garlic, sliced

1 (2-inch) piece fresh gingerroot, thinly sliced

1 cup water

1 tablespoon rice vinegar

1 tablespoon toasted
  sesame oil

⅓ cup tamari (soy sauce)

1 pound firm tofu

2 tablespoons unrefined
  coconut oil

1 large bunch collard greens

½ teaspoon sea salt

1 (8-ounce) soba noodles

¼ cup creamy almond butter

2 teaspoons maple syrup

2 tablespoons tamari
  (soy sauce)

1 tablespoon rice vinegar

1 To make the marinade, in a medium bowl, combine garlic, ginger, water, vinegar, oil, and tamari. Cut the tofu into ½-inch rectangles, and then cut each slab into triangles. Put the tofu slices in the bowl with the marinade, cover, and let it rest for at least ½ hour and up to 8 hours in the refrigerator. The longer it sits, the stronger the flavor.

2 When the tofu has finished marinating, in a skillet over medium-high heat, heat 1 tablespoon of the coconut oil. Remove the tofu from the marinade and pat it dry with a paper towel. This protects you from sputtering oil. Place half of the tofu pieces in the oil and brown both sides, about 1 minute per side. Remove the fried tofu to a paper towel. The heat should be high enough that the tofu browns quickly to give the skin a crispy texture. Repeat with the remaining 1 tablespoon coconut oil and the remaining tofu.

3 To prepare the collards, first pull the leaves away from the stem, discard the stems, and wash the greens carefully. In an 8-quart pot over high heat, bring 2 quarts of water and the salt to a boil. Submerge the collards. Boil until the collards have wilted but still retain a bright green color, 5 to 8 minutes. Sample a piece; the cooked collards should be easy to chew and sweet, not bitter. Pour the collards into a colander in the sink and drizzle cool water over them to halt cooking. When cooled, the collards and squeeze out the excess water with your hands. Chop them into bite-size pieces and set aside.

4 Refill the 8-quart pot with water and bring it to a boil over high heat. Cook the soba noodles according to directions on the package.

5 While noodles are cooking, make the sauce. In a small pan on low to medium heat, put the almond butter, maple syrup, tamari, vinegar, ginger, sesame oil, and water. Using a whisk, mix together until smooth and warm, 3 to 5 minutes. If necessary, add extra water to achieve desired consistency.

6 Serve the noodles with the cooked collards and browned tofu on top. Drizzle the sauce on top.

FOR BABIES 10 MONTHS & OLDER: Reserve some unmarinated tofu, cut up into cubes, and serve it with bite-size pieces of cooked noodles.

VARIATION FOR CHILDREN: Separate the foods. Serve plain noodles, fried tofu, a small pile of collards, and a little bowl of the sauce for dipping.

---

1 tablespoon freshly grated gingerroot

1 teaspoon toasted sesame oil

⅓ cup water

substantial suppers

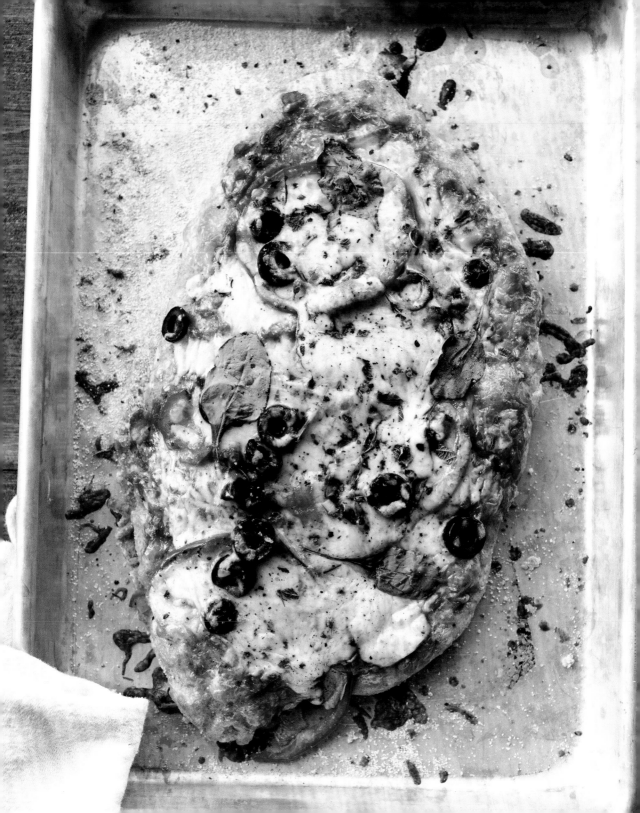

veggie lovers' pizza party

All hands on deck! Get children involved in the tactile fun of making individual pizzas. This recipe yields six (eight-inch) pies, so invite some friends over and make a party of it. Fresh whole grain pizza dough takes about fifteen minutes to make or you can buy premade mixes. Gluten-free packaged pizza dough options are also available.

1 Preheat the oven to 425 degrees F. Place a pizza stone or cast-iron griddle on the lowest rack.

2 In a large bowl, combine the mushrooms, peppers, tomato, oil, oregano, dried basil, and salt and toss well. In a 9-by-13-inch baking dish, roast the vegetable mixture until the vegetables are soft and juicy, about 10 minutes. Remove the baking dish from the oven, stir in the olives and fresh basil, and set aside.

3 On a baking sheet dusted with cornmeal, form the dough into six flat rounds by using your fingertips to make little tapping indentations, flattening and rounding the dough into 8-inch crusts, rather than pulling or stretching.

4 Increase the oven heat to 450 degrees F.

5 Spread 2 to 3 tablespoons of marinara sauce on the surface of each dough round, keeping the sauce toward the perimeter of the round, rather than the center, and leaving ½ inch around perimeter. Cover the sauce with 1 cup of roasted vegetable mix per pizza, again keeping the toppings toward the outside rather than mounding them in the middle to keep pizzas from being too heavy in the center. Divide the mozzarella and Parmesan among the six pizzas. Slide the pizzas onto the prepared pizza stone with a pizza peel or a flat (non-lipped) baking sheet. Depending on the size of your pizza stone,

PREPARATION TIME:
40 to 45 minutes

MAKES SIX 8-INCH PIZZAS

12 ounces (12 to 15) mushrooms, sliced

1 green bell pepper, diced

1 red bell pepper, diced

1 large heirloom tomato, diced

¼ cup extra-virgin olive oil

2 teaspoons dried oregano

2 teaspoons dried basil

1½ teaspoons sea salt

3 to 4 ounces (about 24) pitted kalamata olives, halved

1 cup fresh basil or baby spinach leaves, shredded

Cornmeal or rice flour, for dusting

Marilyn's Best Pizza Dough (page 118) or store-bought

¾ cup marinara sauce

10 ounces mozzarella cheese, shredded (about 4 loose cups)

4 ounces Parmesan cheese, shredded (1½ cups)

substantial suppers

continued

bake the pizzas one or two at a time, until crust edges are golden and cheese is bubbling, about 6 minutes.

6 If using a pizza peel, slip each cooked pizza on the peel, turn on the broiler, and raise the pizza to about 4 inches away from the top of the oven for just a minute or less. This will brown and bubble the top of the pizza in a yummy way.

FOR BABIES 10 MONTHS & OLDER: Pick out some soft roasted mushrooms, puree or mince them, and serve.

VARIATION FOR CHILDREN: Separate the mushrooms, peppers, and tomatoes to roast them. Provide all toppings in small bowls and allow the children to decorate their own pizza before baking.

walnut rice & spice burgers

Pile up a bun with mustard, pickle, tomato, or your favorite condiment and chow down without bothering a single cow. The nut-and-grain combination has enough "stick" to easily form patties.

1 In a small grinder, blender, or food processor, grind the sunflower seeds and walnuts into a fine meal. In a large bowl, put the seed-walnut meal, garlic, cumin, oregano, salt, cayenne, and carrot and mix well. Fold in the cooked rice. Add the tomato sauce a little at a time until you get a stiff but workable texture.

2 Form the rice mixture into patties with moist hands. (Refrigerate the patties for a few hours if possible.) In a skillet over medium heat, heat the oil. Brown the patties on both sides until a light crust forms on the surface and they are warm throughout, about 2 minutes on each side.

3 Serve the patties on whole grain buns.

FOR BABIES 6 MONTHS & OLDER: Puree extra cooked brown rice with a little breast milk or water.

PREPARATION TIME:

15 to 20 minutes

MAKES 4 SERVINGS

¾ cup sunflower seeds

¾ cup raw walnuts

2 cloves garlic, finely chopped

1 teaspoon ground cumin

1 teaspoon dried oregano, or 1 tablespoon fresh oregano

½ teaspoon sea salt

⅛ teaspoon cayenne

1 small carrot or ½ of a large carrot, finely grated

1½ cups cooked brown rice (see page 242 for cooking instructions)

2 tablespoons tomato sauce

2 teaspoons high-heat vegetable oil, such as safflower or peanut

4 sprouted (or other) whole grain buns

substantial suppers

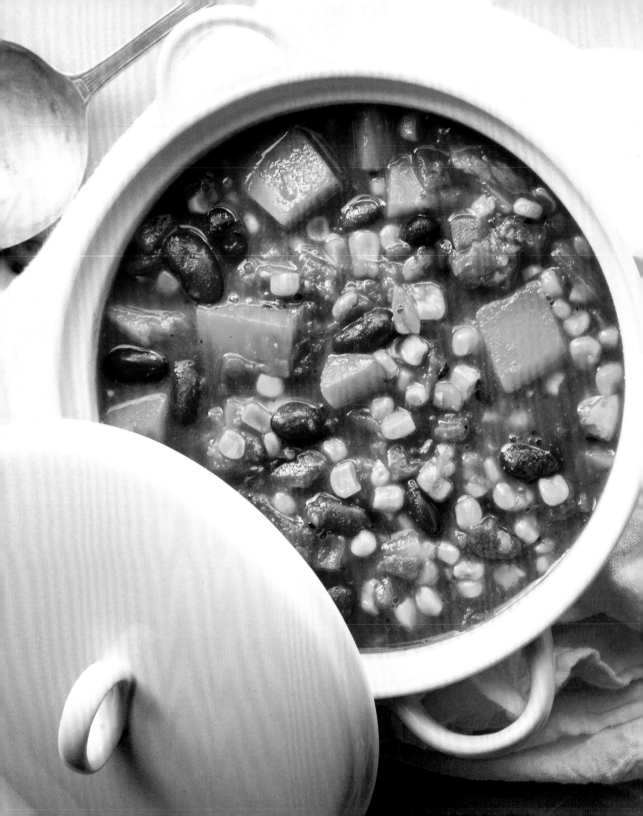

the three sisters (squash, corn, beans) stew

Native Americans grew corn and planted beans at the base. The corn stalks served as a beanpole. The ground space between the stalks was used to grow squash, letting it ramble. The three sisters (corn, beans, and squash) mature harmoniously. If you choose delicata squash (yellow with green stripes), the skin is thin enough that there's no need to peel.

1 In a 4-quart pot over medium-low heat, heat the oil, then add the cumin, oregano, chili powder, and cinnamon and sauté for about 30 seconds. Add the onion, salt, and garlic and sauté until the onion is soft, about 5 minutes.

2 Add the squash and tomatoes, and bring the pot to a simmer. Cover and cook until the squash is fork-tender, about 20 minutes. Add ¼ to ½ cup water if the mixture seems dry.

3 Stir in the cooked beans and corn and simmer until the corn is tender, about 3 to 5 more minute. Taste and add more salt if desired. Starches such as squash and beans can take more salt than you might imagine to bring up the flavor.

4 Serve the stew hot, garnished with cheese.

FOR BABIES 6 MONTHS & OLDER: Reserve some peeled squash cubes, steam or bake them until tender, puree, and serve.

FOR BABIES 10 MONTHS & OLDER: Retrieve some well-cooked squash from the stew, puree and serve.

PREPARATION TIME:

40 minutes

MAKES 6 TO 8 SERVINGS

1 tablespoon extra-virgin olive oil or Homemade Ghee (page 383)

1½ teaspoons ground cumin

1½ teaspoons dried oregano

1 teaspoon chili powder

½ teaspoon ground cinnamon

1 medium onion, finely chopped

2 teaspoons sea salt, plus more if needed

3 cloves garlic, minced

2 pounds winter squash, peeled and cut into 1-inch chunks (2 to 3 cups)

1 (14-ounce) can chopped tomatoes

3 cups cooked pinto or red beans (see page 244 for cooking instructions), or 2 (15-ounce) cans pinto or red beans, drained

1½ cups fresh or frozen corn

½ cup grated Jack or cheddar cheese (optional), for garnish

curried cauliflower dal

Keeping your favorite spice blends handy for Indian, Mexican, or Thai dishes cuts down on time spent hunting for multiple small jars. Since Indian food is a favorite in our house, a jar of Homemade Curry Paste (page 382) resides in the refrigerator. A tablespoon of this aromatic paste replaces the dry spices in this recipe.

PREPARATION TIME:

40 to 45 minutes

MAKES 4 SERVINGS

1 cup dried lentils

1 bay leaf

2¾ to 3 cups water, divided

2 teaspoons Homemade Ghee (page 383) or extra-virgin olive oil

1 medium onion, finely chopped

1 clove garlic, minced

1 teaspoon ground coriander

1 teaspoon ground cumin

1 teaspoon ground turmeric

½ teaspoon ground cinnamon

2 teaspoons sea salt, divided

1 small head cauliflower, cut into small florets

1 cup tomato sauce

1 teaspoon freshly grated gingerroot

3 cups cooked brown rice (see page 242 for cooking instructions), for serving

Yogurt Cucumber Topping (page 364) or plain yogurt, for garnish

½ cup roasted cashews, for garnish

1 Rinse and drain the lentils. In a 2-quart pot over high heat, put the lentils, bay leaf, and 2 cups of the water and bring it to a boil. Reduce the heat to low and simmer, covered, until the lentils are tender and all of the water has been absorbed, 25 to 30 minutes.

2 In a 4-quart pot over medium-low heat, melt the ghee. Add the onion and sauté until golden, about 5 to 7 minutes. In Indian cooking taking the time to fully caramelize the onion is key to developing the flavor in the dish.

3 Add the garlic, coriander, cumin, turmeric, cinnamon, and 1 teaspoon of the salt and stir. Add the cauliflower, tomato sauce, ginger, and the remaining ¾ to 1 cup water and stir well. Simmer, covered, until the cauliflower is tender, 15 to 20 minutes.

4 Stir the cooked lentils into the cauliflower mixture, discarding the bay leaf. Add the remaining salt ¼ teaspoon at a time, until the taste seems right. Serve over rice and garnish with yogurt and roasted cashews.

FOR BABIES 10 MONTHS & OLDER: Pluck out a few cauliflower pieces from the cooked curry and puree it with some water for baby.

lime & chili tempeh tacos

One of my students, Jeff Johnson, presented this dish as part of his final project. I nabbed his creative recipe and serve it as an alternative to beef tacos. Fresh Corn Salsa (page 366) is the perfect condiment.

1 In a medium bowl, put the tempeh. Set aside.

2 In a small bowl, combine 1 tablespoon of the oil, the salt, lime juice, and chili powder and then pour this marinade over the tempeh. Let it marinate for 30 minutes or up to several hours; more time allows the tempeh to absorb more of the flavor.

3 In a large skillet over medium heat, heat the remaining 1 tablespoon oil. Add the onion and sauté until soft, about 3 to 5 minutes. Increase the heat slightly and add the marinated tempeh. Keep the tempeh moving in the pan until it turns golden brown, 4 to 6 minutes. Add the cilantro just prior to serving.

4 Warm the taco shells according to the directions on the package. Fill each shell with the tempeh mixture and top with avocado, cheese, salsa, and lettuce.

FOR BABIES 6 MONTHS & OLDER: Serve the tacos with ripe avocado slices and reserve some of the avocado for baby. Puree or mash well and serve.

PREPARATION TIME:

30 minutes (for marinating); 15 minutes

MAKES 6 TO 8 SERVINGS

2 (8-ounce) packages tempeh, crumbled or chopped into small pieces

2 tablespoons extra-virgin olive oil, divided

1 teaspoon sea salt

¼ cup freshly squeezed lime juice (from 2 large limes)

1 tablespoon chili powder

1 medium onion, finely chopped

¼ cup chopped fresh cilantro

12 taco shells

Avocado slices (optional)

Grated pepper jack or mozzarella cheese (optional)

Salsa (optional)

Shredded lettuce (optional)

middle eastern chickpea falafel

The secret to preparing falafel is to chill the patties before frying. Serve with Lemon Tahini Sauce (page 365).

PREPARATION TIME:

6 to 8 hours (for soaking);
30 minutes (for chilling);
10 minutes (for frying)

MAKES 12 TO 18 PATTIES

1 cup dried chickpeas

2 teaspoons sea salt, divided

1 medium onion, cut into chunks

2 cloves garlic

½ cup fresh Italian parsley

1 tablespoon freshly squeezed lemon juice

1 teaspoon ground coriander

1 teaspoon ground cumin

½ teaspoon baking powder

½ teaspoon freshly ground black pepper

⅛ teaspoon cayenne

¼ to ½ cup unrefined coconut oil, for frying

4 whole grain pitas

Romaine lettuce, shredded

Sliced tomatoes

Lemon Tahini Sauce (page 365) or store-bought

1 In a large bowl, soak the chickpeas in about 5 cups of water with 1 teaspoon of the salt for 6 to 8 hours. Drain the soaked chickpeas and put them in a food processor. Pulse the beans into a crumbly texture, scraping the sides as necessary. Don't overprocess them into a paste!

2 Add the onion, garlic, parsley, lemon juice, coriander, cumin, baking powder, pepper, cayenne, and the remaining 1 teaspoon salt and pulse several more times. Test the mixture. Once it sticks together when you squeeze it with your hand, it's the right consistency.

3 Using your hands, firmly squeeze about ⅓ cup of the chickpea mixture into a 3-inch ball and then slightly flatten the ball into a small patty. Repeat with the remaining chickpea mixture. Place the patties in a pan or on a plate, cover, and refrigerate for at least 30 minutes or up to 8 hours.

4 In a 12-inch frying pan over high heat, heat 3 tablespoons of the coconut oil until it is hot but not smoking. Place half of the patties in the oil until they sizzle and brown, about 2 minutes. Turn each patty over, adding extra oil if needed, and fry until the patties are brown on both sides, 30 to 60 seconds more. If the patties fall apart, the oil is not hot enough. Remove the patties to paper towels until all of the patties have been fried.

5 Divide the falafel among the four pitas and top with the lettuce, tomatoes, and tahini sauce.

FOR BABIES 10 MONTHS & OLDER: Stir a dab of tahini into baby's cereal for added quality fat.

sloppeh tempeh joes

The vegetarian version of the familiar classic was styled after one of my mother's recipes from the '60s. I guess it goes without saying that the same flavorings can be added to cooked ground beef instead of tempeh, which was how my mom made it. Serve with corn on the cob and Creamy Lemon Coleslaw (page 211).

1 Preheat the oven to 175 degrees F.

2 In a 10-inch skillet over medium heat, heat the oil. Add the onion, pepper, garlic, and salt and sauté until soft, 3 to 5 minutes. Add the tempeh to the onion mixture, then raise the heat slightly and let the tempeh brown, stirring occasionally so that all sides are browned, 3 to 5 minutes.

3 In a small bowl, mix together the ketchup, mustard, vinegar, and cloves. Add the ketchup mixture to tempeh mixture, and stir to thoroughly combine. Warm the buns in the oven. Spoon the tempeh mixture onto buns and serve.

FOR BABIES 6 MONTHS & OLDER: If serving corn on the cob as a side dish, skin some cooked corn off of the cob and puree for baby.

PREPARATION TIME:

20 minutes

MAKES 4 SERVINGS

2 teaspoons extra-virgin olive oil

1 medium onion, finely chopped

1 green bell pepper, diced

1 clove garlic, minced

½ teaspoon sea salt

1 (8-ounce) package tempeh, crumbled

⅔ cup Kitchen Ketchup (page 377) or store-bought

2 teaspoons whole grain mustard

1 tablespoon rice vinegar

½ teaspoon ground cloves

4 sprouted whole grain hamburger buns

substantial suppers

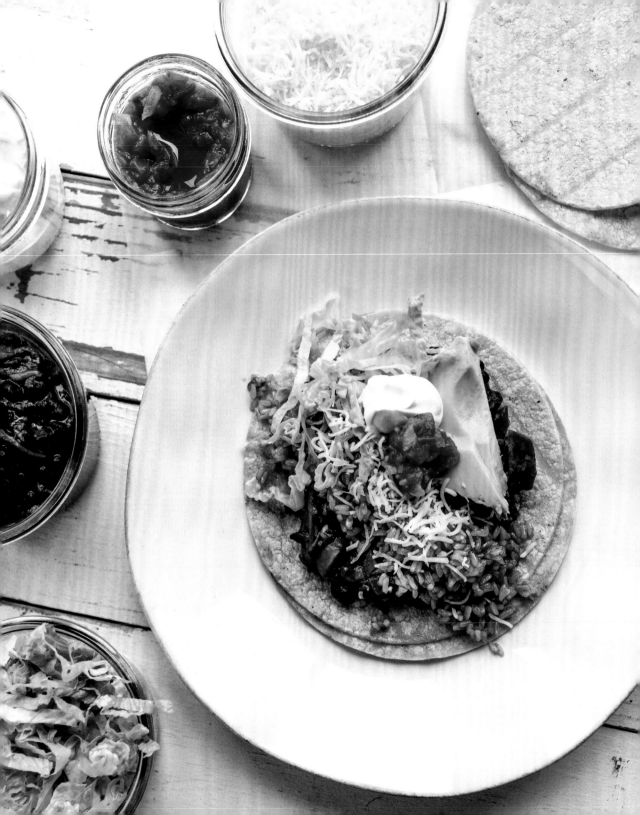

chipotle–black bean tostados

Cooking beans from scratch allows you to infuse the beans with more flavor and control the texture. Canned beans can be lackluster by comparison.

1 In a large bowl, place the beans with 10 cups of water and 2 teaspoons of the salt. Allow the beans to soak for 8 to 10 hours.

2 In a 4-quart pot over medium heat or a pressure cooker, heat the oil. Sauté the onion, garlic, and cumin until onions are soft, about 3 to 5 minutes. Drain the soaking water from the beans. Add the beans, chili, the remaining 2 teaspoons salt, and the stock to onions and spices and bring to boil over high heat.

3 Reduce the heat to low, covered, until beans are tender and all the water has been absorbed, 50 to 55 minutes, or, if using a pressure cooker, bring up to pressure for 40 to 45 minutes. Stir in the cilantro and tomatoes. If the beans are tender but the mixture is still watery, to preserve flavor, uncover and cook off the additional liquid rather than draining it off.

4 Bake or heat the tortillas (per instructions on the package). Serve the tortillas, beans, and your preferred garnishes family style.

FOR BABIES 10 MONTHS & OLDER: Reserve some cooked black beans, mash them well, and serve. Serve the beans in small amounts until baby gets used to digesting them.

PREPARATION TIME:

8 to 10 hours (for soaking); 1 hour (for cooking)

MAKES 12 TO 14 TOSTADOS

2 cups dried black beans

4 teaspoons sea salt, divided

1 tablespoon extra-virgin olive oil

1 medium onion, finely chopped

4 cloves garlic, minced

1 teaspoon ground cumin

1 dried chipotle chili

4 cups Easy Vegetarian Stock (page 168), Simple Chicken Stock (page 165), or water

¼ cup chopped fresh cilantro

½ cup chopped tomatoes

12 to 14 corn tortillas

For garnish/sides:

Avocado slices (optional)

Grated pepper jack or cheddar cheese (optional)

Grated zucchini (optional)

Leaf lettuce, thinly sliced (optional)

Mexican Brown Rice (page 250) (optional)

Sour cream (optional)

Salsa (optional)

substantial suppers

tofu-kale-mustard-dill supper pie

A vegan version of quiche, this dish utilizes super-nutritious kale and carrots. Umeboshi vinegar, the leftover liquid from making umeboshi plums, gives a unique sour-salty zip to the filling but can be replaced with a tablespoon of lemon juice and one-eighth teaspoon of salt.

PREPARATION TIME:

55 minutes

MAKES 8 SLICES

For the crust:

1 cup whole wheat pastry flour

½ teaspoon sea salt

¼ cup (½ stick) cold unsalted butter

2 tablespoons cold unrefined coconut oil

2 tablespoons ice-cold water

For the filling:

2 tablespoons extra-virgin olive oil, divided

1 medium onion, finely chopped

2 carrots, thinly cut into half moons

1 bunch kale leaves, de-stemmed and thinly sliced (chiffonade)

1 pound firm tofu

1 tablespoon *umeboshi* vinegar

1 Preheat the oven to 350 degrees F.

2 To make the crust, in a large bowl, add the flour and salt. Cut the butter and coconut oil into the flour with a pastry cutter or two knives until crumbly. Slowly dribble the water into the flour, blending with a fork. (Alternately, the butter and coconut oil can be incorporated into the flour and salt in a food processor, then water added slowly while pulsing to make the dough.)

3 Gather the dough into a ball; it should be moist and pliable. On a floured surface or a piece of wax paper, roll the dough out into a 9- or 10-inch round. Fold and transfer the dough to an 8- or 9-inch pie pan. Unfold the dough, press it in against the pan, and trim the edges. Prebake the crust for 10 minutes.

4 To make the filling, in a large skillet over medium heat, heat 1 tablespoon of the oil. Add the onion and carrots and sauté until the onion is soft, 3 to 5 minutes. Add the kale ribbons to the onions, turning several times until the kale begins to wilt. Add ¼ cup water to the skillet, reduce the heat to low, and cover while you prepare the tofu filling.

5 In a food processor or blender, puree the tofu, vinegar, mustard, tamari, dill, salt, and the remaining 1 tablespoon of oil until a smooth consistency is created. If using firm tofu, you may need to add a little water. The mixture should be very thick but pourable.

6 To assemble pie, put the onion-carrot-kale mixture in the bottom of the prebaked crust. Pour the tofu mixture over the top, covering the vegetables. Bake until the top of the pie begins to turn beige at the edges, about 30 minutes. Allow the pie to set for 10 minutes, then cut and serve.

1 tablespoon yellow mustard

2 teaspoons tamari (soy sauce)

1½ teaspoons fresh dill, or ½ teaspoon dried dill

½ teaspoon sea salt

FOR BABIES 6 MONTHS & OLDER: Remove softened carrot slices from the skillet and puree.

FOR BABIES 10 MONTHS & OLDER: Remove softened carrot slices and kale ribbons from the skillet and puree with a bit of tofu.

---

substantial suppers

peasant kasha, potatoes & mushrooms

Kasha and potatoes combine here for a rib-sticking dish that works for break-fast or dinner. Perch a Swirling Poached Egg (page 98) and Apple-Fennel Sauerkraut (page 223) on top for a hearty morning meal or serve next to Dr. Bruce's Awesome Grilled Salmon (page 282) at suppertime.

PREPARATION TIME:

25 to 30 minutes

MAKES 6 SERVINGS

1 tablespoon unsalted butter or extra-virgin olive oil

1 small onion, finely
   chopped

2 cloves garlic, minced

1 teaspoon sea salt

1 small red potato, cut into
   ¼-inch dice

3 to 4 mushrooms, cut into
   thin slivers or dice

1 cup kasha

2 cups boiling water

Freshly ground black pepper

1 In a 2-quart pot or straight-sided skillet over medium heat, melt the butter. Add the onions, garlic, and salt and sauté, stirring frequently, until the onion is golden and soft, about 5 minutes. Add the potatoes and mush-rooms and sauté, covered, until they are softened and juicy, 2 to 3 more minutes. Don't hurry this process. Allow each ingredient to have time on the heat before adding the next.

2 Add kasha to mixture and stir, coating the kasha. Pour in the boiling water. Reduce the heat to low. The kasha should be percolating gently, not bubbling. Cover the pot and simmer until all the water is absorbed, about 15 minutes. Remove the pot from the heat, remove the lid, and allow the kasha to rest for 10 minutes.

3 Fluff the kasha and serve garnished with pepper. The dish will likely need more salt; add a little at a time to bring up the flavor.

FOR BABIES 10 MONTHS & OLDER: Remove a baby-size portion, mash the potato with a fork, slice the mush-rooms into tiny pieces, and serve.

sticky szechwan tempeh

In my classes, this dish is used to teach students how to use "reduction" to create a syrupy sauce. We often serve it over cooked quinoa (see page 242 for cooking instructions) with Mango Salsa (page 368) to form a balanced and satisfying meal.

1 In a 10- to 12-inch skillet over medium-high heat, heat 2 tablespoons of the coconut oil until it is hot but not smoking. Place half of the tempeh strips in the skillet and let them quick fry, turning them so that both sides brown, about 1 minute per side. Remove the fried tempeh to a paper towel and repeat the process with the other half of the tempeh strips. Remove the skillet from the heat and let it cool.

2 In a small bowl, whisk together the miso and water until the miso is dissolved. Add the tamari, mirin, vinegar, maple syrup, and sesame oil and whisk again. Put the fried tempeh back in the skillet over medium-low heat. Pour the miso sauce over the tempeh and bring it to a low simmer. The sauce will begin to reduce and thicken.

3 Once the sauce becomes thick and glistening, garnish with green onion and serve immediately.

PREPARATION TIME:

20 minutes

MAKES 3 SERVINGS

¼ cup unrefined coconut oil

1 (8-ounce) package tempeh, cut into ¼-inch strips

2 tablespoons white miso

¼ to ⅓ cup water

2 tablespoons tamari (soy sauce)

2 tablespoons mirin

2 tablespoons balsamic vinegar

2 tablespoons maple syrup

2 teaspoons toasted sesame oil or hot pepper oil

1 green onion, thinly sliced, for garnish

substantial suppers

FOR BABIES 6 MONTHS & OLDER: Serve this dish over cooked quinoa. Reserve some of the cooked grain and puree with water or breast milk to make cereal for baby.

VARIATION FOR CHILDREN: Reserve some of the crispy fried tempeh before adding it to the sauce and serve it with a sprinkle of tamari.

spinach-feta quiche

To create a whole grain piecrust that is flaky and tasty, I find that the best combination of fats for texture and flavor is two parts unsalted organic butter and one part unrefined coconut oil or lard. The crust can be made ahead of time, wrapped tightly in plastic, and stored in the refrigerator to reduce preparation time.

feeding the whole family

PREPARATION TIME:

55 minutes

MAKES 8 SERVINGS

For the crust:

1 cup whole wheat pastry flour

½ teaspoon sea salt

¼ cup (½ stick) cold unsalted butter

2 tablespoons cold unrefined coconut oil

2 tablespoons ice-cold water

1½ cups whole milk or half-and-half

4 eggs

½ teaspoon sea salt

2 cups baby spinach leaves

1 cup crumbled feta cheese

½ ripe tomato, thinly cut into slices

1 Preheat the oven to 375 degrees F.

2 To make the crust, in a large bowl, add the flour and salt. Cut the butter and oil into the flour with a pastry cutter or two knives until crumbly. Slowly dribble the water into the flour mixture, blending with a fork. (Alternately, the butter and oil can be incorporated into the flour mixture in a food processor, and then the water added slowly while pulsing to make the dough.) Gather the dough into a ball; it should be moist and pliable. On a floured surface or a piece of wax paper, roll the dough out into a 9- to 10-inch round. Fold dough in half, then in half again so that you have formed a triangle. Transfer the dough to an 8-inch pie pan, with the point of the triangle dead center, then unfold the dough, press it in against the pie pan, and trim the edges.

3 In a small pan over medium-low heat, scald the milk (this hastens baking time). Let the milk cool until touchable, then, in a medium bowl, whisk the milk, eggs, and salt together. Sprinkle the spinach and feta in the bottom of the crust and pour the egg mixture over the top. Decorate the top with tomato slices in a pleasing arrangement.

4 Bake until the top is golden, 35 to 40 minutes. Insert a knife to test for doneness. It should come out clean. Let the quiche cool slightly before serving.

FOR BABIES 10 MONTHS & OLDER: Remember that egg whites are inappropriate for infants under 1 year of age. Egg yolks, however, are an excellent source of essential fatty acids. Boil an egg for 3 to 4 minutes, peel, discard the white, and serve the warm yolk to baby with a spoon or added to a baked squash or sweet potato.

---

greek shrimp stew *with* feta & dill

To find shrimp from reliable, sustainable sources, check Monterey Bay Aquarium's Seafood Watch guide. Most shrimp caught or farmed using a recirculating aquaculture system in the United States and Canada is a "Best Choice." Oregon pink shrimp, certified sustainable, is a good choice for this stew.

PREPARATION TIME:

30 minutes

MAKES 6 SERVINGS

1 tablespoon extra-virgin olive oil

2 onions, chopped

1 teaspoon sea salt

4 cloves garlic, minced

1 (28-ounce) can chopped or diced tomatoes

1 (8-ounce) can tomato sauce

2 teaspoons Dijon mustard

3 tablespoons fresh dill, or 1 tablespoon dried dill

1 teaspoon honey

1 pound cooked shrimp

¼ to ½ pound feta cheese, crumbled

1 cup chopped fresh Italian parsley

1 In a 4-quart soup pot over medium-low heat, heat the oil, then add the onions, salt, and garlic. Sauté until the onions are soft and golden, about 5 minutes. Add the tomatoes, tomato sauce, mustard, dill, and honey and simmer for 20 minutes.

2 Add the shrimp, feta, and parsley 5 minutes before serving. Stir well and serve once the shrimp is thoroughly warm.

FOR BABIES 10 MONTHS & OLDER: Retrieve one or two cooked shrimp and mince well. Serve mixed into a familiar mashed vegetable such as sweet potato.

caribbean lime halibut

Deceptively simple, this fish delivers tantalizing flavor. In my classes, it is often served with Emerald City Salad (page 135).

1 In a small bowl, put the tamari, 1 tablespoon of the oil, the lime juice, ginger, honey, and garlic and whisk together. Place the fish skin side up in a shallow pan and pour the marinade over it. Be sure that the flesh of the fish is immersed in the marinade. Allow it to marinate 30 to 60 minutes in the refrigerator.

2 Preheat the oven to 400 degrees F.

3 In an ovenproof skillet, cast-iron works well, over medium-high heat, heat the remaining 2 tablespoons oil. Place the halibut in the pan, skin side up, and sear for 1 minute, turn, and then sear the other side for 1 more minute.

4 Leave the fish in the skillet and place it in the oven. Bake until the fish is almost cooked through, 7 to 10 minutes, depending on the thickness of the fish (the rule is 10 minutes total cooking time per inch of fish thickness).

5 Remove the skillet from the oven and place it on the stove. Add any remaining marinade to the hot pan. It will quickly thicken into a sauce surrounding the fish.

FOR BABIES 6 MONTHS & OLDER: This dish is lovely served with a wild rice or quinoa dish. Reserve some of the cooked grain and puree with water to make cereal for baby.

FOR BABIES 10 MONTHS & OLDER: If your baby has some emerging teeth, it might be time to introduce fish. Finely chop a piece of cooked halibut, taking care to remove all tiny bones before serving to baby.

PREPARATION TIME:

30 to 60 minutes (for marinating); 10 to 15 minutes (for cooking)

MAKES 4 SERVINGS

1 tablespoon tamari (soy sauce)

3 tablespoons extra-virgin olive oil, divided

3 tablespoons freshly squeezed lime juice

1 tablespoon freshly grated gingerroot

1 teaspoon honey or sugar

3 to 4 cloves garlic, minced

1 pound halibut fillet

substantial suppers

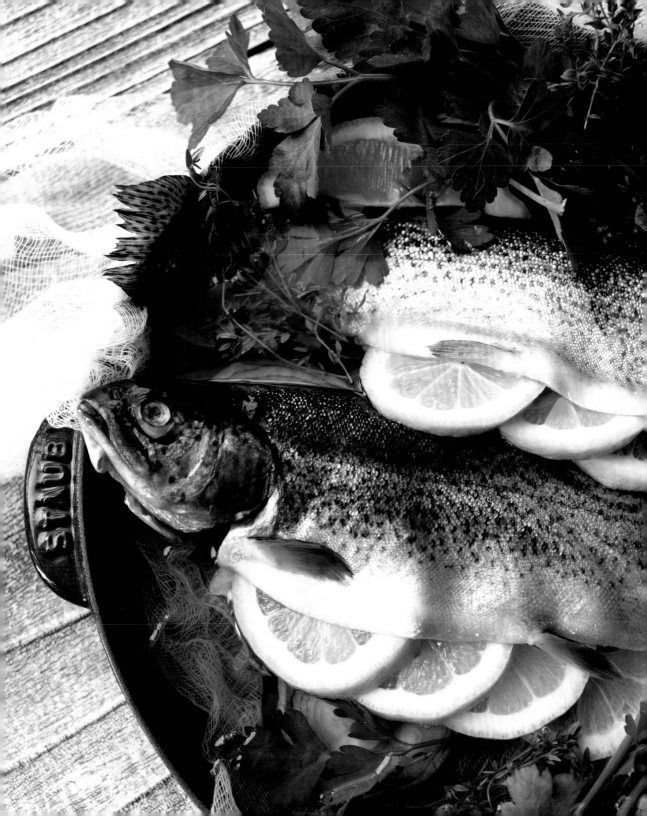

rainbow trout poached *in* herbs

When I was growing up, my family went to southern Colorado every August for vacation. My dad fished the Conejos River and caught fresh rainbow trout. Catching my first trout was a rite of passage. Luckily, the Monterey Bay Aquarium Seafood Watch gives widely available US farm-raised trout a thumbs-up for sustainability.

1 To make the poaching liquid, in an 8-quart pot over medium heat, heat the oil. Add the onion and salt and sauté until soft, about 5 minutes. Add the water, wine, bay leaves, thyme, and parsley. Bring the liquid to a gentle simmer, covered, until tastes are integrated, 5 to 7 more minutes.

2 While the poaching liquid is simmering, prepare the fish. Gently rinse each whole fish. Place the lemon slices in the body of each fish, then wrap each whole fish in cheesecloth, leaving long ends of cloth at the head and tail. Lower both fish into the poaching water, leaving the long ends of the cheesecloth draped over the edge of the pan. Let the fish cook for 6 to 8 minutes, depending on the size of the fish.

3 Using the dry ends of the cheesecloth, remove the fish from the poaching liquid. Remove the fish from the cheesecloth. Open each fillet down the middle and, pulling from the tail, remove the spines. Let the heads come off as well or remove them with a knife. Gently lift out the meat of the fish and serve immediately.

FOR BABIES 10 MONTHS & OLDER: If your baby has some emerging teeth, it might be time to introduce fish. This fish is very tender and mild tasting. Chop it up finely, taking care to remove all tiny bones before serving to baby.

PREPARATION TIME:

20 to 25 minutes

MAKES 4 SERVINGS

2 teaspoons extra-virgin olive oil

1 medium onion, chopped

1 teaspoon sea salt

2 quarts water

1 cup white wine

2 bay leaves

4 to 5 sprigs fresh thyme

4 to 5 sprigs fresh Italian parsley

2 pounds (2 small) whole, fresh rainbow trout

½ medium lemon, thinly sliced

2 to 3 feet of cheesecloth

dr. bruce's awesome grilled salmon

Dr. Bruce Gardner, a family practitioner, prepared this mouthwatering delicacy at a summer picnic. The ginger-lime marinade makes the salmon "awesome." Be sure to purchase wild Alaskan salmon if possible, not farm raised or "Atlantic" (often a pseudonym for farm raised). Wild salmon develop those precious omega-3 fatty acids by having to swim upstream!

PREPARATION TIME:

45 to 60 (for marinating);
10 to 15 minutes
(for grilling)

MAKES 8 TO 10 SERVINGS

2 to 3 pounds salmon fillet

⅓ cup tamari (soy sauce)

2 tablespoons freshly
   grated gingerroot

2 tablespoons freshly
   squeezed lime juice

2 teaspoons toasted
   sesame oil

4 cloves garlic, minced

4 green onions, finely
   chopped

2 red bell peppers, cut into
   thick slices, for garnish

1 Check the flesh of the salmon for pin bones by running your fingers over the surface. Remove any bones with tweezers or needle-nose pliers.

2 In a small bowl, put the tamari, ginger, lime juice, oil, garlic, and green onions and whisk together. Place the fish in a shallow pan and pour the marinade over the top. Allow the fish to marinate for 45 to 60 minutes in the refrigerator, covered.

3 Heat the grill. When your grill is hot, remove the fish from the pan and place it on the grill, skin side down. Place the pepper slices to the side. Brush the top of each fillet with any marinade remaining in the bottom of the pan and grill until the fish flesh facing the grill is well seared, about 5 minutes. (The rule of thumb is to cook fish for 10 minutes per each inch of thickness. It's best to stay slightly under that timing, as the fish will continue to cook once removed from the grill.)

4 Turn the fish and the pepper slices over. Remove the skin with tongs or a metal spatula; it should come off easily. Grill the fish on the other side until the fish is tender and begins to flake when you push it at the thickest part, about 4 more minutes.

5 Serve the fish grilled side up. Garnish with roasted chunks of pepper.

FOR BABIES 6 MONTHS & OLDER: This grilled salmon is delightful served with Lemon-Basil Potato Salad (page 137). Reserve some of the boiled potatoes and mash them with water or breast milk.

FOR BABIES 10 MONTHS & OLDER: A few bites of cooked fish combined with one of baby's regular vegetables are fine. Check the fish carefully and remove any tiny pin bones before serving to baby.

---

orange-glazed salmon kebabs *with* yogurt garlic dip

In this recipe, the salmon is broiled, but these kebabs are yummy grilled too. For extra aromatic flavor, use rosemary stems instead of wooden skewers. Children see small bites on a skewer as manageable to eat compared to facing a large fillet. Serve with Rosemary and Garlic Roasted Potatoes (page 233), which taste yummy with a bite of the drip.

PREPARATION TIME:

30 to 60 minutes (for marinating); 20 minutes (for cooking)

MAKES 4 TO 6 KEBABS

6 wooden skewers

1½ to 2 pounds salmon fillet

For the marinade:

¼ cup thawed orange juice concentrate

2 cloves garlic, minced

2 tablespoons honey

2 tablespoons tamari (soy sauce)

2 teaspoons toasted sesame oil

For the dip:

1 small or ½ large cucumber, peeled, sealed, and grated

1 teaspoon sea salt

1 cup plain whole milk yogurt

1 Soak the skewers in water. Cut the salmon into 1-inch strips. Take the skin off of each strip and then cut into 1-inch cubes. (If preferred, ask your fishmonger to remove the skin of the fillet when you purchase it.) Place the cubes in a shallow dish.

2 To make the marinade, in a small saucepan over low heat, mix the orange juice concentrate, garlic, honey, tamari, and oil and warm until the honey is loosened and incorporated. Pour the orange mixture over the salmon pieces, reserving 1 or 2 tablespoons. Let salmon marinate for 30 minutes or up to 1 hour, turning occasionally.

3 Preheat the oven to broil.

4 To make the dip, in a small bowl, put the cucumber and salt and set aside. In a separate small bowl, combine the yogurt, parsley, lemon juice, and garlic, and set aside.

5 Put four salmon chunks on each skewer. Place the skewers in a baking dish in the oven. Broil for about 3 minutes, then turn the skewers and pour some of the remaining marinade over the salmon. Broil until the flesh begins to flake when pushed, 1 to 2 minutes.

6 Squeeze the grated cucumber to remove excess water and blend it into the yogurt mixture. Place some dip in a small bowl for each diner. Serve the broiled salmon kebabs beside the dip.

2 tablespoons chopped fresh Italian parsley

2 teaspoons freshly squeezed lemon juice

1 clove garlic, minced

FOR BABIES 6 MONTHS & OLDER: A tablespoon of plain whole milk yogurt is good for baby's gut!

FOR BABIES 10 MONTHS & OLDER: These kebabs are delicious served with Rosemary and Garlic Roasted Potatoes (page 233). Smash some roasted potato with 1 teaspoon of plain yogurt and serve.

salmon niçoise salad
with basil gremolata

Any of the salad's components can be prepared in stages throughout the day (or the day before!) so that this cold supper can be quickly arranged for a big family-style platter.

PREPARATION TIME:

45 to 50 minutes

MAKES 4 SERVINGS

For the gremolata:

½ cup loosely packed fresh basil leaves

1 large clove garlic

1 tablespoon lemon zest (from 1 medium lemon)

For the dressing:

1 large clove garlic, pressed

¼ teaspoon sea salt

1 tablespoon champagne or white wine vinegar

1 tablespoon freshly squeezed lemon juice

½ teaspoon Dijon mustard

½ teaspoon sugar, plus more if needed

Freshly ground black pepper

¼ cup extra-virgin olive oil

1 pound baby red or Yukon potatoes

1 green onion, chopped

½ cup plus 2 tablespoons white wine, divided

½ teaspoon sea salt

Freshly ground black pepper

1 bay leaf

1 To make the gremolata, remove any tough stems from the basil. Put the basil, garlic, and zest in a pile on a cutting board. Hold the tip of your knife down on the board with one hand; with the blade poised above the pile and move the blade through your pile, over and over. Make sure the garlic breaks up evenly into the leaves and zest until you have an even texture.

2 To make the dressing, press the garlic into a small bowl and mix it with the salt. Add the vinegar and lemon juice and whisk to combine. Stir in the mustard, sugar, and pepper. Slowly whisk in the oil drop by drop, and then, once the emulsion is stable, add the rest more quickly. Taste the dressing to see if the remaining sugar is needed to tame the acid. Set aside or pour it into a small jar with a lid.

3 In a steamer basket nestled inside a 4-quart pot with 2 inches of water over high heat, put the potatoes. Bring the water to boil, cover the pot, and allow the potatoes to steam until the potatoes are fork-tender, 15 to 20 minutes. Baby potatoes (1 to 1½ inch in diameter) will take about 15 minutes. When the potatoes are warm but can be easily handled, slice them into a medium bowl and add the green onion, 2 tablespoons of the wine, the salt, pepper, and 1 tablespoon of water. Toss gently with your hands so that the potatoes absorb the wine evenly as they cool.

4 In a large skillet over medium heat, put the remaining ½ cup wine, the bay leaf, and a pinch of salt and bring it to a simmer. Lay the salmon fillet flesh side down into the simmering wine, cover, and poach the salmon until the flesh begins to flake when pushed, 6 to 7 minutes. Remove the fillet immediately and transfer it to a plate. Drizzle about 1 tablespoon of the dressing over the top. Once cooled, cover and refrigerate.

5 To make hard-boiled eggs (I like to make a bunch at once, don't you?), put the eggs in a pan of water so that they are submerged. Bring the water to a bubbling boil over high heat, then turn the heat off, cover the pan, and let the eggs sit for 10 minutes. Then run cold water over the eggs to cool them. Store them in a bowl of ice in the refrigerator.

6 To compose the salad, arrange the lettuce in a wreath around the perimeter of a large serving platter. Drizzle a bit of dressing around the lettuce wreath. Mound the potatoes in the center of the platter and give them a splash of dressing. Scatter the tomato around the lettuce wreath to balance the color. Give them a sprinkle of salt, pepper, and dressing. Place the salmon between the tomatoes on one side and the blanched green beans opposite. Peel and halve the hard-boiled eggs and arrange the four halves in two open spots between tomatoes, giving them a sprinkle of salt, pepper, and dressing. Drizzle any remaining dressing over the top of the salad. Scatter the capers artfully and then dust the whole salad with the gremolata. Serve with a salad spoon and fork at the ready for each diner to fill their plate.

½ pound wild salmon fillet

2 eggs

½ head (½ pound) romaine or butter lettuce, cut into bite-size pieces

8 cherry tomatoes, halved, or 1 large heirloom tomato, cut into wedges

1½ cups green beans, blanched

1 tablespoon capers

FOR BABIES 6 MONTHS & OLDER: Several choices here—mashed the steamed potatoes or pureed the blanched green beans.

FOR BABIES 10 MONTHS & OLDER: Finely chop a piece of cooked salmon and remove all tiny bones. Mash the salmon bits into the steamed potato and serve.

nori-wrapped wasabi salmon

By wrapping the salmon in nori before baking, the fish is kept moist and tender. The nori adds unusual flavor and bonus minerals.

PREPARATION TIME:

15 minutes

MAKES 4 SERVINGS

1 tablespoon extra-virgin olive oil

1 tablespoon finely chopped fresh herbs (any combination of thyme, basil, garlic, Italian parsley, and mint)

1 teaspoon sea salt

Freshly ground black pepper

2 (8-ounce) salmon fillets

1 tablespoon Dijon mustard

¼ teaspoon wasabi powder

2 sheets nori

1 Preheat the oven to 450 degrees F and lightly oil a baking dish.

2 In a small bowl, mix together the oil, herbs, salt, and pepper. Rub the non-skin side of the salmon fillets with the herb mixture.

3 In a separate small bowl, mix together the mustard and wasabi. Spread the mustard mixture on each sheet of nori. Place the salmon facedown in the middle of each nori sheet and wrap like a package, folding the sides up and over, so that the fish is fully covered. The nori will stick to itself and the fish.

4 Place the nori-wrapped fish in the prepared baking dish. The general rule for fish is to cook it 10 minutes for each inch of thickness. Since fish continues to cook once removed from the oven, estimate 1 to 2 minutes less than you might think. The nori will lightly flavor the fish and seal in the juices.

FOR BABIES 6 MONTHS & OLDER: The soft, almost-melted nori is full of minerals. Tear off a few pieces from the cooked fish to puree with baby's vegetables or cereal.

goat cheese & kale chicken roulade

When sliced, this dish shows off its pretty pinwheel pattern. This, plus the child-friendly size of the rounds, makes it appealing to all ages. Top with a savory sweet sauce, such as traditional cranberry sauce, fruit chutney, or a savory jam (like red pepper jam) thinned with water. Bread crumbs can be quickly made by buzzing a dry piece of bread in the blender or coffee grinder!

1 Preheat the oven to 375 degrees F.

2 Using a sharp knife, butterfly the chicken breasts by making a lengthwise slit from the thickest side of a chicken breast to within ½ inch of the opposite side. Open the chicken so it lies flat and cover it with plastic wrap. Use a meat mallet to flatten the chicken to ¼ to ½ inch thick. Cut the chicken into two equal pieces. Repeat with second breast, so that you have four pieces.

3 In a medium bowl, put the kale and ¼ teaspoon of the salt. Massage the salt into the kale until the volume has reduced by half as the kale wilts, 2 to 3 minutes. Add the raisins.

4 Spread 1 tablespoon of the goat cheese across the face of each flattened breast piece. Divide the raisins and kale leaves among the pieces. The key to the stuffed chicken breast is to keep the amount of stuffing to a minimum. Firmly roll up each piece, starting at the tapered end.

5 In a shallow bowl, beat the egg. In a separate shallow bowl, put the bread crumbs, thyme, the remaining ½ teaspoon salt, and the pepper.

PREPARATION TIME:

45 minutes

MAKES 4 SERVINGS

2 boneless, skinless chicken breasts (about 1 pound)

2 loose cups lacinato kale, chopped

¾ teaspoon sea salt, divided

¼ cup raisins

2½ to 3 ounces goat cheese

1 egg

½ cup fine dried bread crumbs or cornmeal

½ teaspoon dried thyme

Freshly ground black pepper

¼ cup Autumn Cranberry-Apple Relish (page 375), fruit chutney, or savory jam

substantial suppers

continued

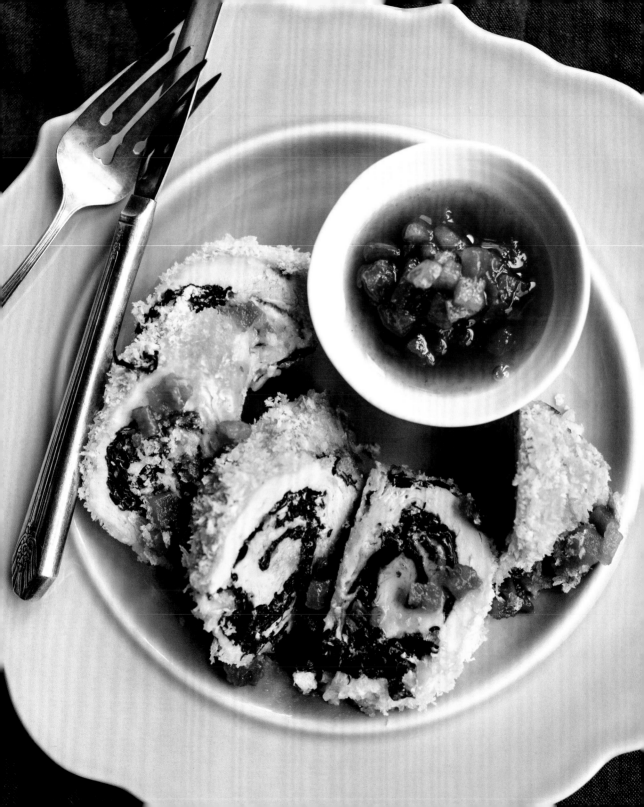

6 Dip each rolled breast in the egg, then roll it in the bread crumb mixture. Place the coated rolls in a dry baking dish and bake until tender or the temperature reads 165 degrees F on an instant-read thermometer inserted at the thickest part, 25 to 30 minutes. Let the roulade rest for about 10 minutes.

7 In a small saucepan over low heat, thin the relish with a few tablespoons of water and warm it. Cut the rolls into ½-inch slices and top with the sauce.

FOR BABIES 6 MONTHS & OLDER: Take some additional chopped kale and steam or sauté it in a few tablespoons of water until soft. Lacinato flavor is milder than other varieties of kale. Puree the kale, with a touch of breast milk or formula, and serve.

asian baked chicken *with* shiitake mushrooms & mirin

The juices emanating from the chicken and mushrooms mingle with the mirin, a sweet cooking wine similar to sherry, to form a savory-sweet sauce.

PREPARATION TIME:

65 to 70 minutes

MAKES 4 SMALL SERVINGS

8 to 10 shiitake mushrooms

½ cup mirin or sake

2 tablespoons tamari (soy sauce)

1 (1-inch) piece gingerroot, peeled and grated

1 pound whole bone-in, skin-on chicken breasts

1 Preheat the oven to 350 degrees F.

2 Wipe the mushrooms clean with a damp towel or rag. In an 8-inch baking dish or a roasting dish, put the mirin, tamari, and ginger. Place the chicken breasts, meaty side down, bony side up, in the dish. Tuck in the whole mushrooms.

3 Cover the dish and bake until the internal temperature of the chicken reaches 165 degrees F on an instant-read thermometer inserted into the thickest part. This may take only 30 minutes if the breasts are small, or up to 50 minutes for larger pieces.

4 Remove the cover and let the chicken breasts rest for 1 to 2 minutes before serving.

FOR BABIES 10 MONTHS & OLDER: Use a little of the juice from the chicken and mushrooms to puree with cooked rice or squash.

gay's mini pot roast *with* many vegetables

My daughter, Grace, always rushed over to her good friend Emi's house for some of her mom's pot roast. Gay keeps the meat to a minimum and the vegetables to the max.

1 Preheat the oven to 350 degrees F.

2 Season the chuck roast liberally with salt and pepper.

3 In a heavy 4-quart pot over medium heat, heat 1 to 2 tablespoons of the oil. Add the roast and brown it on all sides, 1 to 2 minutes per side. Remove the roast from the pot and set aside.

4 Add the remaining 1 to 2 tablespoons oil to the pot, then add ½ of the onion and the celery. Sauté until the onion is caramelized, 5 to 7 minutes, then add the thyme, marjoram, and rosemary. Return the roast to the pot and cover it with the stock and wine. Bring it to a lively simmer over high heat, cover, and place it in oven until meat is tender, about 2 hours.

5 After 2 hours, add the remaining ½ of the onion, the carrot, potatoes, and parsnips. Sprinkle a little more salt and pepper over the vegetables. Continue roasting until vegetables are tender, about 30 more minutes. Add the brussels sprouts. Continue roasting until the sprouts are tender, about 10 more minutes.

FOR BABIES 6 MONTHS & OLDER: Mash up some of those tender roasted parsnips—yum!

PREPARATION TIME:

About 3 hours

MAKES 4 TO 6 SERVINGS

1½ pounds chuck roast

Sea salt and freshly ground black pepper

2 to 4 tablespoons extra-virgin olive oil, divided

1 large onion, chopped, divided

2 stalks celery, diced

1 tablespoon fresh thyme

1 tablespoon fresh marjoram

1 tablespoon fresh rosemary

2 cups beef stock

2 cups red wine

2 large carrots, cut into chunks

3 to 4 small potatoes, cut into chunks

1 to 2 parsnips, cut into chunks

10 to 12 brussels sprouts, halved

substantial suppers

sweet potato & shrimp tempura

Deep-fried tempura can be light and delicate if properly prepared. The frying oil needs to be the right temperature, the batter needs to be cold, and the sweet potato slices can't be too thick or thin.

PREPARATION TIME:

20 minutes

MAKES 4 SMALL SERVINGS

1 medium sweet potato or red garnet yam, cut into ¼-inch rounds

6 to 12 shrimp

1 quart high-heat safflower oil

½ cup whole wheat pastry flour

½ cup rice flour

1 cup ice-cold sparkling water

For the dipping sauce:

½ cup Easy Vegetarian Stock (page 168), Simple Chicken Stock (page 165), or store-bought

2 tablespoons tamari (soy sauce)

1 (1-inch) piece fresh gingerroot, peeled and grated

1 In a 4-quart pot over high heat with a steamer basket inserted in the pot, bring a few inches of water to a boil. Place the sweet potatoes in the basket. Cover and steam until fork-tender but nowhere near falling apart, 2 to 3 minutes. Remove the sweet potatoes, pat them dry with a paper towel, and let them cool.

2 Remove the outer shell from shrimp but not the tail. De-vein the shrimp by making a shallow slit down the middle of the back to expose the black intestine. Remove the black string with the tip of your knife.

3 In a wok over high heat, heat the oil. The oil is ready when the temperature reads 350 to 400 degrees F on an instant-read thermometer.

4 In a medium bowl, put the flours. Add the sparkling water and gently whisk until blended and frothy. Use a minimum of strokes; don't overmix. Prepare a plate or baking sheet with paper towels or a brown paper bag for draining the finished tempura pieces.

5 Take each sweet potato or shrimp piece, dip it into the batter, and shake off the excess. Gently drop it into the hot oil. Pieces should drop to the bottom and then quickly rise to the top. Turn the pieces so that both sides are golden and crispy. Using a slotted spoon, remove each piece, letting the excess oil drip back into the wok, and place it onto the prepared paper towel–lined plate. You can fry three to four pieces at a time. Keep adjusting the heat on the oil so it stays hot.

6 To make the dipping sauce, in a small bowl, stir together the stock, tamari, and ginger. The tempura should be served and eaten right away, although it can be kept warm in the oven for up to 30 minutes if needed.

FOR BABIES 6 MONTHS & OLDER: Reserve some of the steamed sweet potato and puree it with water for baby.

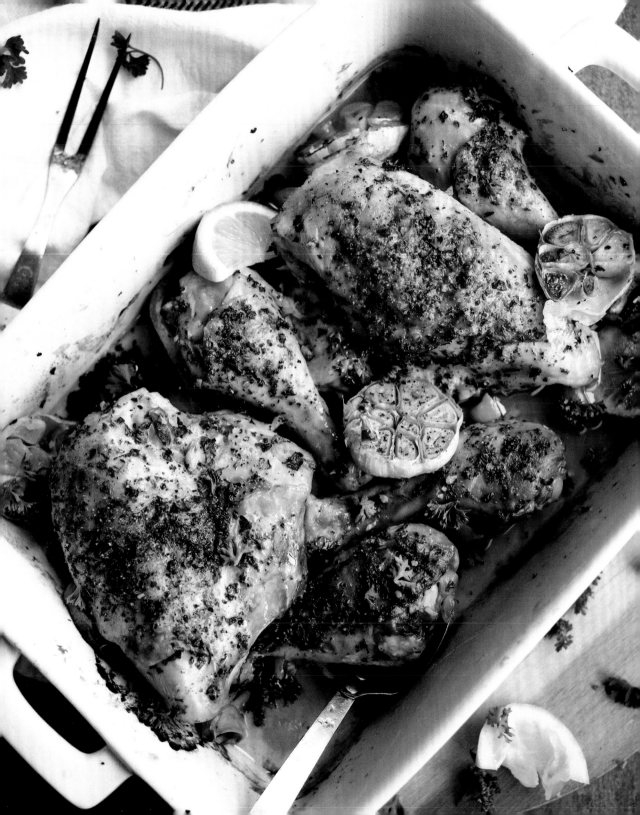

lemony chicken roasted
with garlic & oregano

This recipe uses the whole chicken! Save money, waste less! Plus, you can make stock from the back, right? Preheat the oven to 450 degrees F.

1 Cut chicken into eight parts, discarding the back, neck, and organs. (See How to Cut Up a Whole Chicken on page 166, or ask the store butcher to do this.) Place the chicken pieces in a 9-by-13-inch baking dish.

2 Remove the leaves from oregano and thyme stems and make a pile of the garlic, herb leaves, zest, and salt on a wooden cutting board. Chop together until finely minced. Coat both sides of each chicken piece with the herb mixture by rubbing it on. Get some of the herb mixture under the skin. Make sure the breasts are bone side up and grind pepper over all of the pieces.

3 Put the pan into the oven and immediately lower the temperature to 400 degrees F. Let the chicken roast, uncovered, until outer skin has browned, about 30 minutes. At this point, the smaller pieces (wings and legs) should be done and can be removed. Roast the breast and thighs until the internal temperature at the thickest part reads 165 degrees F on an instant-read thermometer and the skin has browned, 10 to 15 more minutes, depending on the size of the pieces.

4 Remove the pan from the oven and scatter the lemon juice over all of the pieces while they're still hot.

PREPARATION TIME:

80 minutes

MAKES 4 SERVINGS

1 whole free-range chicken (about 4 to 5 pounds)

3 to 4 tablespoons fresh oregano

2 tablespoons fresh thyme

4 to 6 cloves garlic

1 tablespoon lemon zest (from 1 medium lemon)

2 teaspoons sea salt

Freshly ground black pepper

2 tablespoons freshly squeezed lemon juice

297

substantial suppers

FOR BABIES 6 MONTHS & OLDER: To balance the meal, you will need a grain or starchy vegetable and something green. Steamed, pureed broccoli will work for baby, as will some mashed sweet potato.

chicken tikka masala

Chicken Tikka Masala, famous for being the comfort food of the British, is the most commonly requested dish served in Indian restaurants. Once you make it (and it is super easy), the dish will be frequently requested in your home as well. Serve over Golden Spice Rice (page 247) with Blanched Broccoli (page 191).

PREPARATION TIME:

1 to 8 hours (for marinating); 30 minutes (for preparation)

MAKES 4 SERVINGS

For the marinade:

1 cup plain whole milk yogurt

1 tablespoon freshly squeezed lemon juice

2 teaspoons ground cumin

1 teaspoon ground cinnamon

1 teaspoon sea salt

½ teaspoon cayenne pepper

½ teaspoon freshly ground black pepper

1½ pounds boneless, skinless chicken breast, cut into 1½-inch cubes

1 tablespoon unsalted butter or Homemade Ghee (page 383)

1 clove garlic, minced

1 jalapeño, finely chopped

2 teaspoons ground cumin

1 To make the marinade, in a large bowl, combine the yogurt, lemon juice, cumin, cinnamon, salt, cayenne, and black pepper. Stir in the chicken cubes, cover the bowl, and refrigerate it for 1 hour or up to 8 hours.

2 Preheat the oven to broil and place a piece of parchment paper or aluminum foil on a baking sheet.

3 Remove the chicken pieces from the marinade and place them on the prepared baking sheet. Broil for about 5 minutes, then turn the pieces and broil until the edges begin to turn golden, 2 to 3 more minutes.

4 In a large, heavy skillet over medium heat, melt the butter. Sauté the garlic and jalapeño until softened, about 1 minute. Reduce the heat to low and add the cumin, paprika, and salt. Stir in the tomato sauce and cream. Simmer until the sauce thickens, about 10 minutes. Add the broiled chicken and simmer for 10 more minutes. Serve over rice and garnish with the cilantro.

feeding the whole family

2 teaspoons ground paprika

½ teaspoon sea salt

1 (8-ounce) can tomato
sauce

1 cup organic heavy cream

3 cups cooked basmati
brown rice

¼ cup chopped fresh
cilantro

FOR BABIES 6 MONTHS & OLDER: A tablespoon of plain whole milk yogurt added to blended blanched broccoli works well.

VARIATION FOR CHILDREN: Chicken Tikka is basically chicken served in creamy tomato soup. For skeptical young ones, try serving a small bowl of the sauce as a soup with a few broiled chicken pieces on the side.

VARIATION FOR VEGETARIANS

Instead of marinating and broiling chicken, add 3 cups of cooked chickpeas to the creamy tomato sauce.

substantial suppers

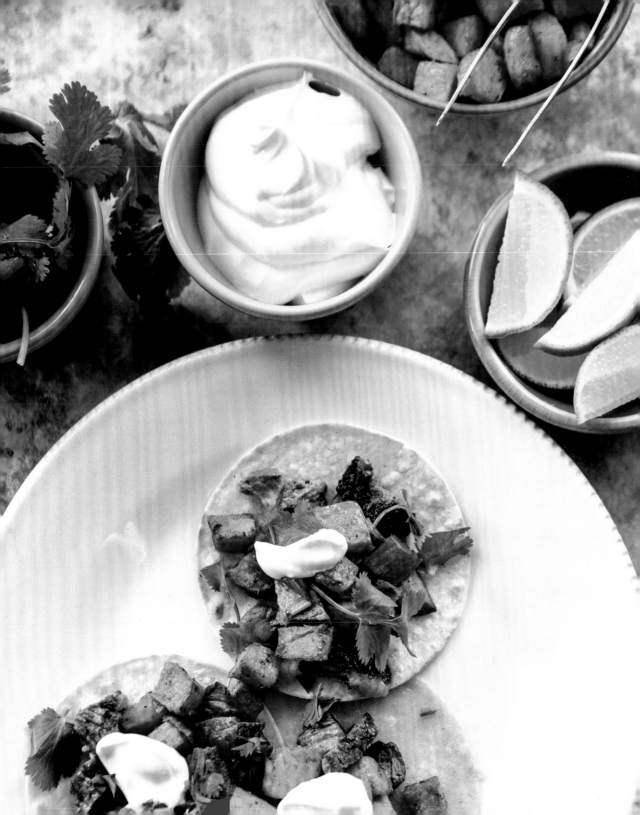

carne asada tacos *with* roasted sweet potatoes & lime crema

Four students, Brooke Erickson, Robyn Kiener, Samantha Waldron, and Michele English, knocked it out of the park by creating a similar version of this for their final presentation.

1 Preheat the oven to 400 degrees F and line a baking sheet with parchment paper.

2 To make the marinade, in a small bowl or jar, combine the cilantro, lime juice, olive oil, chili powder, cumin, and salt. Whisk or shake to emulsify. In a large bowl, toss the sweet potato with 1 to 2 tablespoons of the marinade; add a little extra olive oil if needed to make sure the cubes are coated. Spread the cubes out on the prepared baking sheet. Roast the sweet potatoes until they are tender, golden brown, and you can smash a piece between your thumb and first finger, 20 to 30 minutes. Set aside.

3 Pour the remaining marinade over the beef. Massage the marinade into the beef with your hands, breaking up the muscle fibers on both sides of the beef. Cover and refrigerate for up to 12 hours, or at least 1 hour.

4 Preheat the oven to 400 degrees F.

5 In a cast-iron or oven-safe skillet over high heat, add the vegetable oil. Place the marinated beef in the skillet and sear on each side for 1 minute. Transfer it to the oven for 4 to 6 minutes, depending on the thickness

substantial suppers

PREPARATION TIME:

1 to 12 hours (for marinating); 30 minutes (for preparation)

MAKES 8 TACOS

For the marinade:

¼ cup chopped fresh cilantro

3 tablespoons freshly squeezed lime juice

2 tablespoons extra-virgin olive oil

2 teaspoons chili powder

1 teaspoon ground cumin

½ teaspoon sea salt

1 medium sweet potato, peeled and cubed into ¾-inch cubes

½ pound grass-fed sirloin or rib-eye steak

1 to 2 teaspoons high-heat vegetable oil, such as safflower or peanut

8 corn tortillas

continued

For the topping:

¼ cup sour cream

¼ cup heavy cream

2 teaspoons sugar, plus
more if needed

¼ teaspoon sea salt, plus
more if needed

1 teaspoon freshly squeezed
lime juice, plus more
if needed

of the meat and how rare you would like it. Remove the beef to a cutting board immediately so it does not continue cooking and allow it to rest for 10 minutes. Thinly slice the beef with a serrated knife on a diagonal, against the grain of the meat.

6 Warm the tortillas in the oven in a covered dish for 5 to 10 minutes or warm them by adding a bit of butter to a heated skillet, softening each side. Place the tortillas in another covered dish or wrap them in aluminum foil to keep them warm.

7 To make the topping, in a small bowl, place the creams. Stir in the sugar and salt. Whisk in the lime juice a little at a time until smooth. Taste and add more lime, sugar, or salt to achieve a flavor you like. Fill each tortilla with a few strips of steak, sweet potato, and 1 to 2 tablespoons of the crema topping.

FOR BABIES 6 MONTHS & OLDER: Use some of the tender roasted sweet potatoes; puree them with some water or breast milk and serve.

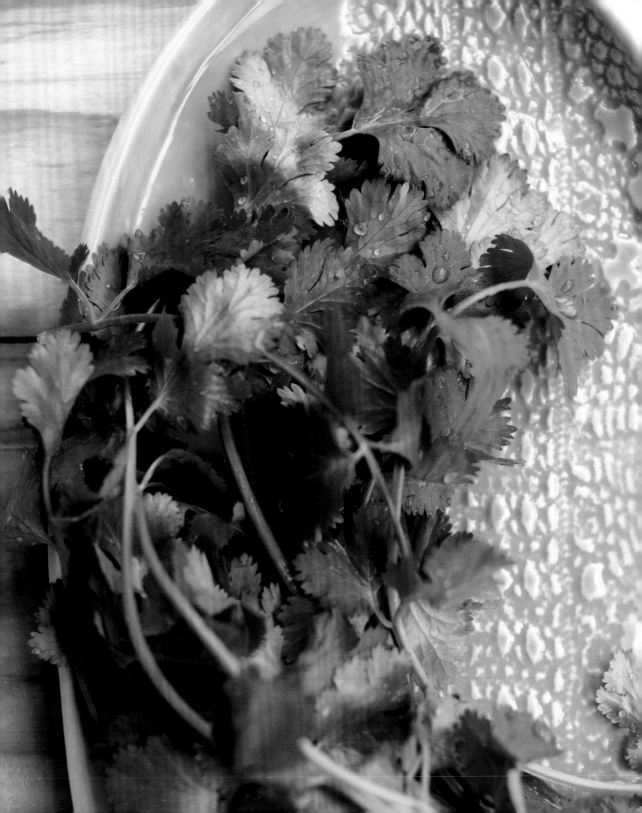

cowgirl bean & beef chili

The chipotle gives this chili the smokiness reminiscent of a campfire, and the cinnamon adds a sweet kiss. This recipe originated from my mom, June, a Kansas native.

PREPARATION TIME:

70 minutes

MAKES 6 TO 8 SERVINGS

1 tablespoon unsalted butter or extra-virgin olive oil

1 small onion, finely chopped

1 clove garlic, minced

1 pound ground grass-fed beef

1½ teaspoons sea salt

1 dried chipotle chili

1 tablespoon chili powder

1 teaspoon ground cumin

1 teaspoon sugar

½ teaspoon ground cinnamon

1 (14.5-ounce) can diced tomatoes with green chilies

1½ cups cooked kidney beans (see page 244, for cooking instructions), or 1 (15-ounce) can kidney beans, drained

1 (8-ounce) can tomato sauce

Grated cheddar cheese, for garnish (optional)

1 In a heavy 4-quart pot over medium heat, melt the butter. Add the onion and garlic and sauté until the onion is soft, about 5 minutes. Add the ground beef, breaking it up into small pieces, until the meat is browned on all sides, 5 to 7 minutes.

2 Add the salt, chipotle chili, chili powder, cumin, sugar, and cinnamon, and stir. Then add the tomatoes, beans, and tomato sauce. Establish a low simmer by bringing the heat up to high, then lowering the heat to low. Cook until mixture is aromatic and has thickened, about 1 hour.

3 Garnish with cheese.

FOR BABIES 10 MONTHS & OLDER: Add a few crumbles of well-cooked ground beef to baby's cereal or vegetable puree.

mom's meatloaf muffins
with kitchen ketchup

Fun shapes sometimes entice young diners. Meatloaf muffins pack well in a lunch box. This meatloaf can also be made loaf style, by baking it for an hour in an eight-and-a-half-by-four-and-a-half-inch loaf pan. You can substitute a teaspoon of dried herbs for 1 tablespoon of fresh herbs listed if fresh are unavailable.

1 Preheat the oven to 350 degrees F and lightly oil twelve muffin tins.

2 In the bowl of a food processor, put the oats and pulse a few times to get a coarse meal. Add the carrot, pepper, onion, garlic, and salt. Pulse fifteen to twenty times more until the vegetables look like confetti. Add the fresh herbs and pulse three to four more times.

3 In a large bowl, put the ground beef. Add the contents of the food processor and the black pepper to the beef. Mix with your hands until uniform. Put the beef mixture in muffin tins, packing it in and smoothing the top.

4 Divide 2 tablespoons of the ketchup among the top of the muffins. Bake the muffins in the oven until the internal temperature of the meat, using an instant-read thermometer, reads 165 degrees F, about 30 minutes. Top meatloaf with remaining ketchup and bake for 5 more minutes.

FOR BABIES 6 MONTHS & OLDER: Steam or roast two to three carrots until quite tender. Puree with some water or breast milk and serve.

PREPARATION TIME:

50 minutes

MAKES 12 MUFFINS

1 cup rolled oats

1 carrot, cut into large chunks

½ green bell pepper, cut into large chunks

½ medium onion, cut into large chunks

3 cloves garlic

3 teaspoons sea salt

1 tablespoon finely chopped fresh basil

1 tablespoon finely chopped fresh thyme

1 tablespoon finely chopped fresh sage

1 tablespoon finely chopped fresh oregano

2 pounds ground grass-fed beef

Freshly ground black pepper

¼ cup Kitchen Ketchup (page 377) or store-bought

substantial suppers

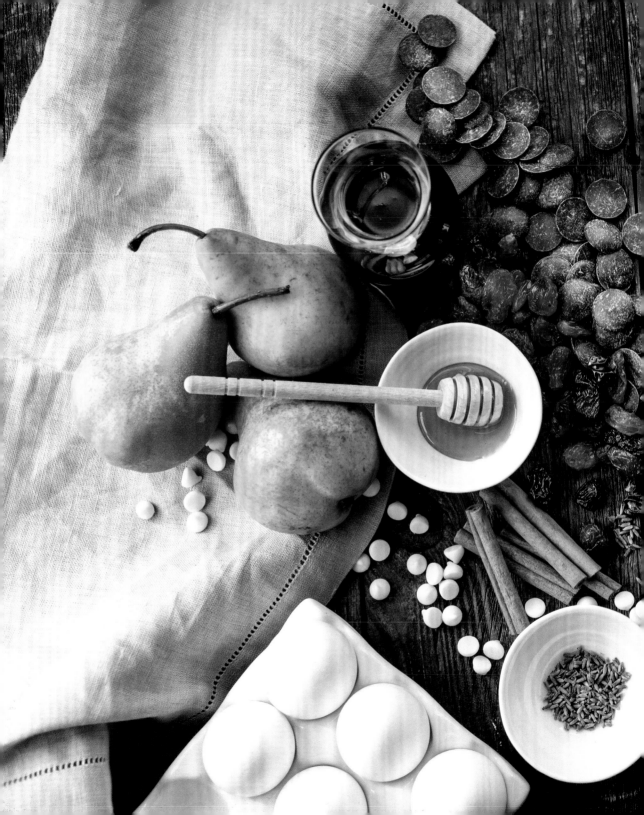

CHAPTER 10

- - - - - - - - -

simple sweet desserts

The Sheltons lived three doors down. The younger daughters were the same age as my sister and me, and we spent a lot of time at their house. They had a big weeping willow in the backyard that created a secret clubhouse with its leafy canopy. The sisters slept in one double bed, not two twins. I could never figure out why Santa visited the Sheltons on Christmas Eve around six p.m. but waited until after midnight to unload presents at our house.

The Shelton coffee tables cradled open bowls of hard candy—in every room—peppermint twists, lemon drops, butterscotch discs, and, my personal jones, cinnamon balls. Despite there being ample soda, candy, ice cream, and chocolate milk at our house, my seven-year-old self was compelled to steal from the Sheltons. I never left their house without a stash of candies tucked into the pockets of my seersucker jumpsuit, sure that no one suspected me.

Now, when I give a lecture on sweeteners it begins with, "My name is Cynthia, and I am a sugarholic." And I wait quietly until the class says, "Hello, Cynthia." Despite my issues, I don't shun desserts. Practicing moderation, which may seem like a dull concept, works.

I have come to understand that I am far from alone in my susceptibility. If one of your children (or you) is "of my ilk," see Sweet Tooth (page 67), where two of the suggestions are schedule whole fruit snack breaks and limit desserts to homemade ones. This recipe chapter supports both. Fruits appear often. Cookies and crusts use whole grain flours to temper any rush. Added nuts, butter, and eggs provide weight to balance any sugar surge.

Make something sweet in your kitchen. Share the joy of homemade dessert with your family. Take some over to the Sheltons in your neighborhood. Find out what time Santa visits their house.

one-trick fruit desserts

These five fruit desserts show off the produce. Heat intensifies the sweetness and softens the texture, resulting in sensuous desserts. Or in the case of mango—it is soft and sweet without heat.

baked apples

1 Preheat the oven to 400 degrees F.

2 Wash the apples and remove the cores. Using a melon baller, dig from the stem down the center, making a well, leaving the bottom intact. Using a carrot peeler, take off a piece of skin round the top to prevent bursting while they bake, but retain the shape.

3 Place the apples in baking dish. Stuff each apple with raisins, sprinkle them with cinnamon, and then fill the well with apple juice. Top each apple with a dab of butter. Bake until a fork pierces the flesh easily, 30 to 40 minutes, depending on how tender you wish to have the apples.

PREPARATION TIME:

45 minutes

MAKES 4 SERVINGS

4 Honeycrisp or Fuji apples

¼ cup raisins

½ teaspoon ground cinnamon

½ cup apple juice

1 tablespoon unsalted butter

pressure-cooked plum sauce

1 In a pressure cooker, place the plums, juice, and salt. Bring the heat to high until the pressure gauge rises. Reduce the heat to low and pressure-cook for 5 minutes.

2 Allow the pressure to come down, then remove the lid. Taste the plums. If you feel the mixture needs to be sweeter, add 1 to 2 teaspoons sugar and reheat, stirring constantly, until the sugar dissolves. Puree the plums in a blender or serve as is, depending on whether you want a smooth or chunky consistency.

PREPARATION TIME:

15 minutes

MAKES ABOUT 2 CUPS

1½ to 2 pounds plums, sliced (4 to 5 cups)

4 to 6 tablespoons apple juice

⅛ teaspoon sea salt

Unrefined cane sugar or brown sugar

continued

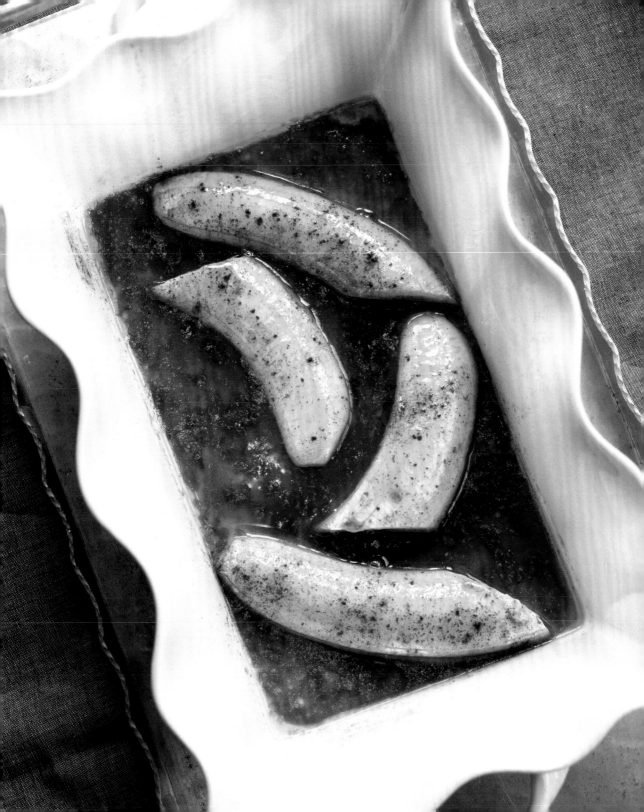

poached pears

1 In a wide pan or skillet over high heat, combine the juice, mirin, and sugar. Bring the contents to a boil, then reduce the heat to medium low and simmer, stirring constantly, until the sugar dissolves completely, about 2 minutes.

2 Add the pears to pan, face down. Simmer, cover, and poach until the pears are tender, about 10 minutes. Using a slotted spoon, remove the fruit from pan and set aside. Keep the poaching liquid in the pan.

3 In a small bowl, combine the water and arrowroot. Bring the poaching liquid to a simmer over low heat. Stir the arrowroot mixture into poaching liquid, stirring constantly. As soon as mixture thickens and clears, remove it from the heat.

4 To serve, place each pear half on a small plate or in a bowl and spoon the sauce over the top.

PREPARATION TIME:

15 minutes

MAKES 4 SMALL SERVINGS

½ cup fruit juice

2 tablespoons mirin or sweet wine

2 tablespoons unrefined cane sugar or brown sugar

2 medium Bosc pears, halved and cored

2 tablespoons water

1 teaspoon arrowroot or kudzu

caramelized bananas

1 Preheat the oven to broil and lightly oil a baking dish.

2 In a small saucepan over low heat, heat the butter, sugar, mirin, vanilla, and nutmeg until butter has melted. Stir to combine.

3 Place the banana halves in the prepared baking dish, cut side down. Pour the sauce over the bananas and broil them until the sugar bubbles and the bananas are lightly browned, about 5 minutes.

PREPARATION TIME:

15 minutes

MAKES 4 SERVINGS

2 tablespoons unsalted butter

2 tablespoons unrefined cane sugar or brown sugar

2 tablespoons mirin or rum

1 teaspoon vanilla extract

⅛ teaspoon ground nutmeg

2 medium ripe bananas, cut lengthwise

continued

broiled peaches

PREPARATION TIME:

40 minutes

MAKES 4 SERVINGS

2 medium peaches, halved
  and pits removed
1 tablespoon unsalted
  butter
1 tablespoon unrefined cane
  sugar or brown sugar

1 Preheat the oven to 350 degrees F and lightly oil a baking dish.

2 Place the peaches, cut side up, in a baking dish. Dot the top of each half with 1 teaspoon butter and then sprinkle them with sugar. Cover the dish and bake the peaches until the face has browned and the flesh can be easily pierced with a fork, about 30 minutes.

3 Turn the oven to broil, uncover the peaches, and move them to the top rack. Broil until the edges start to brown and the sugar caramelizes, 3 to 5 more minutes.

mango lassi

PREPARATION TIME:

5 minutes

MAKES 2 SERVINGS

1 medium ripe mango
1 cup whole milk vanilla
  yogurt
Pinch of ground cardamom
2 to 4 ice cubes

1 The mango has a flat elliptical-shaped seed in its center. Hold the mango vertically and cut from the top down on both sides, just off center, missing the seed. You will have two bowl-shaped halves. Discard the middle section with the seed (or give it to a child to suck the last bits of fruit off!).

2 Using a paring knife, score each half of the mango, creating a crisscross pattern. Push up from the skin side, turning the bowl inside out, and cut the cubes off of the skin.

3 In a blender, put the mango cubes, yogurt, cardamom, and ice and puree until smooth. Using two ice cubes renders a dessert that can be eaten with a spoon. If you want the lassi thin enough to suck through a straw, add all four ice cubes and/or a little water to thin it out.

FOR BABIES 6 MONTHS & OLDER: Easy-as-can-be baby food can be made from cooked fruit. Apply the heat but not the other ingredients to an apple, pear, plum, banana, or peach, and then puree it for baby. Ripe mango blended with a little water is just right for baby.

peanut butter chocolate chunk lunch box cookies

Check out your peanut butter! Make sure there are no added oils or sugar, just peanuts and salt. Also note the saltiness of the nut butter; if it is quite salty, cut back on the amount of salt in the recipe.

PREPARATION TIME:

30 minutes; 30 minutes (for chilling)

MAKES ABOUT 2 DOZEN COOKIES

1 cup chunky peanut butter

¾ cup unrefined cane sugar or brown sugar

2 eggs

1½ teaspoons vanilla extract

¾ cup rolled oats

1 teaspoon sea salt

1 teaspoon baking soda

4 ounces dark baking chocolate (70 percent cacao), chopped into ¼-inch chunks, or ¾ cup semisweet chocolate chips

1 Preheat the oven to 350 degrees F and line a baking sheet with parchment paper.

2 In a large bowl, put the peanut butter, sugar, eggs, and vanilla. With an electric mixer, blend the ingredients until creamy. In a blender or grinder, place the oats, salt, and baking soda and grind them until the dry ingredients resemble coarse flour. Add the oats mixture and chocolate to the peanut butter mixture and fold in well. The dough should easily make balls with moist hands. If not, add a bit more oat flour to the mix.

3 Cookie dough benefits from chilling. Putting cold dough in the oven gives the cookie time to build its structure before the fat begins to melt and spread the cookie. If possible, chill the dough for 30 minutes before baking.

4 Using a measuring tablespoon or moist hands, form 1- to 1½-inch balls and put them on the prepared baking sheet. Bake until edges are golden, 12 to 14 minutes. Allow the cookies 10 minutes or more to cool. Because there is no flour in the recipe, they are delicate when right out of the oven.

FOR BABIES 6 MONTHS & OLDER: The latest research shows that introducing peanuts early may prevent nut allergies. Stir just ¼ teaspoon of the peanut butter between into a mashed banana.

strawberry jam thumbprint cookies

These fun-to-make cookies are perfect with afternoon tea. Variations in flavor can be made by substituting different jams. Try cherry or blackberry!

1 Preheat the oven to 350 degrees F and line a baking sheet with parchment paper. Set aside.

2 In a small grinder or blender, grind the almonds into a fine meal. In a large bowl, combine the almond meal, flour, zest, baking powder, and salt and set aside.

3 In a small pan over low heat, melt the butter. Remove the pan from the heat and whisk in the maple syrup and extracts. Add the wet ingredients to the almond meal mixture and mix well.

4 Form the dough into 1- to 1½-inch balls and flatten them slightly to make discs on the prepared baking sheet. Indent each cookie with your thumb or your child's thumb and put ½ teaspoon of the jam in the imprint.

5 Bake the cookies until the edges turn golden, about 15 minutes.

FOR BABIES 10 MONTHS & OLDER: Add ¼ teaspoon of finely ground almond meal to baby's cereal to increase fat, protein, and fiber value.

PREPARATION TIME:

30 minutes

MAKES 2 DOZEN COOKIES

1 cup almonds

2 cups whole wheat pastry flour

1 tablespoon lemon zest (from 1 medium lemon)

2 teaspoons baking powder

½ teaspoon sea salt

½ cup plus 2 tablespoons unsalted butter

½ cup maple syrup

½ teaspoon almond extract

½ teaspoon lemon extract

¼ cup Old-Fashioned Strawberry-Honey Jam (page 380) or store-bought

simple sweet desserts

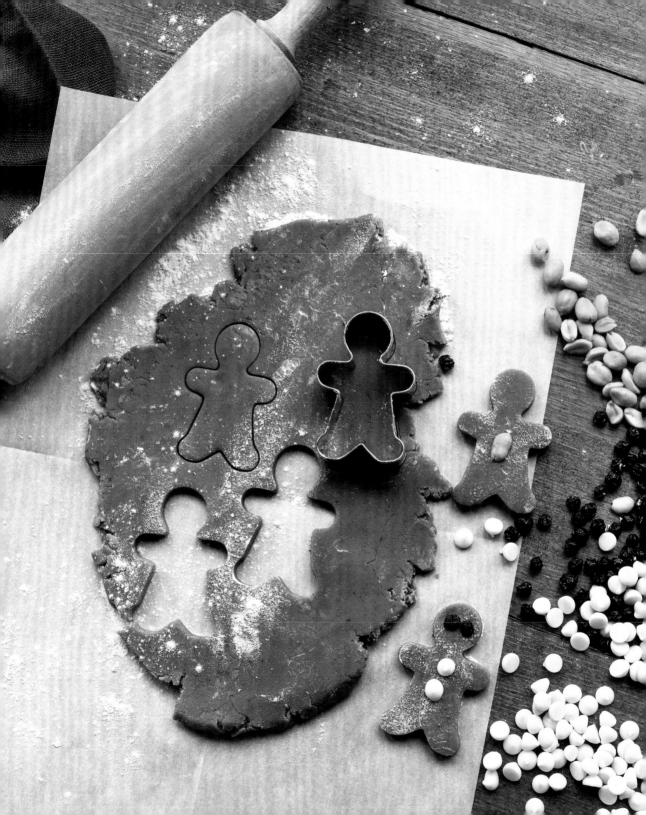

gingerbread people

"Run, run as fast as you can. You can't catch me, I'm the gingerbread man."
Read the story; make the cookies.

1 In a large bowl, put the sugar and butter and beat until smooth and fluffy. This can be done by hand or with an electric mixer.

2 In a small bowl, whisk the egg with a fork. Add the egg to the butter mixture, a little at a time, mixing well with each addition. Add the molasses and ginger and beat again to integrate.

3 In a separate large bowl, combine the flour, cinnamon, allspice, baking soda, cloves, and salt. Add the flour mixture a little at a time to the wet ingredients. The dough will be tackier than some cookie dough, but not overly so. Once most of the flour has been added, start kneading the dough with your hands. If you pick up the dough with moist hands and it sticks to your fingers or palm, add 1 to 2 tablespoons more of the flour mixture until it doesn't stick.

4 Once the dough is formed, line a 9-by-13-inch dish with parchment paper. Flatten the dough on the paper and cover the dish with plastic wrap. Flattening the dough ensures an easier roll out before cutting out shapes and prevents the dough from warming up too much while cutting. Refrigerate for 30 minutes to 1 hour.

5 Preheat the oven to 375 degrees F and grease or line a baking sheet with parchment paper. Set aside.

6 Remove the flattened dough from the refrigerator. Place the dough with the parchment paper beneath it on the counter. Place another piece of parchment paper on top of the dough. Roll out the dough to no less than ¼ inch thick. Use a person-shape cookie cutter to cut

PREPARATION TIME:

40 minutes; 30 to 60 minutes (for chilling)

MAKES 1 DOZEN COOKIES

¾ cup unrefined cane sugar or brown sugar

½ cup (1 stick) unsalted butter, softened

1 egg

1 tablespoon blackstrap molasses

1 tablespoon freshly grated gingerroot

1¾ cups whole wheat pastry flour

½ teaspoon ground cinnamon

½ teaspoon ground allspice

½ teaspoon baking soda

¼ teaspoon ground cloves

¼ teaspoon sea salt

For decorating:

Raisins

Dried cranberries

Peanuts

White chocolate chips

simple sweet desserts

continued

shapes out of the rolled dough. Lift the dough shapes with your bare hand onto the prepared baking sheet. Make sure the dough shapes are at least 1 inch apart from each other. Make eyes, buttons, and smiles with raisins, nuts, and chips.

7 Bake the cookies until the edges turn golden, 8 to 10 minutes.

8 If you need to make the cookies in two batches, be sure to put the remaining dough in the refrigerator until ready to cut out the shapes.

FOR BABIES 10 MONTHS & OLDER: Adding a dot (just a dot; it's bitter) of molasses to baby's pureed vegetables increases the iron value of the food.

rapunzel's triple chocolate brownies

"Rapunzel" is not just the name of the heroine in the classic Grimms' fairy tale—it is also the name of an international, environmentally, and socially responsible food company that produces certified-organic products using sustainable farming practices and global fair-trade programs. Along with other foods, they produce fine chocolate products.

1 In a small pan over low heat, melt the baking chocolate and butter and whisk them together. Set aside and let it cool.

2 Preheat the oven to 350 degrees F and lightly oil an 8-by-8-inch pan.

3 In a large bowl, combine the sugar, flour, cocoa, baking soda, and salt and set aside. In a separate medium bowl, using an electric mixer, beat the eggs until foamy. Combine the cooled chocolate and butter mixture with eggs and beat again.

4 Add the wet ingredients to the sugar-flour mixture and stir to blend. Fold in the chocolate chips and spread the mixture into the prepared pan. Bake until a knife inserted in the middle of the brownies comes out clean, 20 to 25 minutes. Allow the brownies to cool for 15 minutes before cutting them into squares.

PREPARATION TIME:

35 minutes

MAKES 1 DOZEN BROWNIES

2 ounces 65 to 70 percent baking chocolate

¼ cup (½ stick) unsalted butter

¾ cup unrefined cane sugar or brown sugar

½ cup whole wheat pastry flour

¼ cup cocoa powder

½ teaspoon baking soda

Pinch of sea salt

2 eggs

½ cup semisweet chocolate chips

FOR BABIES 10 MONTHS & OLDER: There's not a lot of ingredients in this dessert that are appropriate for baby. Remember that adding ¼ teaspoon of organic butter to baby's pureed vegetables heightens flavor and satisfaction.

chocolate-dipped coconut macaroons

Have problems eating wheat or flour? These fabulous morsels are for you! Be sure to have a good plan for how you will use the precious yolks from the egg. In this recipe, the honey adds sweetness while the rice syrup hardens when cooled, helping the macaroon stay together; however, honey can be used in place of rice syrup (for a softer macaroon).

PREPARATION TIME:

45 minutes

MAKES 18 MACAROONS

¼ cup honey

¼ cup brown rice syrup

About 2½ cups unsweet-
ened shredded coconut

2 egg whites

1 teaspoon vanilla extract

¼ teaspoon almond extract

¼ teaspoon sea salt

4 ounces 65 to 70 percent
baking chocolate

1 Preheat the oven to 325 degrees F. Line a baking sheet with parchment paper.

2 Lightly oil a glass measuring cup and use it to measure the honey and rice syrup. In a 2½-quart pan over low heat, gently heat the honey and rice syrup. Add the coconut and egg whites and stir to combine.

3 Heat the mixture, stirring constantly, until it makes a thick paste, 30 to 60 seconds. Remove the pan from the heat, then stir in the extracts and salt. Let the mixture rest until it is cool enough to touch.

4 With moist hands, squeeze the mixture into small tight mounds, about 1½ inches in diameter. If the mixture is not holding together, add 1 to 2 more tablespoons coconut. Place the cookies side by side on the baking sheet (they will not spread). Bake until the cookies are lightly browned on the edges, 20 to 25 minutes. Allow them to cool to room temperature on the baking sheet.

5 In the top of a double boiler over low heat, melt all but 1 to 2 teaspoons of the chocolate, stirring occasionally. Let the chocolate cool until still quite warm but touchable. Stir in the remaining chocolate. This tempers the

chocolate and helps the chocolate topping have a shiny, rather than a dull, look.

6 Spoon the melted chocolate over the top of each baked and cooled macaroon. Let the chocolate set and harden before serving (brief refrigeration or freezing will hasten this process).

FOR BABIES 10 MONTHS & OLDER: Drop those leftover egg yolks in simmering water for 2 to 3 minutes, then drain or remove them with a slotted spoon. Offer baby some of the soft-cooked yolk.

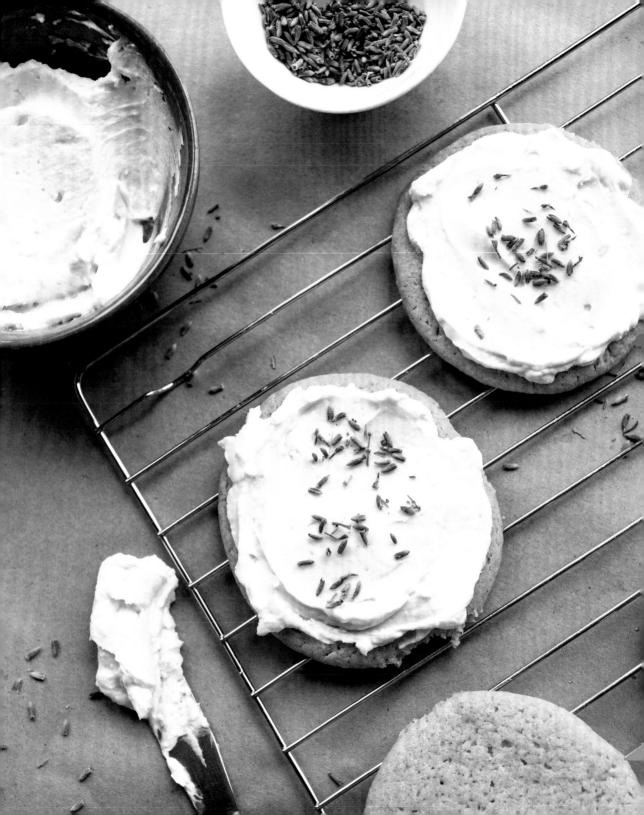

lavender-lemon cutout cookies with lemon cream icing

Children love to participate in cutting out cookie shapes. Grab a stool, tie on an apron, and set those small hands to work! If wheat is not a problem, you can replace the full amount of flour listed below with an equal amount of whole wheat pastry flour. Recently harvested and dried lavender buds will be more potent than those that have aired for months. Use the lesser amount if the aroma of the buds is strong.

1 In a small grinder, combine ¼ cup of the sugar and the lavender buds and pulverize. In a large bowl, place the lavender sugar, the remaining ½ cup sugar, the butter, and the coconut oil. By hand or using an electric mixer, beat the sugar until smooth and fluffy.

2 In a small bowl, whisk the egg with a fork. Add the egg, a little at a time, to the creamed sugar mixture, mixing well with each addition. Add the zest, yogurt, vanilla, and lemon extract and beat again to integrate.

3 In a separate large bowl, combine the flours, baking soda, and salt and stir to thoroughly combine. Gradually add the flour mixture to the wet ingredients; a sticky dough will form. The dough will be tackier than some cookie dough, but not overly so. If the dough sticks to your fingers or palm, cautiously add 1 to 2 tablespoons more flour.

4 Line a 9-by-13-inch pan with parchment paper. Flatten the dough on the paper and cover it with plastic wrap. (Flattening the dough ensures an easier roll out before cutting out shapes and prevents the dough from warming up too much while cutting.) Refrigerate the dough for 30 minutes or up to 1 hour.

PREPARATION TIME:

30 minutes; 30 to 60 minutes (for chilling)

MAKES 1½ DOZEN COOKIES

¾ cup unbleached sugar, divided

2 to 3 tablespoons dried lavender buds

¼ cup (½ stick) unsalted butter

¼ cup unrefined coconut oil

1 egg

2 teaspoons lemon zest

1½ tablespoons plain yogurt, sour cream, or crème fraîche

½ teaspoon vanilla extract

¼ teaspoon lemon extract

¾ cup plus 2 tablespoons sweet potato flour

6 tablespoons tapioca flour

6 tablespoons sorghum flour

¼ teaspoon baking soda

¼ teaspoon sea salt

continued

For the icing:

2 ounces cream cheese

2 tablespoons honey

1 tablespoon unsalted
  butter

1 teaspoon lemon zest

¼ teaspoon lemon extract

Dried lavender buds
  (for decorating)

5 Preheat the oven to 375 degrees F and lightly oil or line a baking sheet with parchment paper.

6 To make the icing, in a medium bowl, put the cream cheese, honey, butter, zest, and lemon extract. Using an electric mixer, blend until the icing is smooth. Set aside.

7 Remove the dough from the refrigerator. Place the dough with the parchment paper beneath it on the counter. Place another piece of parchment paper on top of the dough. Roll out the dough to ¼ inch thick or less. Using a 2-inch-diameter drinking glass with a moistened rim or your favorite cookie cutter, cut shapes out of the rolled dough. Transfer the dough pieces with your bare hand to a the prepared baking sheet. Make sure the dough shapes are at least 1 inch apart from each other.

8 If you need to make the cookies in two batches, be sure to put the remaining dough in the refrigerator until ready to cut out the shapes. Bake the cookies until the edges turn golden, 8 to 10 minutes. Allow the cookies to fully cool, then decorate each cookie with a swirl of icing and a tiny crumble of lavender bud. Alternatively, you can pipe the icing in squiggles onto the cookies for a pretty effect.

FOR BABIES 10 MONTHS & OLDER: Crème fraîche is a lovely cultured dairy product with a milder taste than yogurt. Try adding ½ teaspoon to pureed sweet potato. Be sure to speak in French as you feed baby.

kiwi-banana-
strawberry ambrosia

And here is the summertime version of Winter Fruit Compote (page 329).
Use any fresh berries or other seasonal fruit, but this colorful bright-green,
yellow, and red group is delightful.

1 In a medium bowl, combine the orange juice concentrate and sugar. Add the kiwi, banana, and strawberries, and toss gently to combine.

2 Divide the fruit between four glasses and top it with 1 or 2 tablespoons of the nut cream.

FOR BABIES 6 MONTHS & OLDER: Mashed bananas! Did you know that bananas are a rich source of fructooligo-saccharides, a prebiotic that feeds friendly bacteria in the digestive system?

PREPARATION TIME:

15 minutes

MAKES 4 SERVINGS

¼ cup thawed orange juice
   concentrate

1 tablespoon unbleached
   white sugar

1 kiwi, peeled and sliced

1 cup sliced ripe banana

1 cup fresh strawberries,
   trimmed and halved

Vanilla Nut Cream
   (page 329)

simple sweet desserts

pear-plum crisp

Gather in the autumn fruit harvest to make this warm dessert. The recipe is easily adapted for strawberries and rhubarb in the spring or peaches and blueberries in summer (see variations on the opposite page).

PREPARATION TIME:

80 minutes

MAKES 8 SERVINGS

For the topping:

1 cup rolled oats

½ cup whole wheat pastry flour

⅓ cup chopped walnuts

½ teaspoon sea salt

¼ cup (½ stick) unsalted butter

¼ cup maple syrup

5 cups sliced pears and plums (about 3 pears and 5 plums)

2 tablespoons water

2 tablespoons maple syrup

2 teaspoons vanilla extract

1 teaspoon ground cinnamon

¼ teaspoon ground nutmeg

1 Preheat the oven to 350 degrees F and lightly oil a pie pan or 8-by-8-inch baking dish.

2 To make the topping, in a medium bowl, mix together the oats, flour, walnuts, and salt. In a small pan over low heat, melt the butter. Remove the pan from the heat and stir in the maple syrup. Add the wet ingredients to the oat mixture and stir to incorporate. Set aside.

3 Place the sliced fruit in the prepared baking dish. In a small bowl, combine the water, maple syrup, vanilla, cinnamon, and nutmeg; pour the liquid mixture over the fruit and toss gently.

4 Spoon the oat mixture evenly on top of the fruit. Cover and bake until fruit is soft, 40 to 45 minutes. Uncover and bake 10 more minutes to crisp the topping.

FOR BABIES 10 MONTHS & OLDER: Remove some of the baked pear and plum from the bottom of the crisp. Puree and serve.

VARIATIONS

Strawberry-Rhubarb Crisp

Substitute 1 pint strawberries, trimmed and sliced, and one stalk rhubarb, diced, for the plums and pears. Add 1 tablespoon tapioca to the fruit mixture before spreading the topping on. The tapioca will absorb and thicken the juices from the berries. Bake for 30 minutes covered, or 10 minutes uncovered.

- -

Peach-Blueberry Crisp

Substitute 1 pint blueberries and 3 cups sliced peaches for the plums and pears. Add 1 tablespoon tapioca to the fruit mixture before spreading the topping on. The tapioca will absorb and thicken the juices from the berries. Bake for 35 to 40 minutes covered, or 10 minutes uncovered.

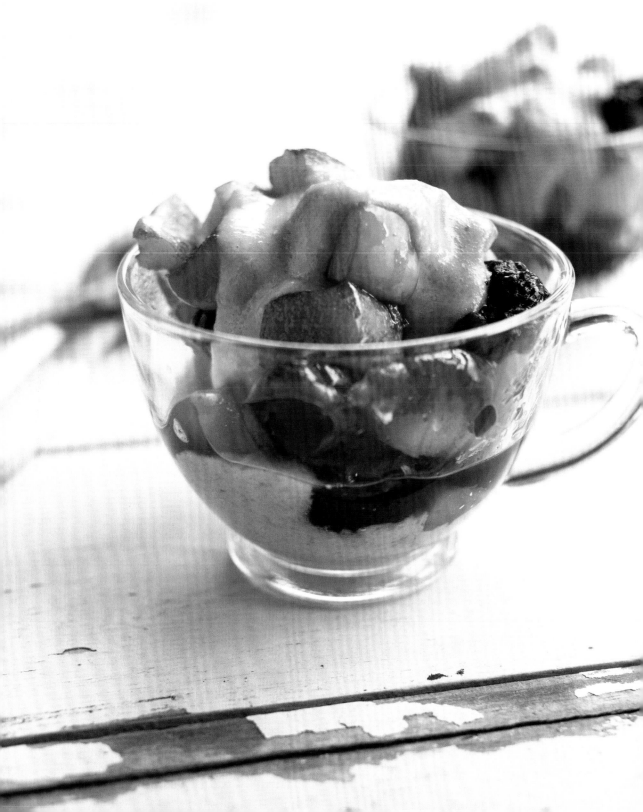

winter fruit compote
with vanilla nut cream

Dried fruit has traditionally been used in winter when fresh fruit was unavailable. This compote is a tummy-warming treat that's perfect for cold weather. Nut cream also makes a wonderful topping for cakes and gingerbread.

1 In a 2-quart pan over medium-high heat, add the juice, apricots, prunes, apple, pear, cinnamon stick, and nutmeg and bring it to a boil. Reduce the heat to low and simmer, covered, until all the fruit is soft, 20 to 30 minutes. Remove the cinnamon stick.

2 To make the vanilla nut cream, in a blender, grind the cashews into a fine meal. Add the maple syrup and vanilla and pulse a few times. With the blender running, add the water a little at a time until you have a thick and creamy but pourable consistency.

3 Divide the compote into four individual serving bowls and top it with 1 or 2 tablespoons of nut cream.

FOR BABIES 10 MONTHS & OLDER: Reserve some of the cooked fruit and puree. Serve just ½ teaspoon (it's sweet and intense) with your baby's cereal.

PREPARATION TIME:

35 minutes

MAKES 4 SERVINGS

1 cup apple juice

½ cup dried apricots

¼ cup pitted prunes

1 medium apple, sliced

1 medium pear, sliced

1 cinnamon stick

⅛ teaspoon ground nutmeg

For the vanilla nut cream:

½ cup raw, unsalted cashews

3 tablespoons maple syrup

2 teaspoons vanilla extract

2 to 3 tablespoons water

simple sweet desserts

apple pie *with* whole grain butter crust

One year, when my daughter was turning ten, she requested a coed birthday party at the skating rink. Instead of traditional cake, she wanted apple pies. I will never forget her blowing out candles on a pie and all those overheated kids happily eating big slices between rounds on the rink.

PREPARATION TIME:

1 hour (for preparing and baking); 30 minutes to 8 hours (for chilling dough)

MAKES ONE 9-INCH PIE

For the crust:

1 cup whole wheat pastry flour

1 cup unbleached white flour

½ teaspoon sea salt

½ cup (1 stick) cold unsalted butter

¼ cup cold unrefined coconut oil

¼ cup ice water

For the filling:

4 to 5 large apples (about 2½ pounds)

½ cup unrefined cane sugar or brown sugar

1 tablespoon arrowroot

½ teaspoon ground cinnamon

⅛ teaspoon ground nutmeg

⅛ teaspoon sea salt

1 To make the crust, in a medium bowl, put the flours and salt. Grate the butter on the large holes of a box grater. Add the butter and coconut oil to the flour mixture and, using a pastry cutter or fork, incorporate the fat into the flour until the mixture resembles coarse meal. Add the ice water, drop by drop, until the dough forms into a ball and holds together. Remove the dough from the bowl and transfer to a lightly floured surface.

2 Give the dough two or three quick kneads until it becomes smooth. Divide it in half and shape it into two balls; flatten each ball slightly to make a disk. Wrap each disk in plastic wrap. Refrigerate for at least 30 minutes and up to 8 hours before using.

3 Preheat the oven to 350 degrees F.

4 Peel apples if they are not organic. Quarter, core, and cut the apples into thin slices and put them into a large bowl. In a small bowl, combine the sugar, arrowroot, cinnamon, nutmeg, and salt and sprinkle it over the apples. Amounts of sweetener and spice can vary to taste. The amounts given make for a mildly sweet, lightly spiced pie. Toss gently until the fruit is evenly coated.

5 Roll out half of the chilled dough on a floured surface into a circle an inch or two larger than your pie pan. Fold the dough in half and in half again. Gently place the point of the folded dough in the center of the pie pan, then unfold it, and press in gently against the pan. Place the apples in the bottom of the pie shell. Roll out the remaining half of the dough, and fold it in half and in half again. Gently place the point of the folded dough in the center of the fruit, and then unfold it. Press the edge of the two crusts together and trim excess off of the edge of the pie pan with a knife. Prick the top of the pie three or four times so that steam can release. Bake until the edges of the crust are golden, 45 to 50 minutes.

FOR BABIES 6 MONTHS & OLDER: Buy extra apples to make Homemade Applesauce (page 376) for baby.

coconut maple crème

This smooth and silky dessert works on its own or with a few slices of brightly colored fruit on top.

PREPARATION TIME:
About 40 minutes

MAKES 4 SERVINGS

½ teaspoon unrefined coconut oil or other vegetable oil

2 eggs

1 cup coconut milk

1 tablespoon sugar

1 teaspoon vanilla extract

Pinch of sea salt

½ cup maple syrup

1 Preheat the oven to 350 degrees F. Lightly grease the entire inside of four ramekins with the oil.

2 With a whisk or an electric mixer, in a medium bowl, beat the eggs for 1 minute. Then add the coconut milk, sugar, vanilla, and salt and mix until well combined.

3 Pour a little maple syrup into the bottom of each ramekin, enough to just cover the bottom, about 2 teaspoons per ramekin. Now pour the egg mixture into each ramekin up to three-quarters full. (Do not stir—the syrup will naturally remain at the bottom of the ramekin.)For a smoother texture, strain the egg mixture through a fine mesh strainer to remove any egg bits before pouring it into the ramekins.

4 Fill an 8-by-8-inch baking dish with ¼ inch hot water. Place the ramekins in the water, and then put the dish in the oven. Bake until an inserted knife or toothpick inserted into the center of the ramekins comes out clean, 25 to 35 minutes. Do not overbake. Allow the ramekins to cool, and then put them in the refrigerator until ready to serve.

5 To serve, run a knife around the outer rim of the custard. Overturn the ramekins onto individual dessert plates. The pudding should fall out easily, with the syrup naturally dripping down over the coconut custard. This dessert will keep, covered, in the refrigerator for up to 5 days.

FOR BABIES 10 MONTHS & OLDER: Top pureed fruit with a ½ teaspoon of coconut milk for added healthy fat.

mary's buttermilk chocolate cake

For a dairy-free version, substitute the buttermilk with one cup soy milk or nut milk (see page 351) plus one tablespoon lemon juice, and use an equal amount of melted coconut oil in place of the butter.

1 Preheat the oven to 375 degrees F and lightly oil two 8-inch cake pans.

2 In a large bowl, mix together the flour, cocoa, baking powder, baking soda, and salt.

3 In a small saucepan over low heat, melt the butter, then remove the pan from the heat. Once cooled, in a separate bowl, combine the buttermilk, maple syrup, butter, and vanilla. Gently fold the wet ingredients into the flour mixture until well combined.

4 Divide the batter between the prepared cake pans. Bake until a knife or toothpick inserted in the center of the cake comes out clean, 30 minutes.

PREPARATION TIME:

45 minutes

MAKES ONE 2-LAYER CAKE

2½ cups whole wheat pastry flour

¼ cup cocoa powder

1 teaspoon baking powder

1 teaspoon baking soda

½ teaspoon sea salt

½ cup (1 stick) unsalted butter

1 cup buttermilk

1 cup maple syrup

1 tablespoon vanilla extract

simple sweet desserts

FOR BABIES 10 MONTHS & OLDER: This cake is divine topped with broiled peach slices (see Broiled Peaches, page 312). Serve baby pureed broiled peaches.

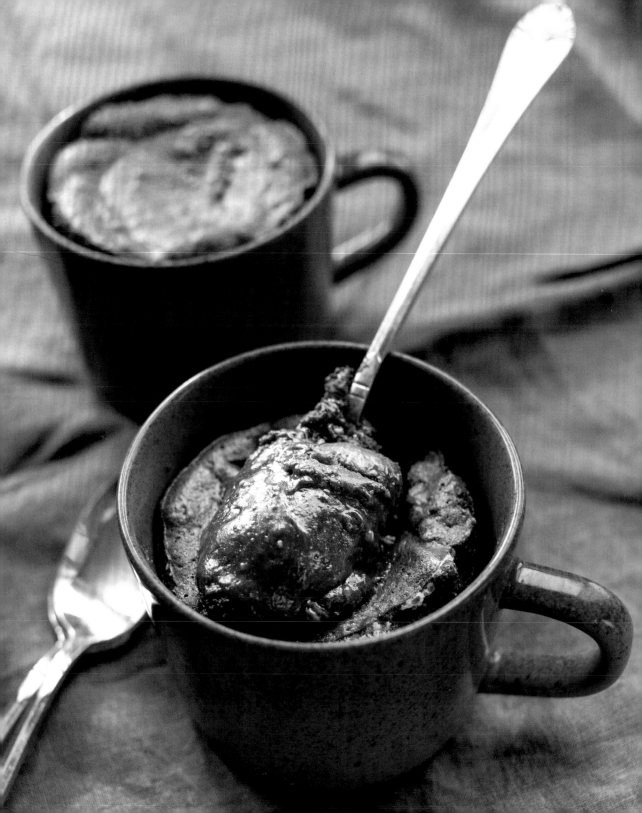

mini chocolate lava cakes _with_ salted caramel

These mini cakes are quick to make, gluten-free, and travel well to parties and potlucks.

1 Preheat the oven to 450 degrees F. Butter the insides of four 4-ounce mason jars, ramekins, or mugs and set aside.

2 In a small bowl, put the chocolate and almond butter and put the bowl over a pot of simmering water. Stir until melted.

3 In a separate bowl, combine the eggs, sugar, and salt. Using an electric mixer, beat the egg mixture until it is pale and light in color and the volume has doubled. Gently fold in the flour and then the chocolate–almond butter mixture.

4 Divide two-thirds of the batter between the jars, reserving one-third of the batter. Cut each caramel into two pieces. Drop one piece on top of the batter in each jar. Cover the caramel piece in each jar with the remaining batter.

5 Fill an 8-by-8-inch baking dish with ¼ inch hot water. Place the jars or ramekins in the water, then put the dish in the oven. Bake until the outer edges just barely begin to pull away from the jar or ramekin, the top surface of the cake is less shiny, and when you tap the surface it feels firm, not sticky, 8 to 10 minutes. Do not overbake. The cakes will be soft and gooey, so eat them with a spoon!

PREPARATION TIME:

20 minutes

MAKES 4 MINI CAKES

½ teaspoon unsalted butter, for buttering

¾ cup (4 to 5 ounces) dark chocolate

2 tablespoons creamy almond butter

2 eggs

¼ cup unrefined cane sugar or brown sugar

Pinch of sea salt

1 tablespoon sweet potato or millet flour

2 pieces chocolate-covered salted caramels

simple sweet desserts

FOR BABIES 10 MONTHS & OLDER: Has your baby been introduced to scrambled eggs? Around 10 to 12 months, this simple food works. See Green Eggs, No Ham (page 99) for tips.

carrot cake *with* walnuts, currants & apricot glaze

This familiar cake looks quite festive when you decorate the top with fresh raspberries alternated with date halves. This cake is also delicious crowned with Yummy Yam Frosting (see opposite page) instead of the apricot glaze. Double the recipe to make a two-layer cake.

PREPARATION TIME:

1 hour

MAKES 8 SERVINGS

1¼ cup whole wheat pastry flour

1 teaspoon baking soda

1 teaspoon sea salt

1 teaspoon ground cinnamon

¼ teaspoon ground cloves

½ cup (1 stick) unsalted butter

½ cup honey

2 eggs

1 large carrot, grated (about 1 cup)

⅓ cup chopped walnuts

⅓ cup currants

1 tablespoon lemon zest (from 1 medium lemon)

For the glaze:

1 tablespoon arrowroot or kudzu

½ cup apricot juice or nectar

1 tablespoon freshly squeezed lemon juice

1 tablespoon honey

1 Preheat the oven to 350 degrees F. Lightly oil a 9-inch cake pan.

2 In a large bowl, combine the flour, baking soda, salt, cinnamon, and cloves and set aside.

3 In a small saucepan over low heat, melt the butter and honey. Remove the pan from the heat, let it cool, then add the eggs and whisk to combine. Add the wet ingredients to flour mixture and mix well. Fold in the carrots, nuts, currants, and zest. Pour the batter into the prepared cake pan; tap it on the counter to release air bubbles and bake until a knife inserted in center of the cake comes out clean, about 30 minutes. Remove and let cool.

4 To make the glaze, in a small pan, dissolve the arrowroot in the apricot juice. Heat mixture on medium to high heat, stirring constantly, until it becomes clear and thick, about 5 minutes. Remove the pan from the heat, add the lemon juice and honey, and stir well. Once cooled slightly, spread the glaze over the top of the cake.

FOR BABIES 6 MONTHS & OLDER: Buy an extra carrot. Slice it and place it in a small covered baking dish to bake while the cake is baking. Mash or puree it and serve.

yummy yam frosting

This naturally sweet, golden-orange frosting can be used to top cookies, cupcakes, quick breads, graham crackers, or gingerbread people. This recipe makes enough to frost two-dozen cookies or a one-layer cake.

1 In a medium bowl, put the yam, cream cheese, maple syrup, and juice and beat with an electric mixer until smooth. Add the melted butter and salt to the yam mixture and beat it again. The goal is a smooth, spreadable consistency. Add a few more teaspoons of juice if needed.

FOR BABIES 6 MONTHS & OLDER: Reserve some extra baked yam. Mash well and serve.

PREPARATION TIME:

5 minutes

MAKES 1¼ CUPS

1 cup baked yam or sweet potato, skin removed (from 1 large sweet potato or yam)

¼ cup softened cream cheese

2 tablespoons maple syrup

1 teaspoon freshly squeezed lemon or orange juice

1 tablespoon unsalted butter, melted

¼ teaspoon salt

337

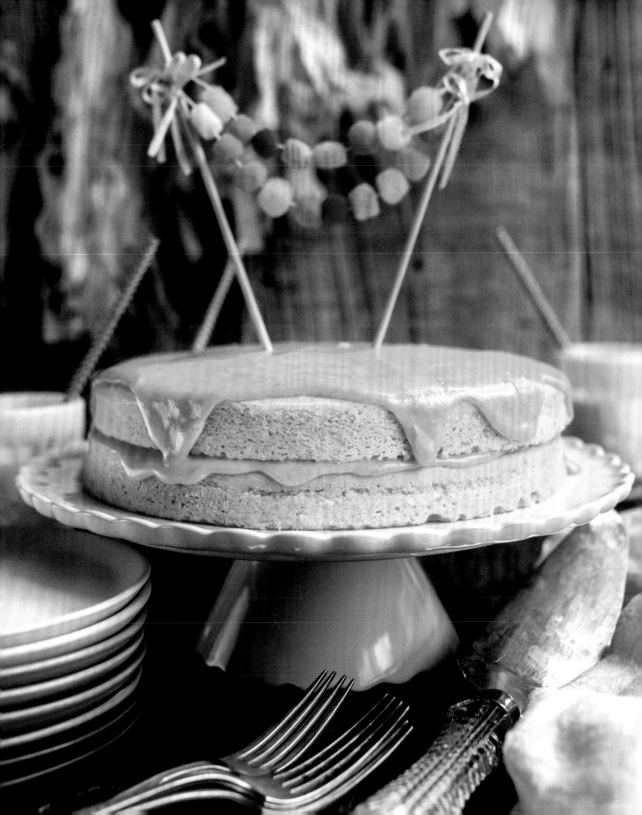

gracie's yellow birthday cake

Cooked millet gives this cake its yellow color and dense, moist texture, making it similar to pound cake. When my daughter was little, she loved it served on a pool of Strawberry Sauce (page 340) with fresh sliced strawberries on top.

1 Preheat the oven to 350 degrees F. Lightly oil and dust with white flour two 8-inch cake pans.

2 In a large bowl, combine the flours, baking powder, baking soda, and salt and set aside.

3 In a blender, put the millet and orange juice and blend until smooth. Add the butter, maple syrup, and vanilla and pulse briefly. Separate the eggs, reserving the whites in a separate bowl. Add the egg yolks to millet puree and pulse again. Add the millet puree to the flour mixture and mix well.

4 With an electric mixer, whip the egg whites until peaks form. Fold the egg whites into the batter. Pour the batter into cake pans. Bake until the cake begins to pull away from edge of pan, 30 to 40 minutes. Let the cake cool in the pans for 10 minutes before removing.

FOR BABIES 6 MONTHS & OLDER: Reserve some extra cooked millet to puree with water. Warm before serving.

PREPARATION TIME:

50 to 55 minutes

MAKES ONE 2-LAYER CAKE

1½ cups unbleached white flour, plus more for dusting

½ cup whole wheat pastry flour

1 teaspoon nonaluminum baking powder

1 teaspoon baking soda

½ teaspoon sea salt

1½ cups cooked millet

1¼ cups freshly squeezed orange juice (from 4 oranges) or store-bought

½ cup (1 stick) unsalted butter, melted

½ cup maple syrup

2 teaspoons vanilla extract

2 eggs

339

simple sweet desserts

strawberry sauce

Serve cake slices on a red strawberry pool of sauce or put the sauce in a squeeze bottle and swirl out a design on top of your favorite cake, pudding, or frozen dessert.

PREPARATION TIME:

10 minutes

MAKES 1 CUP

1 pint fresh strawberries, trimmed

1 teaspoon freshly squeezed lemon or orange juice

1 tablespoon honey or maple syrup

1 In a blender, place all but four or five strawberries, the juice, and the honey and blend until smooth. Use the sauce immediately or refrigerate in a sealed container. The sauce will keep several days in the refrigerator. Use the remaining strawberries for decorating.

FOR BABIES 10 MONTHS & OLDER: The tiny seeds in strawberries can be difficult to digest for tiny babies. Wait until baby is closer to 1 year old and serve ripe, sliced strawberries as a finger food.

---

feeding the whole family

fruitsicles

You can buy ice pop molds in the summertime at most stores that carry toys or kitchenware. Dream up an endless variety of frozen treats to delight sun-soaked children and adults.

1 Note how much liquid it will take to fill your fruit pop molds. Each of these recipes makes 1 cup of liquid, which fills four of the common cylindrical-style molds.

2 Choose a fruit pop variation. In a blender, blend all the ingredients for that variation until smooth, then pour the liquid into the fruit pop molds and freeze for at least 2 hours.

3 Run warm water on the outside of the holder until the fruit pop pulls out easily.

FOR BABIES 10 MONTHS & OLDER: Use ice cube trays to make iced fruit cubes. A few pieces of fruity ice can soothe gums sore from teething. Choose the simple melon pops to start.

PREPARATION TIME:

5 minutes; 2 hours (for freezing)

MAKES 4 POPS

For creamy orange-vanilla pops:

¾ cup freshly squeezed orange juice (from 3 medium oranges)

¼ cup vanilla yogurt

1 teaspoon vanilla extract

For banana-raspberry pops:

1 banana

½ cup water

⅓ cup fresh raspberries

For melon pops:

2 cups of melon chunks (like cantaloupe, honeydew)

¼ cup water

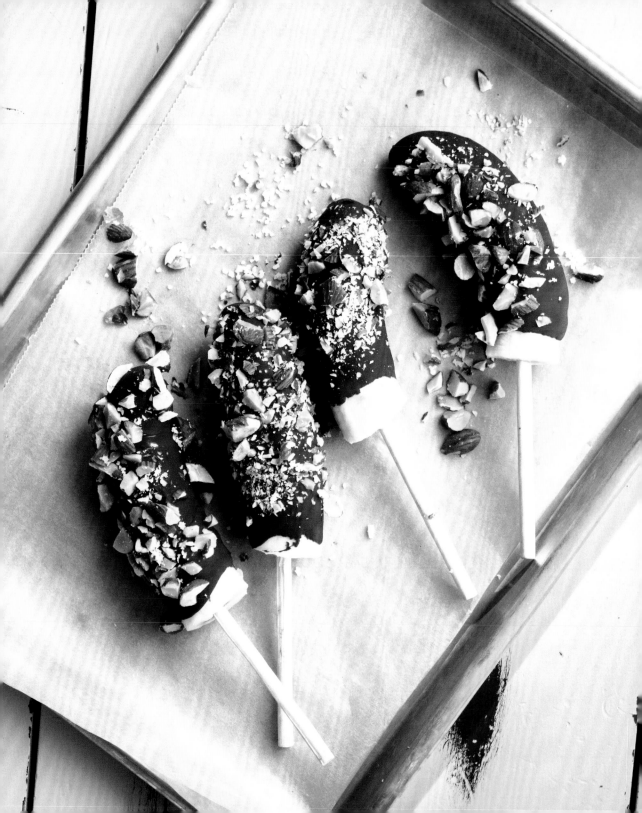

salted almond–dark chocolate banana pops

A tip of the hat goes to one of my nutritionist heroes, Ellie Krieger, who created the inspiration recipe for these fruity treats.

1 Preheat your oven to 325 degrees F.

2 Place the almonds in a dry baking dish and toast them until the color has darkened and a nutty aroma is present, about 25 minutes.

3 Insert a craft stick into the cut end of each banana half. Place them on a tray, cover it with plastic wrap or a plastic bag, and freeze them for 3 hours.

4 Break up the chocolate into small pieces. In the top of a double boiler over low heat, put the chocolate, reserving one 1-inch piece. Melt the chocolate, stirring constantly. As soon as the chocolate is melted, remove the pan from the heat and let it cool to just warm enough to touch comfortably. Now stir in the reserved piece of chocolate. This is a quick way to temper the chocolate.

5 Pour the chocolate into a pint jar or tall glass. Finely chop the almonds and put them on a large plate. Add the salt to the almonds and mix until even.

6 Dip each frozen banana half into the chocolate, tipping and turning to coat it. Then immediately roll it in the salty nuts and place it on wax paper. Repeat with the remaining banana halves.

7 Serve immediately or put the chocolate banana pops in a sealed container and keep them in the freezer.

PREPARATION TIME:

30 minutes; 3 hours
(for freezing)

MAKES 8 POPS

¼ cup almonds

4 medium ripe bananas, halved

8 wooden craft sticks

6 ounces 70 percent baking chocolate

½ teaspoon coarse sea salt

343

simple sweet desserts

FOR BABIES 6 MONTHS & OLDER: A slice of frozen banana sans chocolate and nuts can be a sweet treat. The icy cold can soothe gums sore from teething.

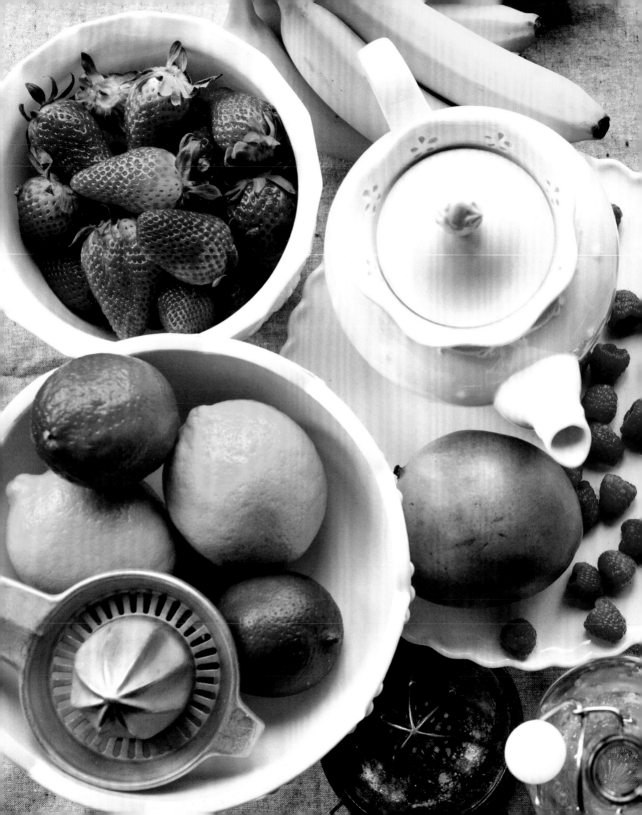

daily drinks & brews

When a teary, upset child comes rushing for comfort, try this method of uncovering the problem. After a solid hug, grab a small glass of water. Ask the child to count and drink ten slow sips. Count along, keeping the pace slow. Assure the child that you need to hear what happened but that drinking water will help them tell the story better.

One.
Two.
Three.

Deep inhale.

Four.
Five.
Six.

Big exhale.

Seven.
Eight.
Nine.

Another hug.

Ten.

"What happened?"

Time and hydration will slow the adrenaline rush, offer a tiny speck of perspective, and afford a clearer telling of the story. My daughter's first-grade teacher, Tricia Walker, used this ritual with major success.

lemon water

Keep a pitcher of lemon water in the refrigerator during hot weather to quench thirst.

1 Put the lemon slices in a pitcher of water. Let it set 10 to 20 minutes. Refrigerate or drink at room temperature.

PREPARATION TIME:

1 minute

MAKES 1 QUART

½ lemon, sliced

1 quart water

> It's important to keep the attention at mealtime on eating, not drinking. Save juices, milks, and other caloric drinks for between-meal snacks. For everyday meals, serve water to drink.
>
> Infants under one year of age do not require any liquids besides breast milk or formula and water. Only two of the following recipes give suggestions for giving babies a part of the recipe.

bubbly fruit tea

This fruit tea is a delicious way to dilute fruit juice for youngsters.

PREPARATION TIME:

10 minutes

MAKES 1 QUART

1 fruity hibiscus herbal
    tea bag
1 cup boiling water
1 teaspoon honey
1½ cups fruit juice
1½ cups sparkling water

1 In a cup, add the hibiscus tea bag and cover it with the boiling water. Allow it to steep for 3 to 4 minutes, then remove the tea bag. Add the honey and stir. Allow the tea to cool.

2 In a pitcher, combine the brewed tea with the juice and sparkling water; serve cold.

banana milk

School-aged children can make this drink by themselves.

1 In a blender, put the banana, milk, and vanilla. Puree until thoroughly combined and serve.

PREPARATION TIME:

5 minutes

MAKES 2½ TO 3 CUPS

1 ripe banana

2 cups milk

2 teaspoons vanilla extract

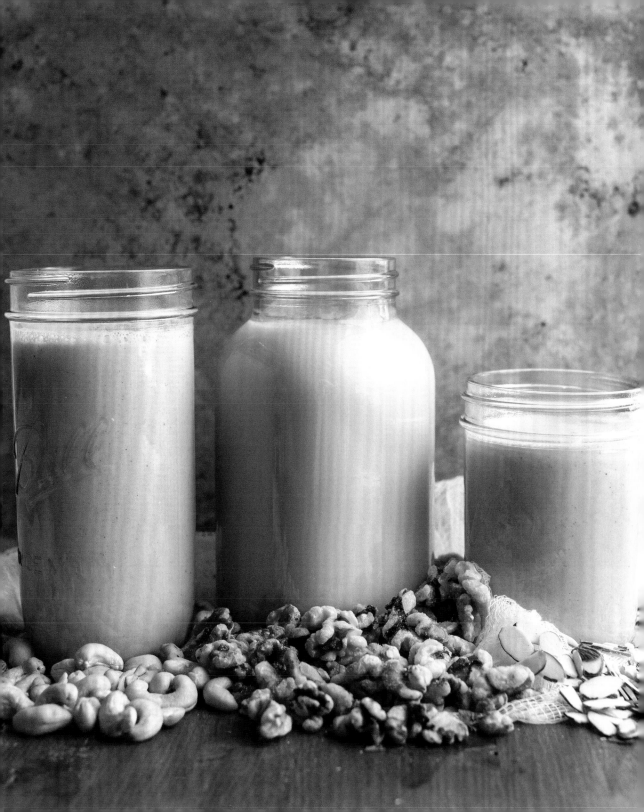

nut milks

Nut milks, a nutritious and versatile beverage, taste good on cereals or fruit desserts. You can use them to replace cow's milk in any recipe. Nut milks can be kept in the refrigerator for a couple of days, although they may separate and need to be reblended. Here are ideas for three nut milks, although the possibilities are limitless.

Nut milk bags are available online. They make straining the pulp out of the milk easy; worth the investment (ten or twelve dollars for two) if you make nut milk often.

almond-sesame milk

Almonds are noted for their monounsaturated fats, the same type of health-promoting fats as are found in olive oil. In addition to healthy fats and vitamin E, a quarter cup of almonds contains 62 milligrams of magnesium plus 162 milligrams of potassium.

1 In a blender, put the almonds and seeds and grind into a fine powder. Add a few tablespoons of the water and blend until you have a paste. Add the rest of the water and the maple syrup and blend until thoroughly combined.

2 Pour the contents of the blender through a fine mesh strainer lined with cheesecloth resting in a large bowl to remove the nut pulp. Pick up the ends of the cheesecloth and squeeze the pulp to remove all the milk. A nut milk bag can also be used.

PREPARATION TIME:
5 to 10 minutes

MAKES 2 CUPS
¼ cup almonds
¼ cup sesame seeds
2 cups water
1 tablespoon maple syrup

continued

almond-cashew milk

PREPARATION TIME:

5 to 10 minutes

MAKES 2 CUPS

¼ cup almonds

¼ cup cashews

2 cups water

3 pitted dates

Cashews not only transform water into a creamy milk but also have bragging rights for their monounsaturated fats, magnesium, and copper.

1 In a blender, place the almonds and cashews and grind into a fine powder. Add a few tablespoons of the water and blend until you have a paste. Add the rest of the water and the dates and blend until thoroughly combined.

2 Pour the contents of the blender through a fine mesh strainer lined with cheesecloth resting in a large bowl to remove the nut pulp. Pick up the ends of the cheesecloth and squeeze the pulp to remove all the milk. A nut milk bag can also be used.

nut butter milk

PREPARATION TIME:

5 to 10 minutes

MAKES 2 CUPS

2 cups water

2 tablespoons creamy almond, sesame, or cashew butter

1 tablespoon honey

Using nut butters hastens the process of making nut milk, as no pre-grinding or straining is necessary.

1 In a blender, place the water, nut butter, and honey. Blend until smooth.

FOR BABIES 10 MONTHS & OLDER: Adding a few tablespoons of nut milk to baby's cereal adds flavor and nutrients.

cranberry-ginger cider

Serve this warming beverage in glass mugs so folks can appreciate the beautiful deep-red color.

1 In a medium saucepan, add the juice, cider, ginger, and zest. Bring heat up to a near boil, then reduce, cover, and simmer 15 minutes. Simmering longer will increase the ginger flavor.

2 Remove pieces of ginger and ladle the warm beverage into mugs. Float an orange slice on top.

PREPARATION TIME:

20 minutes

MAKES 4 CUPS

2 cups cranberry juice

2 cups apple cider

1 (2-inch) piece gingerroot, cut ¼ inch thick

1 teaspoon orange zest

Orange slices, for garnish

353

daily drinks & brews

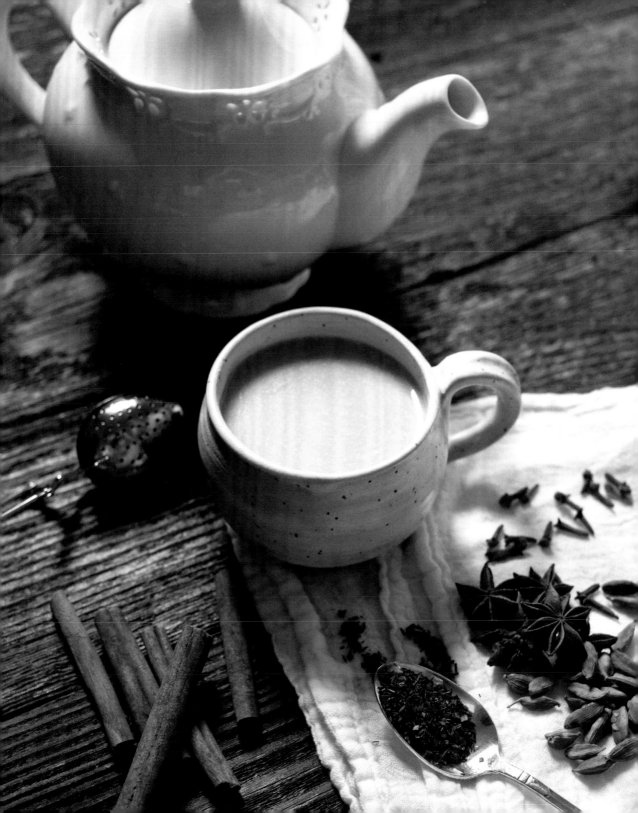

rooibos chai tea

This drink (which I was first introduced to as "Yogi Tea") is filled with many warming spices, which are welcome on cold winter days. Children love its sweet taste. Traditionally this tea is made with black tea. I have omitted it because children don't need the caffeine. Rooibos (red tea) is free of caffeine and contains aspalathin, a flavonoid present in medicinal herbs used to treat skin and circulatory disorders. Any preferred milk can be added, including nut milks.

1 By hand or with a mallet, break up the cinnamon sticks. In a coffee grinder, put the cinnamon pieces, cloves, cardamom seeds, peppercorns, and star anise and give them a pulse or two to roughly break them up.

2 In a 4-quart pot over high heat, put the water, spice mixture, and ginger, and bring the water to a boil. Reduce the heat to medium low and simmer (covered) for 30 to 60 minutes. The longer the tea simmers, the more potent it will be. Taste it after 30 minutes. Add the rooibos during the last 5 minutes.

3 After the taste is to your liking, add the milk. If using cow or goat milk, bring the tea to a boil again for 1 minute. Otherwise, just reheat. Strain the tea into cups and stir in honey to taste.

FOR BABIES 10 MONTHS & OLDER: Adding a few tablespoons of brewed rooibos tea to baby's sippy cup of water is fine. The taste is mild. In South Africa, rooibos tea is given to infants mixed with breast milk to soothe colic and eczema.

PREPARATION TIME:

About 45 minutes

MAKES 4 TO 5 CUPS

2 cinnamon sticks

15 whole cloves

20 whole cardamom seeds

20 whole black peppercorns

1 star anise

4 cups water

1 (2-inch) piece fresh ginger-root, sliced ¼ inch thick

1 tablespoon rooibos (red) tea

1 cup milk

Honey

daily drinks & brews

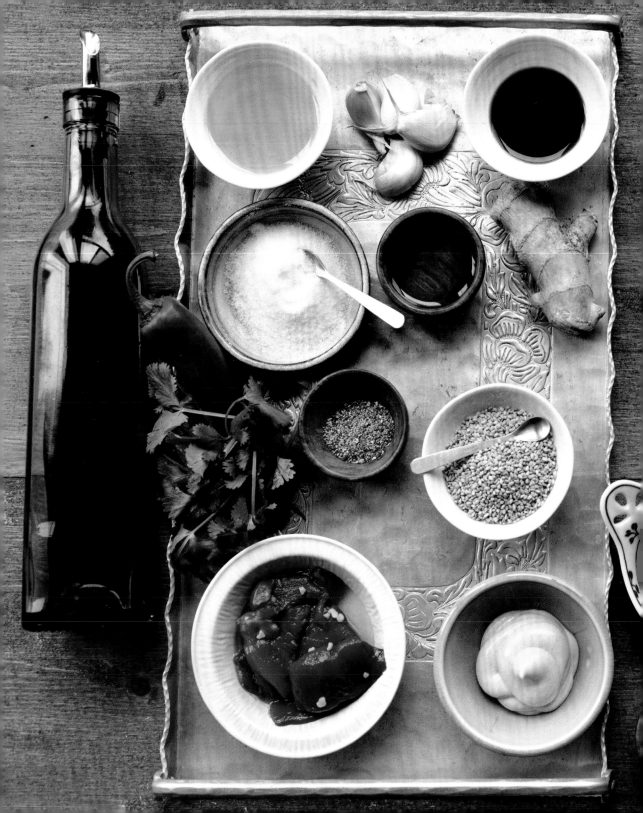

CHAPTER 12

refreshing relishes & convenient condiments

Mom put a dab of mayonnaise on a canned pear and set it on an iceberg lettuce leaf as a frequent side dish. I found the look and taste of it nauseating, and as an adult, the combination still baffles me. Dousing cheesy scrambled eggs with ketchup, however, was more than acceptable. Neither my brother, sister, or I would eat scrambled eggs without it. I still like it.

My daughter's high school boyfriend tossed hot sauce on everything he ate. I always wondered when and why that preference started. Show me a slice of cheddar, and I must have some Dijon mustard. Dill pickle goes with my peanut butter and toast.

My daughter and I crave kasha for breakfast when chilly mornings roll around. We like it with a poached egg on top, a plop of sauerkraut or kimchi on the side, and just an itty drizzle of something called Thai chili sauce. The folks who made this sauce weren't aware of our dependency. It just disappeared from the grocer's shelf. We got a little desperate. Grace found some online and paid more in shipping for the four bottles than she paid for the sauce. Now we can't even find it online and have attempted to make it ourselves, with little success.

Everybody's got their compulsory condiments. What's your thing? Making condiments and sauces may seem like just another extra, nonessential step, but don't underestimate their dazzle. Having some on hand will change how you cook. Sure plain brown rice sounds boring, but what if it had Coconut Peanut Sauce (page 361) on it? Oatmeal is for old people with no teeth, right? Maple-Glazed Walnuts (page 371) on top change the game.

Next time your child refuses a food, ask them—what would make it yummier? A little salsa? A teaspoon of jam? (Please, not a dab of mayo.)

sweet pepper relish

This relish makes a colorful, crunchy addition to sandwiches or bean soups; it is a good topping for fish too.

1 In a clean 1-pint jar, put the peppers and jalapeño. Add the sugar, vinegar, and salt and stir to mix. Allow the mixture to marinate for at least 10 to 15 minutes before serving.

2 Put a lid on the jar and keep it in the refrigerator, where it will keep for about 1 week.

FOR BABIES 10 MONTHS & OLDER: Try some of this relish on a sandwich made with French Lentil Dijon Spread (page 159). When making the spread, reserve plain cooked lentils and puree with a little water for baby.

PREPARATION TIME:

15 to 20 minutes

MAKES 1 CUP

1 cup finely diced red, orange, or yellow bell pepper

1 jalapeño, finely diced

3 tablespoons sugar

3 tablespoons unfiltered apple cider vinegar

Pinch of sea salt

almond-ginger drizzle

This sensuous sauce may be used to top grains or vegetables. It's especially nice over kasha or cooked greens. You can substitute different nut butters to create slight variations in taste.

PREPARATION TIME:

5 minutes

MAKES 1 CUP

⅓ cup water

¼ cup creamy almond butter

2 tablespoons tamari
(soy sauce)

1 to 2 teaspoons hot
pepper oil

1 tablespoon rice vinegar

2 teaspoons maple syrup

1 teaspoon freshly grated
gingerroot

1 In a small saucepan over low heat, add the water almond butter, tamari, oil, vinegar, maple syrup, and ginger and bring the mixture to a light simmer. Using a whisk, mix the ingredients until smooth. Simmer on low for 3 to 4 minutes with a lid on, or until ingredients are integrated and creamy looking, then remove the pan from the heat.

2 Once removed from heat, the mixture may thicken. Thin it with a little more water and re-warm if needed. Serve the drizzle immediately over grains, beans, or cooked vegetables.

FOR BABIES 10 MONTHS & OLDER: Stir ½ teaspoon of almond butter into baby's warm cereal or pureed vegetables for added calories and other nutrients.
VARIATION FOR CHILDREN: Omit the hot pepper oil. Use the drizzle as a dipping sauce for raw vegetables.

coconut peanut sauce

A simple variation on the previous recipe gives this sauce more of a "Thai" touch. This sauce is yummy on cooked greens or noodles and essential for dipping Thai Fresh Vegetable Rolls (page 157). Be sure to buy peanut butter with no sugar or additives—keep it real.

1 Taste the peanut butter. If it is salty, you may need to reduce the amount of tamari added to the sauce. If it is not salty tasting, leave the amount as is.

2 In a small saucepan over medium heat, add the peanut butter, tamari, vinegar, ginger, maple syrup, and oil and bring it to a light simmer. Whisk in the coconut milk until smooth. Simmer on low, covered, until flavors integrate and mixture becomes creamy, 3 to 4 minutes.

3 The mixture may thicken if left to stand. Thin it with a little water and re-warm if needed. Serve immediately over grains, beans, or cooked vegetables.

FOR BABIES 10 MONTHS & OLDER: Stir 1 to 2 teaspoons of coconut milk into baby's warm whole grain cereal or pureed vegetables for added fats.

PREPARATION TIME:

5 minutes

MAKES 1 CUP

¼ cup creamy peanut butter

2 tablespoons tamari (soy sauce)

1 tablespoon rice vinegar

2 teaspoons freshly grated gingerroot

2 teaspoons maple syrup

1 to 2 teaspoons hot pepper oil

1 small (5.46-ounce) can coconut milk (about ⅔ cup)

361

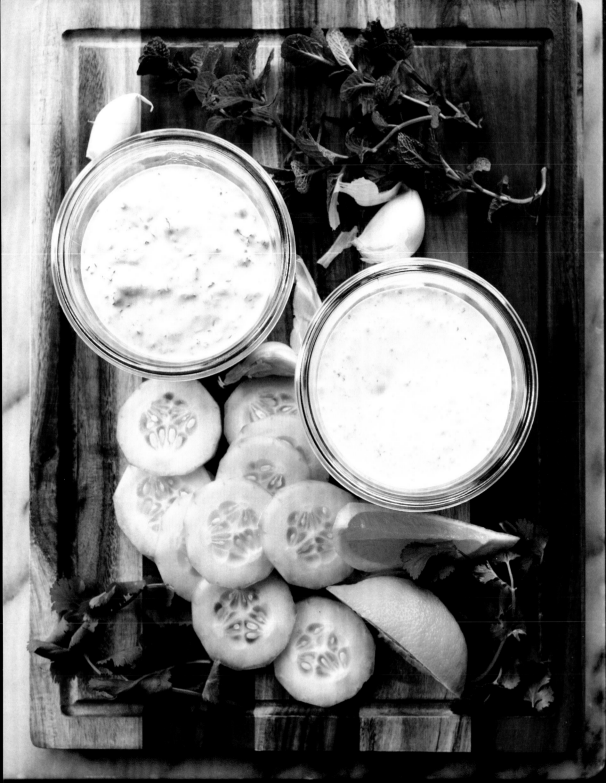

tzatziki sauce

Yogurt toppings appear in several ethnic cuisines. Raita is typically used with Indian foods, while tzatziki (more garlic and more lemon) is paired with Greek dishes.

1 In a small bowl, combine the garlic and cucumber with the yogurt, lemon juice, mint, and salt. Chill for at least ½ hour or up to overnight to allow flavors to marry.

2 Store covered in the refrigerator where it will keep for about 1 week.

FOR BABIES 10 MONTHS & OLDER: Adding ½ teaspoon of chopped green herbs to baby's vegetables or cereal boosts the vitamin content of the food.

PREPARATION TIME:

10 minutes; 30 minutes (for marinating)

MAKES 1 CUP

3 to 4 cloves garlic, minced

¼ of a large cucumber, peeled, seeded, and diced

1 cup plain whole milk yogurt

2 tablespoons freshly squeezed lemon juice

2 teaspoons finely chopped fresh mint or Italian parsley

Pinch of sea salt

yogurt cucumber topping (raita)

Be sure to buy organic yogurt that has active cultures and no added fillers (i.e., nonfat milk solids or pectin).

PREPARATION TIME:

5 minutes; 30 minutes (for marinating)

MAKES 1½ CUPS

1 cup plain whole milk yogurt

½ cucumber, peeled, seeded, and diced

2 tablespoons finely chopped fresh mint or cilantro

1 clove garlic, minced

½ teaspoon ground cumin

Pinch of cayenne

Pinch of sea salt

1 In a small bowl, combine the yogurt, cucumber, mint, garlic, cumin, and cayenne. Sprinkle in the salt to bring out the flavors. Chill for about ½ hour or up to overnight before serving.

2 Store covered in the refrigerator where it will keep for about 1 week.

FOR BABIES 10 MONTHS & OLDER: Serve baby a teaspoon of plain yogurt mixed with cooked vegetables.

---

lemon tahini sauce

This dressing is so versatile it is worth making regularly to use as a topping on brown rice, soba noodles, or as a lively salad dressing. Tahini is a creamy paste made of crushed, hulled sesame seeds. Look for it with other nut butters or Middle Eastern foods.

1 In a blender, put the tahini, oil, lemon juice, garlic, tamari, cayenne, and ¼ cup of the water and puree until smooth.

2 Continue adding water to get desired consistency; it can be the consistency of thick cream or thinner if using as a salad dressing. Taste for salt and add more tamari if needed. Allow the mixture to set for 30 minutes to allow the flavors to meld.

3 The sauce will keep in the refrigerator for 10 to 14 days.

FOR BABIES 10 MONTHS & OLDER: Add a little tahini to baby's cereal or pureed vegetables for added high-quality fat.

PREPARATION TIME:

5 minutes; 30 minutes
(for marinating)

MAKES 1½ CUPS

½ cup tahini

¼ cup extra-virgin olive oil

¼ cup freshly squeezed
   lemon juice (from
   1½ small lemons)

1 clove garlic

2 teaspoons tamari
   (soy sauce)

Pinch of cayenne

About ¾ cup water

fresh corn salsa

This salsa shines in late summer when sweet corn is in season. Put it on a taco. Just do it. Or some black bean soup.

PREPARATION TIME:

5 to 10 minutes; 20 minutes (for marinating)

MAKES 4 SMALL SERVINGS

1 ear of corn, shucked, kernels removed with knife (about 1 cup corn)

1 jalapeño, seeded and minced

½ ripe avocado, cut into cubes

¼ medium red onion, diced

2 tablespoons fresh cilantro

1 to 2 tablespoons freshly squeezed lime juice, plus more if needed

½ teaspoon ground cumin

½ teaspoon freshly ground black pepper

¼ teaspoon sea salt

1 In a medium bowl, put the corn, jalapeño, avocado, onion, cilantro, lime juice, cumin, pepper, and salt. Stir gently. Taste and add more lime juice and salt if desired. Allow the mixture to marinate for at least 20 minutes.

2 This salsa can be made in advance and stored in a sealed container in the refrigerator for 3 to 4 days. Drain off any excess liquid before serving.

FOR BABIES 6 MONTHS & OLDER: Tried-and-true mashed avocado makes perfect baby food.

---

thai cucumber-jalapeño relish

This relish adds big flavor to bland grains, noodles, or tofu. Control the heat factor by tasting a tiny piece of the jalapeño, noting the heat and adding it a little at a time.

1 In a medium bowl, combine the cucumber, jalapeño, green onion, onion, cilantro, sugar, lime juice, vinegar, and salt. Gently stir until sugar has dissolved. Taste and add more lime, sugar, and salt if desired. Allow the mixture to marinate for at least 20 minutes.

2 The relish can be made in advance and stored in a sealed container in the refrigerator for up to 1 week.

VARIATION FOR CHILDREN: The jalapeño gives this topping a lot of heat! Replace the jalapeño with more cucumber for a less fiery version.

PREPARATION TIME:

5 minutes; 20 minutes (for marinating)

MAKES 4 SMALL SERVINGS

½ medium cucumber, peeled, seeded, and diced

1 small jalapeño, seeded and minced

1 green onion, minced

¼ medium white onion, diced

¼ cup chopped fresh cilantro

2 tablespoons sugar

1 tablespoon freshly squeezed lime juice

1 tablespoon rice vinegar

Pinch of sea salt

mango salsa

This salsa is fabulous served as a garnish with Huevos Rancheros (page 102) or Caribbean Lime Halibut (page 279).

PREPARATION TIME:

10 minutes; 30 minutes
(for marinating)

MAKES 6 SMALL SERVINGS

2 medium ripe mangos

1 bunch green onions, thinly
sliced on the diagonal

2 jalapeños, finely diced

¼ cup finely chopped fresh
cilantro

2 tablespoons freshly
squeezed lime juice (from
about 2 limes)

Pinch of sea salt

1 The mango has a flat elliptical-shaped seed in it. Hold each mango vertically and cut from the top down on both sides just missing the seed. You will have two bowl-shaped halves. Discard the middle section with the seed. Score the meat of the mango in a ¼-inch crisscross pattern on each half. Push up from the skin side, turning the bowl inside out, and cut the cubes off of the skin.

2 In a medium bowl, put the mango cubes, green onions, jalapeño, cilantro, and lime and stir to combine. Fold in the salt and taste. Add more lime and salt if desired. Let the mixture sit about 30 minutes in the refrigerator to mingle flavors.

3 This salsa will keep in the refrigerator for 3 to 4 days.

FOR BABIES 6 MONTHS & OLDER: Blend some of the ripe mango pieces to serve as a perfect beginner food.

tofu ginger-garlic dressing

Need to go dairy-free? Here's creaminess without the cream. Try it as a dip for Deep-Fried Millet Croquettes (page 248).

1 In a blender, put all of the ingredients and process until smooth. Add more water if you prefer a thinner dressing.

2 This dressing will keep in the refrigerator for 4 to 5 days.

FOR BABIES 10 MONTHS & OLDER: Cut up extra tofu into small cubes. Steam or drop the cubes into boiling water for a few seconds. Let them cool and serve as a finger food.

PREPARATION TIME:

5 minutes

MAKES 1 CUP

½ pound tofu

¼ cup water

2 tablespoons extra-virgin olive oil

2 tablespoons freshly squeezed lime juice

2 teaspoons tamari (soy sauce)

1 teaspoon freshly grated gingerroot

2 cloves garlic, minced

369

pumpkin seed & parsley garnish

This garnish adds a crunchy texture and exciting flavor to smooth dishes like Rosemary Red Soup (page 175), or use it instead of sesame seeds on Sweet Rice Timbales (page 255). The fresh parsley adds nice dark leafy green nutrients.

PREPARATION TIME:

5 minutes

MAKES ABOUT ¾ CUP

½ cup pumpkin seeds

¼ cup fresh Italian parsley

3 to 4 tablespoons
    extra-virgin olive oil

¼ teaspoon sea salt

2 cloves garlic

1 Heat a dry skillet over medium heat. Add the pumpkin seeds and keep them moving with a wooden spoon. After a few minutes, they will begin to pop, puff up, and give off a nutty aroma. Remove the seeds from the heat. Taste one. They should be crunchy.

2 In a food processor, put the toasted pumpkin seeds with the parsley, oil, salt, and garlic and pulse three or four times until you have a coarse mixture. (The toasted seeds, garlic, and parsley can also be finely chopped by hand.)

3 Store in a covered container in the refrigerator for up to 1 week.

FOR BABIES 10 MONTHS & OLDER: Grind a few toasted pumpkin seeds before adding other ingredients, then add to any food you are pureeing for baby for healthful fiber and minerals.

maple-glazed walnuts

These walnuts are yummy on hot cereal, in a fresh green salad, or tucked in a lunch box compartment. They satisfy the desire for sweets and fats in a nutritious way.

1 Preheat the oven to 325 degrees F and lightly oil a baking dish.

2 In a small bowl, combine the walnuts, maple syrup, salt, pepper, and cayenne and toss to coat. Spread the nut mixture into baking dish.

3 Bake until nuts are golden and maple syrup bubbles, 8 to 10 minutes, stirring occasionally to break up clumps. Remove the baking dish from the oven, and cool the nuts on the baking dish. Remove them while slightly warm with a spatula.

4 Store in a covered container in the refrigerator for up to 1 month.

FOR BABIES 10 MONTHS & OLDER: Toast one or two walnuts without the syrup and spices. Grind them up and add them to baby's cereal or pureed vegetables. (They're especially nice on baked sweet potato.)

PREPARATION TIME:

20 minutes

MAKES ⅔ CUP

Extra-virgin olive oil or
    unsalted butter, for oiling
⅔ cup walnuts
2 tablespoons maple syrup
Pinch of sea salt
One grind of black pepper
Tiny pinch of cayenne

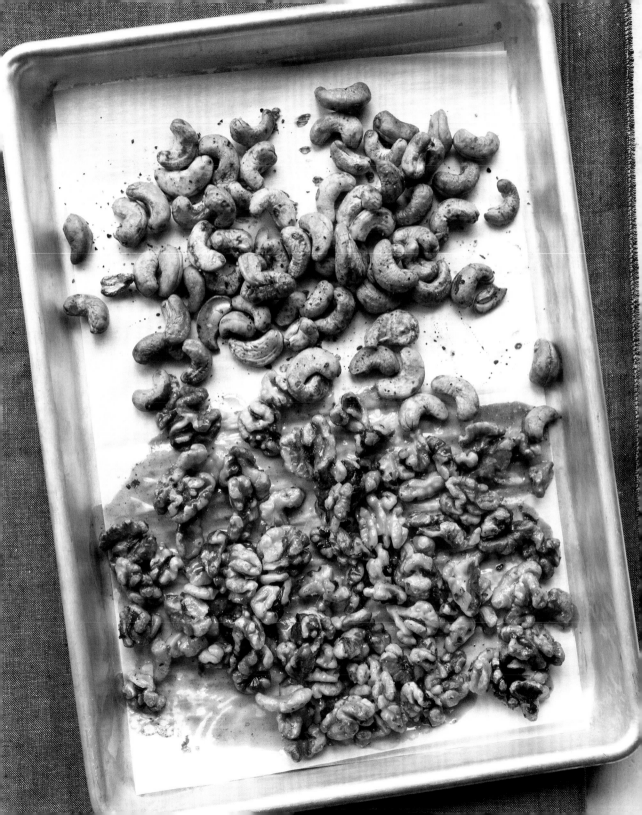

tamari-roasted cashews

Tamari-roasted nuts make a crunchy addition to any lunch box. Sprinkle a few on salads or grains to liven up the flavor and texture. A jar of these nuts makes a welcome gift as well.

1 Preheat the oven to 325 degrees F.

2 Place nuts in a dry 8-by-8-inch baking dish. Toast the nuts in the oven until they begin to turn golden and give off a nutty aroma, 12 to 15 minutes.

3 While the nuts are toasting, in a small bowl, mix the tamari, cumin, coriander, and cayenne together. Remove the nuts from oven and sprinkle the spice mix over the nuts, then stir and return the pan to oven to dry out for 10 more minutes. Once the nuts seem dry, turn the oven off but leave the pan in the oven as it cools off, at least 10 minutes.

4 Store the toasted nuts in a sealed container or jar, where they will keep for at least 1 month.

PREPARATION TIME:

30 minutes

MAKES 2 CUPS

2 cups whole raw cashews

1 to 2 tablespoons tamari (soy sauce)

½ teaspoon ground cumin

½ teaspoon ground coriander

Pinch of cayenne (optional)

FOR BABIES 10 MONTHS & OLDER: Remove a few of the toasted nuts before sprinkling them with tamari and spices. Grind the nuts to a fine meal and stir tiny amounts into baby's cereal or vegetables for a new flavor.

---

refreshing relishes & convenient condiments

< (top) Tamari-Roasted Cashews, (bottom) Maple-Glazed Walnuts

strawberry-blueberry sauce
for pancakes & waffles

Cooking berries with a bit of sugar and serving over pancakes (or hot cereal) helps satisfy the one and a half to two cups of daily fruit recommended for children in a welcome way.

PREPARATION TIME:

10 minutes

MAKES 2 CUPS

¼ cup unrefined cane sugar

¼ cup water

½ pint fresh blueberries, or
  1 cup frozen

½ pint fresh strawberries,
  hulled and halved, or
  1 cup frozen

1 teaspoon freshly squeezed
  lemon juice

1 In a small saucepan over medium heat, combine the sugar and water. Stir to dissolve the sugar.

2 Add the blueberries and simmer, covered, until the blueberries are tender or have started to burst, about 15 minutes. Add the strawberries and simmer 10 more minutes. Remove the pan from the heat, add the lemon juice, and allow mixture to cool for 5 minutes.

3 In a blender, puree the berry mixture; or, if you prefer a chunkier texture, press it with a potato masher. Add a touch of water if mixture appears too thick.

FOR BABIES 6 MONTHS & OLDER: Reserve some fresh blueberries, puree them with a little water, and serve.

feeding the whole family

autumn cranberry-apple relish

This relish is the perfect topping for Goat Cheese and Kale Chicken Roulade (page 289) and a natural served at the Thanksgiving or Christmas dinner table.

1 In a 2-quart saucepan over medium-high heat, put the cranberries, apples, juice, currants, maple syrup, zest, and salt and bring it to a boil. Reduce the heat to low, cover, and simmer, stirring frequently, until the cranberries have burst and mixture has thickened, 20 to 25 minutes. Remove the lid and cook off any excess liquid to thicken, if desired, though the mixture will thicken as it cools.

2 Remove the pan from the heat. Once cooled slightly, stir in the walnuts. Serve at room temperature.

3 This relish will keep in a sealed container in the refrigerator for 1 week.

FOR BABIES 10 MONTHS & OLDER: If your baby has teeth, reserve some apple slices, steam until soft, let cool, and serve as finger food.

PREPARATION TIME:

30 minutes

MAKES 2½ CUPS

1½ cups fresh, whole cranberries

1 cup chopped apple

1 cup apple juice or water

½ cup currants

¼ cup maple syrup

1 teaspoon orange zest

¼ teaspoon sea salt

¼ cup chopped walnuts

375

homemade applesauce

There are many excellent brands of jarred applesauce, but there is nothing quite as satisfying as freshly made applesauce from seasonal apples. There's no need to peel the apples if they are organic.

PREPARATION TIME:

20 minutes

MAKES 2 CUPS

4 medium apples (about 1½ pounds), cut into 1-inch chunks

½ to ⅔ cup apple juice or apple cider

2 cinnamon sticks

½ teaspoon ground allspice

¼ teaspoon sea salt

1 tablespoon unrefined cane sugar or brown sugar (optional)

1 In a 2-quart pot over medium heat, add the apples, juice, cinnamon, allspice, and salt. Taste a slice of apple to decide if and how much sugar you will add (none if this will become food for baby), and add your desired amount of sugar. Bring the pot to a boil, reduce the heat to low, and simmer, covered, until the apples are tender and some of the liquid has cooked off, about 15 minutes. (Alternately, applesauce can be made in the pressure cooker. Once the pressure cooker is up to pressure, only 5 minutes of cooking time is required.)

2 Remove the cinnamon sticks and puree the apple mixture in the blender or mash it with a potato masher, depending on whether you want a smooth or chunky consistency.

FOR BABIES 6 MONTHS & OLDER: This is it—the perfect food for baby, mommy, and all. Omit the unrefined cane sugar for these wee ones.

kitchen ketchup

No fillers, cheap sweeteners, or unknown ingredients are present when you make ketchup at home; plus, the flavor is richer and the texture thicker (not watery!).

1 In a medium bowl, put the tomato paste, vinegars, honey, sugar, garlic, salt, and allspice and stir well until smooth and uniform.

2 Taste and add more honey, sugar, salt, or vinegar to get a taste you like.

3 The ketchup will keep in a closed container in the refrigerator for 1 to 2 weeks.

FOR BABIES 6 MONTHS & OLDER: Nothing is better than ketchup on Rosemary and Garlic Roasted Potatoes (page 233). Puree several chunks of roasted or steamed potatoes with a little water or breast milk for baby.

PREPARATION TIME:

6 to 8 minutes

MAKES 1 CUP

1 (6-ounce) can tomato paste

3 tablespoons apple cider vinegar, plus more if needed

1 tablespoon balsamic vinegar, plus more if needed

3 tablespoons honey, plus more if needed

1 tablespoon brown sugar, plus more if needed

1 clove garlic, pressed

½ teaspoon sea salt, plus more if needed

¼ teaspoon ground allspice

refreshing relishes & convenient condiments

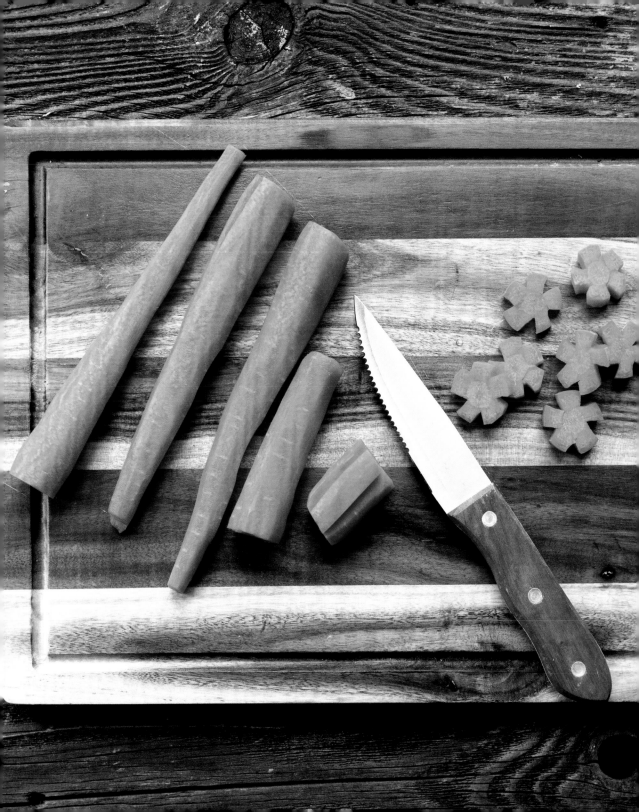

carrot flowers

Add beauty to any dish or lunch box by decorating it with pretty flower-shaped orange carrots.

1 Using a sharp paring knife, make a lengthwise slit into each 4-inch length of carrot, about ⅛-inch deep. Make another lengthwise slit at a 45-degree angle to the first. Remove the *V*-shaped strip from the carrot. Cut out four more *V*-shaped strips at equal intervals around the carrot. Repeat this process on each piece of carrot.

2 Slice the grooved carrot lengths into ¼-inch rounds, creating flower-shaped slices. In a 2-quart pan over high heat, bring 2 cups of water and the cinnamon to a boil. Add the carrot flowers and reduce the heat to medium. Blanch the carrots a few minutes until tender. Drain, then cover the carrots in ice-cold water for 2 to 3 minutes. Drain again and store the carrots in the refrigerator, where they will keep for 3 to 4 days.

FOR BABIES 6 MONTHS & OLDER: Leave some carrots in the boiling water several minutes longer until soft enough to puree, and serve to baby.

PREPARATION TIME:

10 minutes

MAKES 1 CUP

1 pound (about 4 or 5) carrots, trimmed and cut into 4-inch lengths

1 cinnamon stick

379

refreshing relishes & convenient condiments

old-fashioned strawberry-honey jam

Here's a full-circle recipe involving the bees, the honey they make from flower nectar, and the evolution of the strawberry flower into fruit. Always choose organic when it comes to strawberries, as they are listed on the Environmental Working Group's Dirty Dozen list of most pesticide-laden foods.

PREPARATION TIME:

1½ hours

MAKES 6 TO 7 HALF-PINTS

4 pounds fresh organic
    strawberries

2¼ cups honey

½ cup sugar

1 tart apple, grated

1 tablespoon freshly
    squeezed lemon juice

1 To prepare the jars, run six to seven pint-size jars and their lids through the dishwasher to sterilize them. If you don't have a dishwasher, you can fill an 8-quart pot with water and put a rack or a towel on the bottom. Once the water is at a full boil, add the jars. Turn off the heat. Leave everything in the water for about 15 minutes, then remove them and put them on a baking sheet lined with a towel to air dry.

2 To make the jam, clean and trim the strawberries. Cut each strawberry into two to three pieces; quarter the large ones.

3 In a heavy 8-quart pot over high heat, combine the strawberries, honey, sugar, apple, and lemon juice. Bring the pot to a boil, stirring frequently.

4 Reduce the heat to low and establish a low bubble. Continue to stir every so often, scraping the sides of the pot where the fruit has thickened and stuck. Break up the strawberries with a potato masher as they soften. Let the mixture bubble for 45 to 60 minutes; it will reduce by almost half.

5 To test for doneness, put a small plate or ramekin in the freezer for 5 minutes. Spoon a bit of the jam onto the cold plate and put it back in the freezer for 1 minute. When you push the jam with your finger, does it set up and leave a clean space where you pushed it? When you spoon the jam onto the plate, does the jam coat the back of the spoon? Has the mixture reduced by about half? Is the temperature of the berry mix up to 220 degrees F? If you answered yes to most of these questions, your jam is ready.

6 To preserve the jam, fill the jars with hot jam, leaving ¼-inch headspace. A widemouthed canning funnel works well.

7 Wipe the rims with a clean, lint-free towel. Put the lids and bands on the jars, turning the band so the lid is secure but not overly tight.

8 Place a canning rack or extra jar bands on the bottom of a large pot filled two-thirds to three-quarters full of water (this can be done in an 8-quart pot or a 10- to 12-quart canning pot). Bring the water to a full boil over high heat. Lower the jars into the water so that they are fully immersed. Process for 10 minutes, then remove each jar to a towel on the counter and let it cool. You will hear a "plink" when the processed jar has sealed!

9 This jam will be thick but much softer (easier to spread!) than jams that use commercial pectin.

FOR BABIES 10 MONTHS & OLDER: If your baby has teeth, reserve two or three soft, ripe berries cut into slices for finger food.

---

homemade curry paste

My life is so much easier with a jar of this in the refrigerator. My friend Jeff Basom created this multiuse flavoring for soups, beans, and all sorts of Indian-flavored dishes. This handy product for busy cooks makes a unique Christmas gift.

PREPARATION TIME:

20 to 25 minutes

MAKES 1 CUP

1 cup extra-virgin olive oil

1 pound onions, finely chopped

¼ cup cumin seeds

¼ cup coriander seeds

2 tablespoons whole mustard seeds

2 teaspoons whole black pepper

1 teaspoon fenugreek seeds

1 teaspoon whole cloves

¼ cup ground turmeric

¼ cup gingerroot, peeled and finely chopped

4 teaspoons ground cinnamon

2 teaspoons ground allspice

2 teaspoons cayenne

1 teaspoon ground cardamom

1 teaspoon sea salt

1 In a 2-quart pot over low heat, heat the oil. Add the onions and sauté until very soft.

2 While the onions are cooking, in a coffee or spice grinder, grind the cumin, coriander, mustard seeds, pepper, fenugreek, and cloves to a fine powder. Add the freshly ground spices to onions.

3 Add the turmeric, ginger, cinnamon, allspice, cayenne, cardamom, and salt to the onion mixture; cook, stirring continuously, until spices are no longer powdery, about 5 minutes.

4 Store the curry paste in a sealed jar in the refrigerator, where it will keep for several months.

FOR BABIES 10 MONTHS & OLDER: Use this paste to make Curried Lentil and Potato Stew (page 186). Remove some of the cooked potatoes and carrots from the soup, puree, and serve.

homemade ghee

In the East, ghee is thought to take on and magnify the properties of food it is combined with, making the food more nutritious. Ghee is sometimes used in place of oil, especially in dishes that contain Indian spices. Ghee imparts a buttery flavor but can hold a much higher temperature than butter without scorching.

1 In a 2-quart saucepan over medium-low heat, heat the butter until it begins to bubble, 4 to 5 minutes, and then turn the heat to low.

2 White foam (from the milk solids) will begin to accumulate on the top. Use a fine mesh strainer and begin gently skimming the milk solids off the top without disturbing the bottom. As you continue this process, the liquid in the bottom of the pan will begin to appear clear and golden.

3 When all the water is boiled out of the butter, the cooking fat will sound like hissing and the bubbling will stop. Remove the pan from the heat and let it cool a few moments. Pour the ghee into a clean 8-ounce jar. It will solidify as it cools.

4 Store the ghee in the refrigerator, covered, where it will keep for several months.

PREPARATION TIME:

15 minutes

MAKES ABOUT 1 CUP

½ pound unsalted butter

FOR BABIES 6 MONTHS & OLDER: Use ghee to make Curried Cauliflower Dal (page 266). Reserve a small portion of soft-cooked cauliflower from the dal. Don't be afraid that it will have traces of spice. Puree with a little water or breast milk and serve to baby.

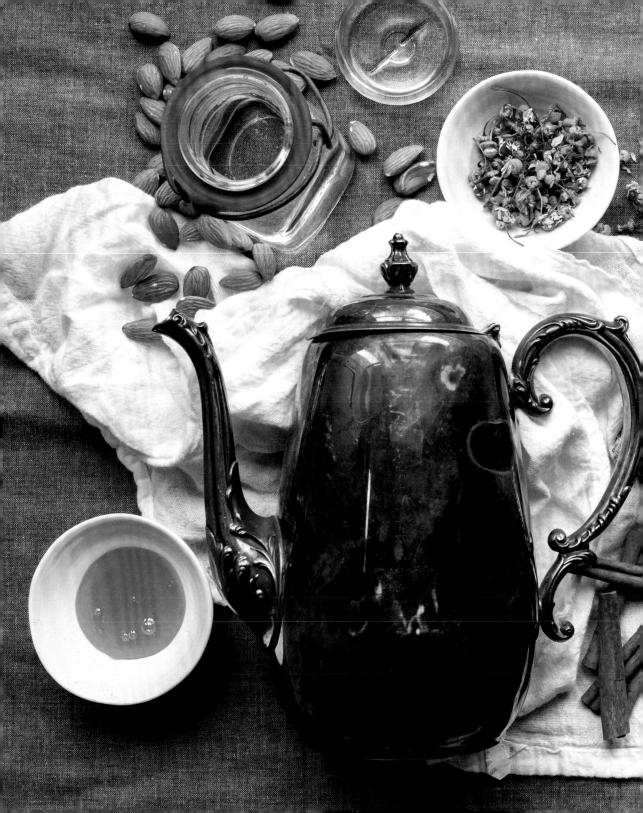

- - - - - - - - -

kitchen remedies *for* children

While whole food eating habits have provided the foundation of sound health for me and my family, we have also benefited from using alternative therapies such as acupuncture, herbs, homeopathy, and home remedies.

For the past half-dozen years, I have regularly visited a gifted practitioner, Teri Adolfo, MS, MTCM, who combines acupuncture with Ayurvedic medicine to provide the best of both traditional therapies. Naturally, I sought her help to put together a chapter of kitchen remedies for children with minor maladies.

Warning: Using these remedies is in no way a substitute for a call or visit to the doctor. If your child has a fever, swelling, rash, or earache, or diarrhea lasting more than a day, contact your pediatrician. The following tonics are meant for alleviating minor discomforts. Remember, too, that sleep and fluids (water) form the primary tools for recovery.

In a recent book giveaway on my blog, I asked contest entrants to write in what foods they were given as a child when feeling ill. Two people mentioned bacon-and-peanut-butter sandwiches (hard to fathom!). For the most part, there was predictability in the responses. Chicken noodle soup and ginger ale comments were numerous, also tea and toast. Both the Vietnamese Pho Ga Soup (page 181) and the Miso Soup with Tofu and Bok Choy Ribbons (page 171) make excellent recuperative foods. Teri and I have put together a few more concoctions to address specific maladies.

When a child doesn't feel good, the parent wants to feel useful, as well as being a conduit to someone with more expertise. Preparing these gentle remedies can be comforting for both the child and the caregiver.

soothing tea *for* colic *or* tummy ache

This combination of herbs and spices is useful for many digestive issues, including gas or bloating. If you are nursing, have a cup of tea before or while you are nursing and pass it on to baby.

1 In a small, dry skillet, lightly toast the seeds to awaken their flavor. Stir continuously until their aroma reaches your nose and the seeds start to crackle, 3 to 4 minutes. Crush the seeds with a rolling pin or pulse in a small grinder.

2 Prepare the tea by pouring 1 cup boiling water over 1 teaspoon of the crushed seed mixture (save the remainder in a sealed container for later). Steep the tea for 10 minutes and then strain.

PREPARATION TIME:

20 minutes

MAKES 3 CUPS

1 teaspoon fennel seeds
1 teaspoon cumin seeds
1 teaspoon coriander seeds

DOSAGE FOR BABIES 6 MONTHS & OLDER: 3 teaspoons brewed tea in ½ cup warm water, twice a day.

DOSAGE FOR CHILDREN: ½ cup tea, twice a day.

ginger tea *for* nausea

Ginger tea is a soothing drink for someone with an upset stomach or nausea. It's also the perfect remedy for a cold, as gingerroot warms the body and increases circulation. If using this tea to alleviate cold symptoms, you may want to triple the recipe and sip tea throughout the day.

PREPARATION TIME:

30 minutes

MAKES 2 CUPS

2 cups water

A piece of gingerroot the size of the patient's thumb, thinly sliced

Freshly squeezed lemon juice

Maple syrup or honey

1 In a small pot over medium-low heat, simmer the water and ginger until the water has reduced to 1 cup, 20 to 30 minutes. This is strong tea! Strain and pour the tea into a cup. Add a squeeze of fresh lemon to each cup. Stir in sweetener as desired.

DOSAGE FOR BABIES 10 MONTHS & OLDER: 1 teaspoon tea in ½ cup of warm water, once a day.

DOSAGE FOR CHILDREN: Suitable in a cup for child.

kudzu root broth *for the* runs

Kudzu, or kuzu, root resembles broken chalk. The root of this plant has appreciable healing properties. For more than two thousand years, kudzu root has been used as an herbal medicine for the treatment of fever, acute dysentery, diarrhea, diabetes, and cardiovascular diseases. Look for kudzu root in small packages in the Asian or macrobiotic section of the health food store or at a store selling medicinal herbs.

1 In a small pan, dissolve the kudzu in the water. Put the pan with the mixture over medium heat, stirring constantly. As the mixture comes to a simmer, it will become clear and thick. Once this happens, remove the broth from heat. Add the tamari, then mix well. Serve immediately. This can be drunk or sipped from a spoon.

PREPARATION TIME:

5 minutes

MAKES 1 CUP

1 tablespoon kudzu

1 cup cold or room-
temperature water

2 teaspoons tamari
(soy sauce)

389

DOSAGE FOR BABIES 1 YEAR & UNDER: Not appropriate.

DOSAGE FOR CHILDREN: ½ cup served in a small bowl with a spoon.

fennel tea *for* constipation

This recipe creates a small quantity of dry mix that can be made into many cups of tea. Buying herbs in bulk at a natural pharmacy or herb store is usually more economical.

PREPARATION TIME:

25 minutes

MAKES TEA BLEND FOR 8 CUPS

4 teaspoons fennel seeds

2 teaspoons spearmint leaves (or 2 tea bags)

1 teaspoon psyllium seed powder

½ teaspoon ground cinnamon

½ teaspoon orange zest

1 To make the tea blend, in a small bowl, combine the fennel, spearmint leaves (if using tea bags, remove the spearmint and discard the bags), psyllium seed, cinnamon, and zest. Stir to blend and store it in a sealed container. The zest will dry out, and that's fine.

2 To make 1 cup of tea, pour 1 cup of boiling water over 1 teaspoon of tea blend, cover, and steep for 15 to 20 minutes.

DOSAGE FOR BABIES 10 MONTHS & UNDER: Nursing moms can drink a cup of tea, and baby will benefit.

DOSAGE FOR BABIES 10 MONTHS & OLDER: 2 teaspoons brewed tea in ½ cup of warm water, twice a day.

DOSAGE FOR CHILDREN: ½ cup, up to three times a day.

honey thyme cough syrup

Thyme has a long history of use in natural medicine in connection with chest and respiratory problems, including coughs, bronchitis, and chest congestion. The volatile oil components of thyme are known for inducing antimicrobial activity.

1 In a 2-quart pot over high heat, add the water and thyme. Bring the water to a bubbling boil, then reduce the heat to medium low to simmer for 12 minutes.

2 Let the tea cool slightly, then strain the tea into a bowl or jar, pressing the mixture to squeeze out all of the liquid. Add the honey and stir until it is fully dissolved. Transfer the tea to a clean glass container and store in the refrigerator. Take 1 teaspoon at a time for cough, sore throat, and colds.

PREPARATION TIME:

15 minutes

MAKES 1½ CUPS

1 cup water
¼ cup dried thyme
½ cup local honey

DOSAGE FOR BABIES 1 YEAR & UNDER: Not appropriate.

DOSAGE FOR CHILDREN: 2 teaspoons, every 4 hours.

391

kitchen remedies for children

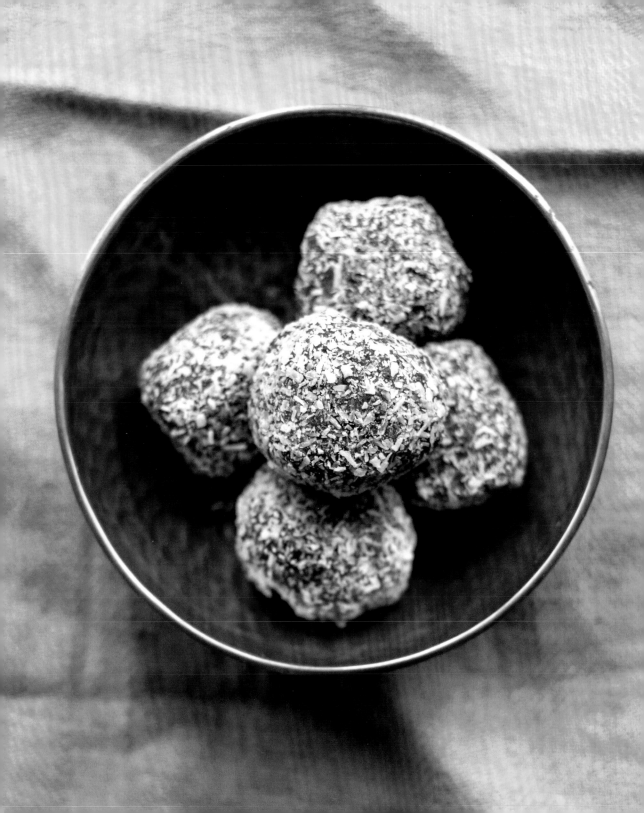

smooth move prune balls

Did you know that dates actually have more fiber than prunes? Plus, they are sweeter! The combination of prunes, dates, and psyllium seeds provides the fiber needed to get things moving for constipated children (and adults!).

1 In a food processor, put the prunes, dates, and nut butter and pulse until the dried fruits are piecemeal in the nut butter. Add the maple syrup, seeds, and salt and pulse again until the mixture begins to collect into one mass.

2 With moist hands, form the mixture into ¾- to 1-inch balls. Spread coconut on a plate and roll each ball in coconut. Store the prune balls in a sealed container in the refrigerator.

DOSAGE FOR BABIES 1 YEAR & UNDER: Not appropriate.

DOSAGE FOR CHILDREN: ½ ball, every 12 hours until movement occurs.

PREPARATION TIME:

15 minutes

MAKES 14 TO 18 BALLS, DEPENDING ON SIZE

½ cup pitted prunes

½ cup pitted dates

¼ cup peanut or almond butter

2 teaspoons maple syrup

1 tablespoon psyllium seeds (or powder)

1 tablespoon chia seeds

¼ teaspoon sea salt

2 tablespoons shredded unsweetened coconut

393

kudzu pudding *for* sugar blues

The kudzu root has long been researched as a treatment for alcohol abuse. In the East, the name for kudzu tea is xing-jiu-ling, which translates as "sober up." Since sugar addiction and alcohol addiction have similar biochemical pathways, it makes sense that the root might work for both issues. When sugar cravings feel relentless, I make a cup of this pudding. The juice satisfies the sweet tooth, the tahini fat slows down any rush, and the kudzu has its own magic.

PREPARATION TIME:

5 to 10 minutes

MAKES 1 SERVING

1 tablespoon kudzu

1 cup apple juice, cold or room temperature

1 teaspoon tahini

½ teaspoon vanilla extract

1 In a small pan, dissolve the kudzu in the juice. Heat the mixture over medium heat, stirring constantly. As mixture comes to a simmer, it will become clear and thick. Once this happens, after 2 to 4 minutes, remove the pan from the heat.

2 Add the tahini and vanilla to the pan and stir to combine. Serve immediately; the mixture will get rubbery if allowed to cool to room temperature.

DOSAGE FOR BABIES 1 YEAR & UNDER: Not appropriate.

DOSAGE FOR CHILDREN: ¼ to ½ cup served in a bowl with a spoon

congee *for* recovery

Children displaying little or no appetite, upset stomach, or the first sign of cold and flu need easily digestible nourishment. Congee is one of the traditional Chinese foods used for thousands of years to help the ill recover. Congee can be made sweet or savory. According to Teri Adolfo, Ayurvedic acupuncturist, children find this version appealing.

1 In a small grinder or food processor, break up the rice grains by pulsing once or twice.

2 In a 2- or 3-quart pot, over high heat, combine the rice, water, and ginger and bring the mixture to a boil. Reduce the heat to low to simmer, cover, and cook for 40 minutes, or until rice is soft porridge-like. Stir in the dates and zest during the last 15 minutes of cooking time.

DOSAGE FOR BABIES 10 MONTHS & OLDER: ¼ cup, 3 times a day.

DOSAGE FOR CHILDREN: ½ to 1 cup served in a bowl with a spoon, 3 times a day.

PREPARATION TIME:

45 minutes

MAKES 2½ CUPS

½ cup of short-grain white rice

3 cups water

2 teaspoons freshly grated gingerroot

3 dates, cut into small pieces

1 teaspoon lemon zest

kitchen remedies for children

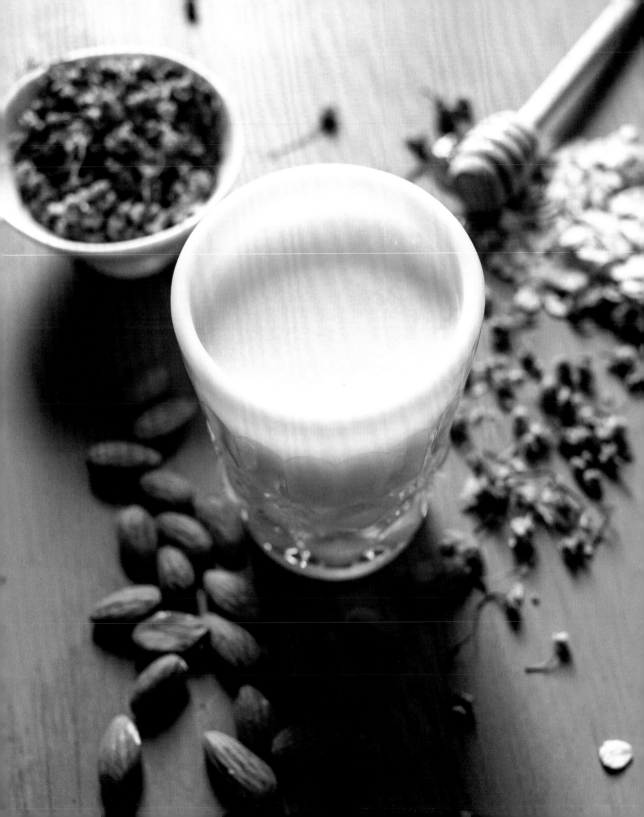

goodnight sleep tight milk

Chamomile and oat straw plus the calcium inherent in almond milk help relax the muscles and mind for a good night's sleep. Oat straw is a known nervine, meaning that it soothes and nourishes the central nervous system.

1 In a teapot or pan, put the chamomile and oat straw. Pour the boiling water over the herbs and steep for 10 minutes. Allow the tea to cool.

2 In a blender, place the almonds and grind into a fine powder. Then add a few tablespoons of the tea and blend until you have a paste. Add the rest of the tea and the honey and blend again.

3 Pour the contents of the blender through a fine mesh strainer lined with cheesecloth into a large bowl to remove the nut pulp. Pick up the ends of the cheesecloth and squeeze the pulp to remove all the milk. A nut milk bag can also be used.

4 Store the herbal milk in a sealed jar in the refrigerator. Warm ½ cup and serve to your child during your bedtime ritual. Maybe while you're reading a favorite book?

PREPARATION TIME:

20 minutes

MAKES 4 SERVINGS

4 teaspoons chamomile tea (or 2 tea bags)

4 teaspoons oat straw or rolled oats

2 cups boiling water

½ cup almonds

1 tablespoon honey

397

DOSAGE FOR BABIES 1 YEAR & UNDER: Not appropriate.

DOSAGE FOR CHILDREN: ½ cup before bed. Alternately, steeped herbal tea can be combined with cow's milk and warmed.

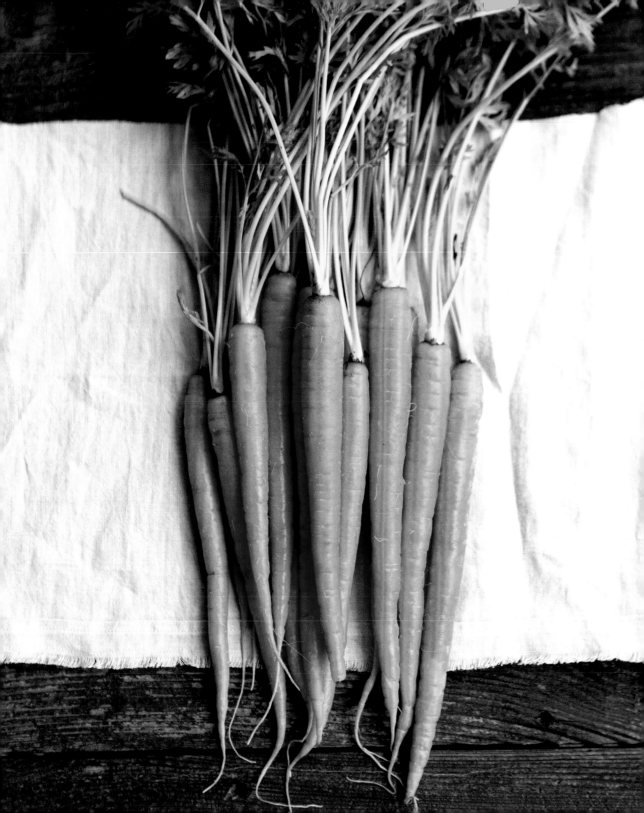

acknowledgments

The faculty and staff at Bastyr University's School of Nutrition and Exercise Science have shaped my working life by giving me a place to teach and learn for over two decades. In particular, I wish to acknowledge my friends and mentors Debra Boutin, Patrice Savery, Dr. Mark Kestin, Chef Jim Watkins, and Chef Jeff Basom.

I have gleaned much from the people who run Seattle's own chain of high-quality natural foods markets: Puget Consumers Co-op (PCC) where I have been a teacher for the PCC Cooks program, off and on, for a couple of decades. Their nationally recognized cooking program is stellar thanks to the work of their former leader, and my friend, Marilyn McCormick.

Thank you to Annemarie Colbin, founder of the Natural Gourmet Institute. Annemarie passed away April 2015 and left behind a legacy as my mentor, colleague, and a champion of the real foods movement.

My heartfelt thanks to my mother-in-law, Lura Geiger, who was brave enough to give this book its start. And bless my sister Cathy, who supports me in all endeavors.

My second family, The Edge, keeps me sane. Oh dear heavens, what would I do without you?

I would also like to thank the following people for their various contributions of sage advice and recipe ideas: Matt Smith, Jamie Lopez, Emma McLeod, Jennifer Adler, Gay Stielstra, and Siona Sammartino.

The fine people at Sasquatch Books have supported *Feeding the Whole Family* for nearly a decade. I'm proud to have my book as a part of their fine offerings.

And, finally, I would never have started this book journey without Michael and Grace and their ceaseless support of who I am and who I will be. I'm such a lucky person.

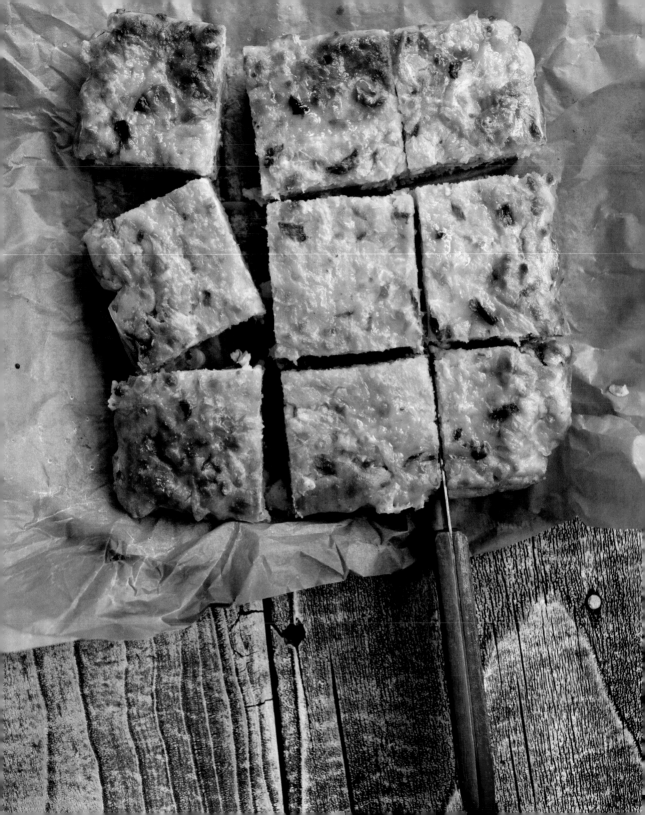

have it your way

- - - - - - - - - - - - - - - -

FLOURS

whole grain flour

Whole grain flour contains bran and tends to absorb more liquid than white flour. If you replace white flour with whole grain flour in equal amounts, your dish may come out too dry. Replace 1 cup white flour with ⅞ cup whole grain flour.

gluten-free flour

Wheat, Kamut, spelt, rye, and barley flours all contain gluten. For the family member that is gluten intolerant or gluten sensitive, you'll need to substitute a gluten-free flour. I find the formulas with bean flours give baked goods a funny beany taste and prefer one of these. Each is formulated by ratios. If you use gluten-free flour often, make a lot and store flour blends in a sealed container.

1 part sweet potato flour
1 part sorghum flour
½ part tapioca flour

1 part brown rice flour
¼ part potato starch
⅛ part tapioca flour
¹⁄₄₈ part xanthan gum

1 part sweet brown rice flour or rice flour
1 part almond flour
¼ part tapioca flour

FATS

Notice whether the fat in your recipe is solid or liquid. When you replace a liquid fat with a solid fat (for example, canola oil with butter), melt the solid fat to get the correct measurement. It is tricky to replace a solid fat with a liquid fat (for example, replacing Crisco with olive oil). You will need to examine how the fat is used in the recipe and experiment.

If you need to make a dairy-free recipe that calls for butter, you can some-times substitute coconut oil. Be aware that coconut oil can make the final product a little greasy.

MILKS

Soy, rice, or nut milk (see page 351) can be substituted for cow's milk in any recipe.

SWEETENERS

To replace a granulated sweetener with a liquid sweetener (e.g., replace white sugar with maple syrup), reduce each cup of the liquid content in the recipe by ¼ cup. If no liquid is called for in the recipe, add 3 to 5 tablespoons of flour for each ¾ cup of liquid-concentrated sweetener. Warm sticky syrups before working with them by setting the jar in hot water for five to ten minutes and oil the measuring utensils.

Due to the presence of a natural starch-splitting enzyme, the malted sweeteners (brown rice syrup and barley malt) may liquefy the consistency of the mixture. This is more likely if the recipe calls for eggs. Boiling the malt syrup for 2 to 3 minutes before using can prevent this. Let it cool slightly before adding to recipe.

To replace a liquid sweetener with a granulated sweetener (e.g., replacing honey with unrefined cane sugar), increase each cup of the liquid content (the sweetener or any other liquid) of the recipe by ¼ cup or reduce the flour by 3 to 5 tablespoons. The dried or granulated natural sweeteners tend to absorb liquid. Check your dough or batter to see if it resembles the texture you are used to and consider adding an extra tablespoon of water or fat if the mixture seems dry. Adding extra moisture is especially important if you are also substituting white flour with whole grain flour in the recipe. Whole grain flours, because of their fiber, also absorb moisture.

EGGS

Eggs are unequal in their ability to bind. They also add high-quality protein and fat to baked goods and desserts, which help balance the high-carbohydrate content. I don't recommend replacing eggs in a recipe unless there you are working with an egg allergy or have a commitment to eating vegan. If you do need to replace eggs, two eggs equal approximately ½ cup of liquid and fat.

Egg substitution options (for two eggs):

• Try ½ cup of fruit or vegetable puree. Dates, bananas, applesauce, sweet potato, or yam are a few choices. The texture will be softer than if the dish were made with eggs.

• Grind 2 tablespoons of flaxseed, add 6 tablespoons boiling water, let mixture set for fifteen minutes, then whisk it with a fork. The flax will also significantly increase the fiber content.

• Use 6 tablespoons of the water from an unsalted can of chickpeas, also known as "aquafaba." It sounded odd to me, but the website Food52 swears this substitution works best.

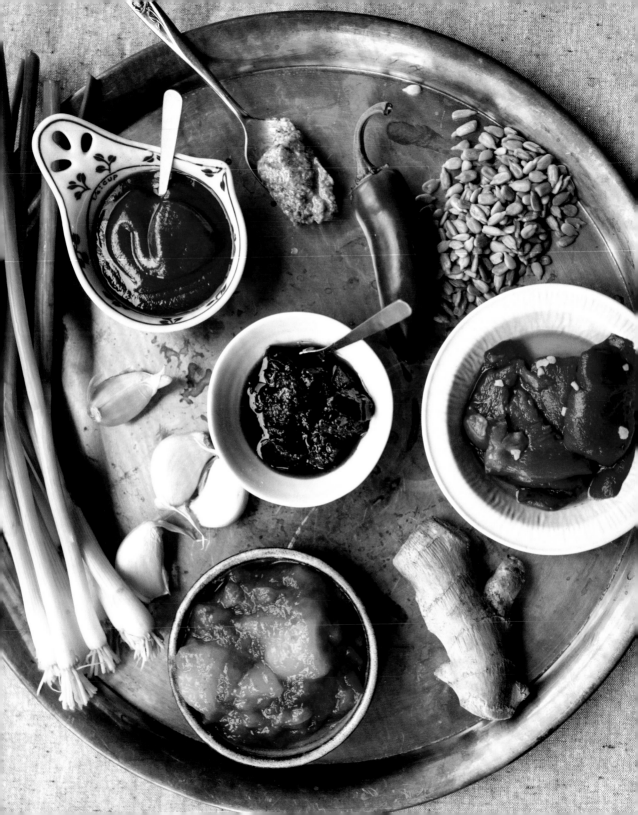

books about food
for children

- - - - - - - - - - - - - - - -

BOARD BOOKS
(PRE-K TO KINDERGARTEN)

Carle, Eric. *My Very First Book of Food*. New York: Philomel Books, 2007.
Gibbons, Gail. *The Vegetables We Eat*. New York: Holiday House, 2008.

PICTURE BOOKS
(KINDERGARTEN TO FOURTH GRADE)

Butterworth, Chris. *How Did That Get in My Lunchbox?* Somerville, MA:
    Candlewick Press, 2013.
Curtis, Andrea. *What's for Lunch?* Markham, ON: Red Deer Press, 2012.
Martin, Jacqueline Briggs. *Alice Waters and the Trip to Delicious*. Bellevue,
    WA: Readers to Eaters, 2014.
Mora, Pat. *Yum! Mmmm! Qué Rico! Americas' Sproutings*. New York: Lee &
    Low Books, 2007.

Pryor, Katherine. *Sylvia's Spinach*. Bellevue, WA: Readers to Eaters, 2012.

Robbins, Ken. *Food For Thought*. New York: Flash Point, 2009.

CHAPTER BOOKS
(FOURTH GRADE AND UP)

Katzen, Mollie, and Ann Henderson. *Pretend Soup and Other Real Recipes*. San Francisco: Tricycle Press, 1994.

Knisley, Lucy. *Relish: My Life in the Kitchen*. New York: First Second, 2013.

Lair, Cynthia. *Feeding the Young Athlete*. Bellevue, WA: Readers to Eaters, 2012.

Larkin, Eric-Shabazz. *A Moose Boosh: A Few Choice Words on Food*. Bellevue, WA: Readers to Eaters, 2014.

Pollan, Michael. *Food Rules*. New York: Penguin Press, 2009.

Pollan, Michael. *The Omnivore's Dilemma: Young Readers Edition*. New York: Dial Books, 2015.

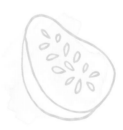

index

Note: Photographs are indicated by *italics*.

conversion chart

VOLUME

UNITED STATES	METRIC	IMPERIAL
¼ tsp.	1.25 ml	
½ tsp.	2.5 ml	
1 tsp.	5 ml	
½ Tbsp.	7.5 ml	
1 Tbsp.	15 ml	
⅛ c.	30 ml	1 fl. oz.
¼ c.	60 ml	2 fl. oz.
1/3 c.	80 ml	2.5 fl. oz.
½ c.	125 ml	4 fl. oz.
1 c.	250 ml	8 fl. oz.
2 c. (1 pt.)	500 ml	16 fl. oz.
1 qt.	1 l	32 fl. oz.

LENGTH

UNITED STATES	METRIC
⅛ in.	3 mm
¼ in.	6 mm
½ in.	1.25 cm
1 in.	2.5 cm
1 ft.	30 cm

WEIGHT

AVOIRDUPOIS	METRIC
¼ oz.	7 g
½ oz.	15 g
1 oz.	30 g
2 oz.	60 g
3 oz.	90 g
4 oz.	115 g
5 oz.	150 g
6 oz.	175 g
7 oz.	200 g
8 oz. (½ lb.)	225 g
9 oz.	250 g
10 oz.	300 g
11 oz.	325 g
12 oz.	350 g
13 oz.	375 g
14 oz.	400 g
15 oz.	425 g
16 oz. (1 lb.)	450 g
1½ lb.	750 g
2 lb.	900 g
2¼ lb.	1 kg
3 lb.	1.4 kg
4 lb.	1.8 kg

TEMPERATURE

OVEN MARK	FAHRENHEIT	CELSIUS	GAS
Very cool	250–275	130–140	½–1
Cool	300	150	2
Warm	325	165	3
Moderate	350	175	4
Moderately hot	375	190	5
	400	200	6
Hot	425	220	7
	450	230	8
Very Hot	475	245	9